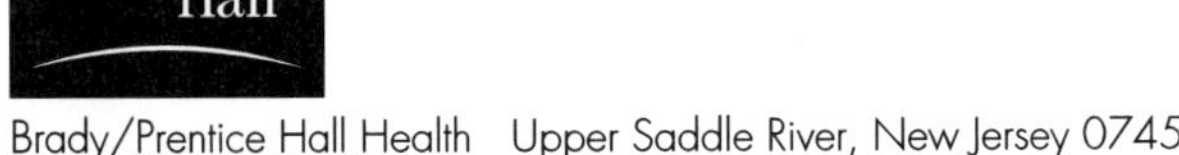

Brady/Prentice Hall Health Upper Saddle River, New Jersey 07458

MedReview for EMT-B

Bob Elling

The Student Workbook Companion to

MedEMT

A Learning System for Prehospital Care

Mark G. Wills
Grant B. Goold
K. Lee Watson

Acquisitions Editor: Laura Edwards
Publishing Consultant: Elena Mauceri
Production Editor: Diane Gonciarz, Navta Associates
Director of Manufacturing and Production: Bruce Johnson
Managing Editor: Patrick Walsh
Manufacturing Manager: Ilene Sanford
Art Director: Marianne Frasco
Marketing Manager: Tiffany Price
Editorial Assistant: Jeanne Molenaar
Cover Design: Maria Guglielmo
Cover Photo: Victory Technology, Inc.
Interior Design: Judine O'Shea, Navta Associates
Composition: Judine O'Shea and Carrie Schuler, Navta Associates
Printing and Binding: Banta Company, Harrisonburg, VA

Prentice-Hall International (UK) Limited, *London*
Prentice-Hall of Australia Pty. Limited, *Sydney*
Prentice-Hall Canada Inc., *Toronto*
Prentice-Hall Hispanoamericana, S.A., *Mexico*
Prentice-Hall of India Private Limited, *New Delhi*
Prentice-Hall of Japan, Inc., *Tokyo*
Prentice-Hall Singapore Pte. Ltd.
Editora Prentice-Hall do Brasil, Ltda., *Rio de Janeiro*

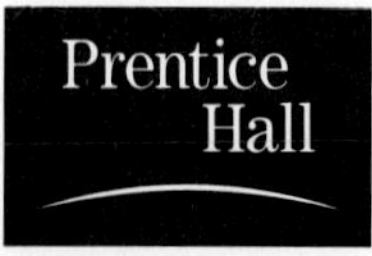

10 9 8 7 6 5 4 3 2 1
ISBN 0-13-093986-2

MedReview

TABLE OF CONTENTS

Table of Contents *continued*

Module 6 INFANTS AND CHILDREN

Module 7 OPERATIONS

APPENDICES:

Introduction

Welcome to MedReview! This workbook was designed to compliment the MedEMT textbook and CD-ROM, and follows the same chapter format.

We know that many students learn best by using a combination of media, or "multimedia." Using MedReview along with the other components of the MedEMT package will help you achieve success in your EMT-Basic course. An example of using this multimedia approach is in the self-testing capabilities of the MedEMT package. As you proceed through the course, you will want to test yourself frequently to be sure that you are learning all the objectives of becoming an EMT-Basic. Using the CD-ROM, an electronic medium, will provide you with opportunities for testing and immediate feedback.

MedReview was also prepared to provide you with additional practice in a more traditional, "non-computerized" format. You need not be sitting at your computer to use this workbook. EMS instructors who utilize the MedEMT package may assign homework from MedReview as well.

FEATURES

Each chapter has the following features that are designed to enrich your learning experience.

Summary

At the beginning of each chapter there is a chapter summary that hits the high points of the chapter as written in the MedEMT textbook. This is a good way to help you begin to review the general areas of knowledge that you should have picked up when reading the text chapter. If one of these points discussed in the summary seems new to you, perhaps you may not have fully understood the point when it was covered in the chapter.

Review Questions

This section of MedReview provides you with plenty of practice, with both true/false questions, as well as multiple-choice questions. Many of these questions are written in a manner that is typical of both State and National Registry examinations that EMT-Basic students need to pass in order to be issued a certification or license. Each of these questions has a reference to the page(s) in the MedEMT textbook where the topic is discussed. Answers are provided in the back of the book so you can check your work.

CD-ROM Links

In each of the chapters of MedReview, there are a number of links to the CD-ROM where you can view videos and animations. You can view videos containing full-color scenes from EMS, or animations that help reinforce the content and make learning much more interesting.

Case Studies

Each chapter includes case studies that provide a transition into the field. The case studies allow you to take the factual information that you have learned and apply it to a real-life scenario. This is the place where you are required to think critically and use good judgement based on the concepts you have learned in the MedEMT package. Many of the cases reflect actual calls that the authors themselves have responded to over the years.

Key Terms Matching

Becoming an EMT-Basic involves learning the language of this specialized field of medicine. Understanding anatomical terms, physiological terms, terms that describe positions of the body, and names of diseases or conditions your patients may have are all a part of the role of an EMT-Basic. You need to become familiar with the language of medicine in order to effectively work in the field of EMS. The Key Terms Matching section provides a way for you to practice using the new terms that were introduced in the textbook chapter.

Labeling Diagrams

Many of the chapters include diagrams for you to label with the appropriate captions. These exercises provide a more visual way to apply the content you've learned.

Skills Checklists

Many chapters include a listing of EMT-Basic skills that incorporate national standards or the Department of Transportation EMT-Basic Curriculum descriptions of a method of doing each skill. These checklists have been reprinted from the *Pocket Reference for the EMT-B and First Responder* by Bob Elling, MPA, REMT-P. This handy, pocket-sized reference contains not only all of the steps of each of the EMT-B skills, but also many of the medical terms, abbreviations, anatomical charts, and reference tools used in the field. This text is available from Brady/Prentice Hall.

D.O.T. Objectives Checklists

A very important part of each chapter is the objectives. Your EMT-Basic course covers and enriches the Department of Transportation's objectives as taken directly from the training curriculum. The authors of the MedEMT text have included in a number of areas additional objectives to enrich the curriculum. Each chapter of MedReview lists the actual cognitive (knowledge) D.O.T. objectives. One way to be sure that you understand the EMT-Basic course is to read the objectives as if they are sentences with a question mark at the end of each objective. Then answer the question. If you have any difficulty answering the question, then you must go back to the actual chapter where the objective was covered and be assured that you learn about the objective. Most state and national examinations reference their questions to the D.O.T. objectives, rather than a specific EMT-Basic textbook since there are so many textbooks available to the student and instructors. We've included MedEMT page references so that you can go back and study more if needed.

STRATEGY FOR SUCCESS

MedReview provides a simple—but effective—strategy for studying the EMT-Basic material using the complete package.

1. Read each chapter in the MedEMT textbook.
2. As you read the text, follow along using the CD-ROM.
3. Use MedReview as an additional learning tool. Read over the chapter summary to be sure you understand the key points of the chapter.
4. If you recall all the key points in the summary, then proceed to the Review Questions to be sure that you can apply the chapter content to specific questions.
5. Next, answer the review questions. If you have any trouble finding an answer, use the page reference provided to review that section of the MedEMT textbook. After completing the entire set of questions, go to the Answer Key at the back of MedReview and check your answers. If there are any questions that you get wrong, look up the reference and review the material right away.
6. If you come across a CD-ROM Link, follow that link to learn more on the topic. The sights and sounds on the CD will help to reinforce the content. It always makes a concept easier to understand when you utilize multiple senses.

7. Next, do the labeling diagram(s). These are helpful to put the detailed information into a different perspective.

8. Use the skill checklists to review your knowledge of important EMT-B skills. They list the steps of the skills that you will be practicing in your lab sessions.

9. The final test of how well you have learned the content of the EMT-Basic course is to review the D.O.T. objectives as if they had a question mark after each of them. Ask yourself, "Can I answer this question?" and if you can correctly, then move on to the next objective. By using these simple strategies, you should be able to thoroughly learn the material in the course and easily identify areas where you should spend more time studying.

A final word of advice: have fun while learning. EMS can be a very serious business and the EMT-Basic's job carries with it some very serious responsibilities. However, no one ever said you couldn't have fun becoming an EMT-Basic. Lighten up and enjoy the ride—you are about to embark on one of the most rewarding careers around: helping others in need!

ABOUT THE AUTHOR OF MEDREVIEW

Bob Elling, MPA, REMT-P

Bob is Program Coordinator for the Institute of Emergency Medicine at Hudson Valley Community College in Troy, NY. He has been involved in EMS since 1975 and is currently a paramedic with the Town of Colonie, NY EMS Department. He is a member of the Regional Faculty for the New York State Department of Health EMS Bureau. Bob is also a Professor of EMS with the American College of Prehospital Medicine, a member of the JEMS editorial review board, a co-author of the National First Responder, Paramedic, and EMT-Intermediate curricula. Bob's e-mail address is bobelling@usa.net.

CHAPTER 1

Introduction to Emergency Medical Care

Chapter 1 Summary

The Emergency Medical Services (EMS) system has many elements, including the caller who recognizes the emergency, the telecommunicator or dispatcher, the First Responder, the EMS providers, the hospital staff, and others involved in the patient's recovery. All these elements must work together to provide the highest quality of patient care.

There are four primary levels of training involved in an EMS system. First Responders are trained to provide care until an ambulance arrives. EMT-Basics are trained to provide basic lifesaving care on the scene of an emergency and in an ambulance during transport to an appropriate facility. EMT-Intermediates and EMT-Paramedics provide advanced medical care.

The National Highway Traffic Safety Administration (NHTSA), a part of the U.S. Department of Transportation (D.O.T.), is the federal agency that oversees the development of training standards and curriculum for EMS personnel. NHTSA also provides guidelines and support to each state in defining the ten key EMS system standards.

The EMT-Basic has many roles and responsibilities. In most states, the EMT-Basic (EMT-B) is the minimum level of education for personnel staffing an ambulance. You, the EMT-B, must ensure your personal safety, as well as the safety of the crew, patient, and bystanders. You must perform a patient assessment so you can provide the appropriate care based upon your assessment findings. You have to be able to lift and move patients safely. You must provide safe transport and transfer care of the patient to an appropriate health care facility. You must collect data and keep accurate records, as well as be a patient advocate. In some EMS systems, EMT-Basics may be trained in advanced skills such as endotracheal intubation. That is why this material is included as an optional section of the training program.

Quality assurance or improvement is essential to providing the best prehospital care. Reviewing patient care reports is a common method of quality assurance. Often, the medical direction physician is involved in quality improvement. The medical direction physician also supports EMT-Basics by providing standing orders, protocols, and direct contact during emergency calls. The EMT-Basic operates as an extension of the medical direction physician.

REVIEW QUESTIONS

Please circle the best answer for each question.

1. All of the following are responsibilities of the EMT-Basic EXCEPT:
A) interacting with other health care providers.
B) assuring safety of crew, patient, and bystanders.
C) designing the emergency medical services system.
D) participating in quality improvement committees.
[Reference text pages 21-23, 25]

2. What functions of the Emergency Medical System does the state control?
A) Regulation of providers through licensure, certification, or registration.
B) Regulation of agencies through licensure, certification, or registration.
C) Develop policies, procedures, and rules for all EMS components in the state.
D) All of the above.
[Reference text page 14]

3. Aeromedical transportation, as well as ground transportation is an important part of many EMS systems
A) True **B)** False
[Reference text page 16, 732]

4. Public involvement in the EMS system should be avoided.
A) True **B)** False
[Reference text page 17]

5. The task of caring for sick and injured patients is delegated to prehospital providers by:
A) physicians. **B)** state agencies.
C) local government. **D)** 911 Centers.
[Reference text page 17]

6. 9-1-1 is often called the ________ access number.
A) Instrumental **B)** Universal
C) Experimental **D)** National
[Reference text page 17]

7. By dialing 9-1-1, a caller can usually access:
A) law enforcement. **B)** the fire department.
C) emergency medical services. **D)** all of the above.
[Reference text page 17]

8. There are three nationally recognized levels of Emergency Medical Technician including Basic, _______ and _______.

A) Integral and Paramedic. **B)** Intermediate and Advanced.
C) Integral and Advanced. **D)** Intermediate and Paramedic.
[Reference text page 18-19]

9. Starting intravenous lines and inserting an endotracheal tube is part of the training of the:

A) First Responder. **B)** EMT-Basic.
C) EMT-Intermediate. **D)** EMT-Paramedic.
[Reference text page 19]

10. A First Responder is trained to care for a patient during ambulance transport.

A) True **B)** False
[Reference text page 18]

11. Part of an EMT-Basic's duty is to decide on the facility to which the patient should be transported. Which site would be most appropriate to receive a 52 year-old man with severe burns?

A) A rural hospital emergency department ten minutes away
B) A pediatric clinic across the street staffed by a physician
C) The university hospital and burn center fifteen minutes away
D) The city hospital's trauma center fifteen minutes away
[Reference text pages 16, 21, 30]

12. EMD is an abbreviation for Emergency Medical:

A) Department. **B)** Dispatcher.
C) Documentation. **D)** Direction.
[Reference text page 20]

13. When responding to an emergency situation, the primary concern of the EMT-Basic is to:

A) make sure the media knows the truth.
B) assist in rescuing victims from danger.
C) ensure his or her own personal safety and the safety of others.
D) determine the cause of the injury or illness.
[Reference text page 22]

14. Sometimes it may be necessary to risk injury to yourself in order to properly care for, move or lift a patient.

A) True **B)** False
[Reference text pages 21, 22]

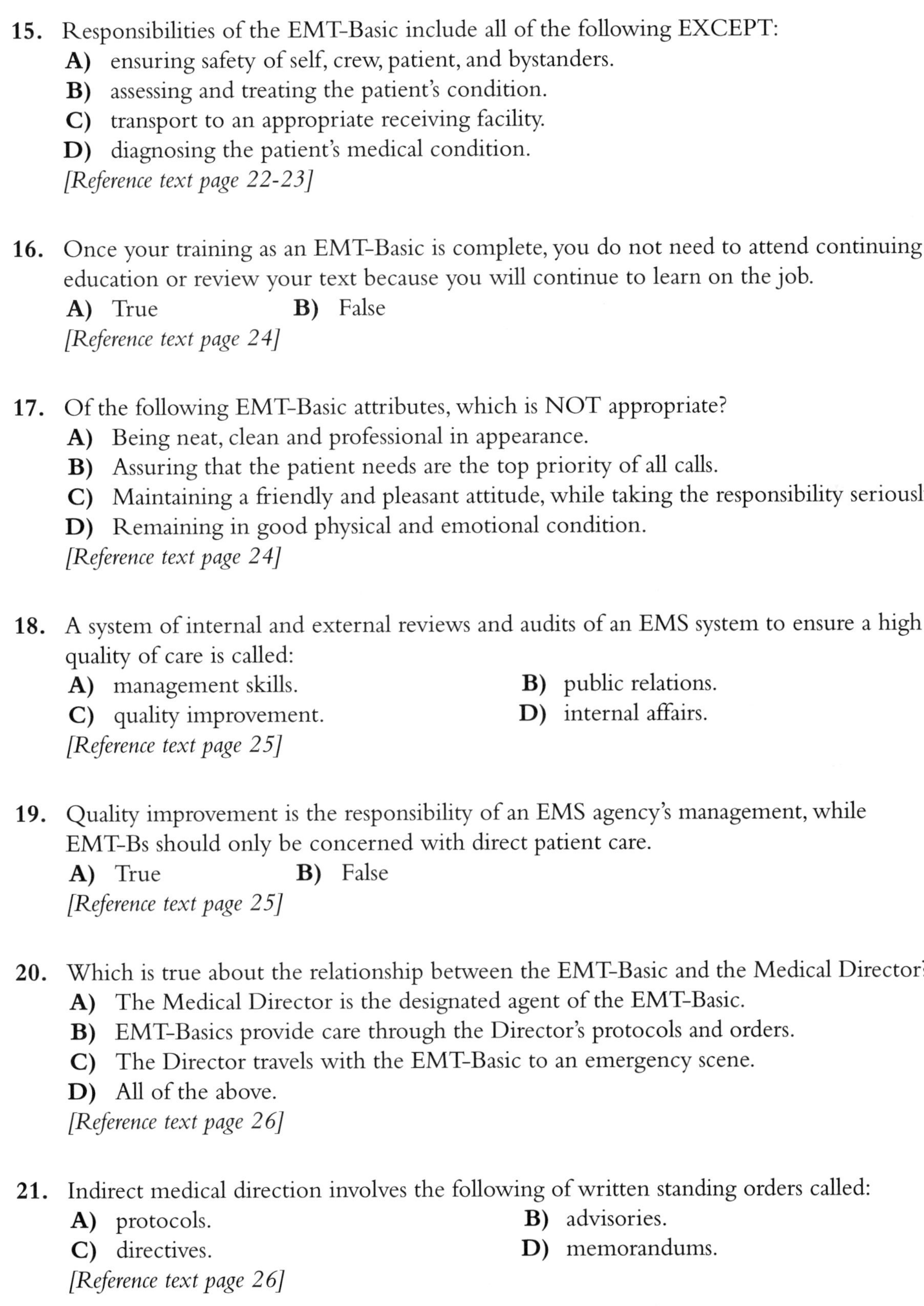

15. Responsibilities of the EMT-Basic include all of the following EXCEPT:
A) ensuring safety of self, crew, patient, and bystanders.
B) assessing and treating the patient's condition.
C) transport to an appropriate receiving facility.
D) diagnosing the patient's medical condition.
[Reference text page 22-23]

16. Once your training as an EMT-Basic is complete, you do not need to attend continuing education or review your text because you will continue to learn on the job.
A) True **B)** False
[Reference text page 24]

17. Of the following EMT-Basic attributes, which is NOT appropriate?
A) Being neat, clean and professional in appearance.
B) Assuring that the patient needs are the top priority of all calls.
C) Maintaining a friendly and pleasant attitude, while taking the responsibility seriously.
D) Remaining in good physical and emotional condition.
[Reference text page 24]

18. A system of internal and external reviews and audits of an EMS system to ensure a high quality of care is called:
A) management skills. **B)** public relations.
C) quality improvement. **D)** internal affairs.
[Reference text page 25]

19. Quality improvement is the responsibility of an EMS agency's management, while EMT-Bs should only be concerned with direct patient care.
A) True **B)** False
[Reference text page 25]

20. Which is true about the relationship between the EMT-Basic and the Medical Director?
A) The Medical Director is the designated agent of the EMT-Basic.
B) EMT-Basics provide care through the Director's protocols and orders.
C) The Director travels with the EMT-Basic to an emergency scene.
D) All of the above.
[Reference text page 26]

21. Indirect medical direction involves the following of written standing orders called:
A) protocols. **B)** advisories.
C) directives. **D)** memorandums.
[Reference text page 26]

22. Which of the following is NOT a general responsibility of an EMT-Basic?
A) Assess the patient and provide emergency medical care.
B) Secure crime scenes and provide testimony in court.
C) Keep accurate records and collect necessary data.
D) Safely lift and move the patient to the ambulance.
[Reference text pages 22, 28, 31]

23. Upon arrival at the scene, it is important to evaluate for scene safety, mechanism of injury or nature of illness and the need for additional help.
A) True **B)** False
[Reference text page 27]

24. Which of the following individuals should not handle traffic control at the scene of an automobile collision?
A) An EMS provider not directly involved with patient care.
B) A law enforcement officer investigating the crash.
C) Concerned citizens who are available and willing but who appear agitated
D) None of the above.
[Reference text page 27]

25. Upon arriving at an emergency facility with a patient, the EMT-Basic should:
A) stay in the ambulance and complete the written report.
B) assist with unloading the patient, then restock the unit.
C) unload the patient and transfer care to facility staff.
D) do none of the above.
[Reference text page 23]

26. An EMT-Basic is responsible for assisting with the maintenance and upkeep of the ambulance.
A) True **B)** False
[Reference text page 31]

27. In addition to the classroom sessions required for EMT-Basic certification, the trainee should participate in field and clinical experiences, such as volunteering at the local emergency department and performing "ride-alongs" with local ambulance services.
A) True **B)** False
[Reference text page 5]

28. Which of the following groups are part of the EMS system?

1) EMS providers
2) Hospital staff
3) Emergency Medical Dispatchers
4) Rehab center staff

A) 1,2
B) 1,2,3,4
C) 1,3
D) 1,2,3

[Reference text pages 19-21]

29. Which federal agency is responsible for assisting states in EMS system design and EMS training standards?

A) Occupational Health and Safety Administration
B) Department of Health and Human Services
C) National Highway Traffic Safety Administration
D) Office of Emergency Medical Services

[Reference text page 14]

30. The state lead EMS agency is responsible for:

A) determining how prehospital care will be provided.
B) establishing and updating EMS legislation.
C) setting guidelines for certification and recertification.
D) all of the above.

[Reference text page 14]

31. The EMS system is responsible for transporting ill or injured persons to the closest, most appropriate hospital.

A) True **B)** False

[Reference text page 30]

32. The NHTSA EMS system standards describe all of the following, EXCEPT:

A) transportation and resource management.
B) facilities and communications.
C) record keeping and donor programs.
D) evaluation and trauma systems.

[Reference text page 14]

33. One whose training emphasizes immediate care and scene control is called a/n:

A) EMT-Paramedic. **B)** First Responder.
C) EMT-Basic. **D)** EMT-Intermediate.

[Reference text page 18]

34. Conditions that can be dangerous to the EMT-Basic include:
A) patient's blood and body fluids.
B) hazards in or around the location.
C) violent patients or family members.
D) all of the above.
[Reference text page 21]

CD-ROM LINK: *Refer to the* BSI Precautions *video in Chapter 1 of the MedEMT CD-ROM where an EMS instructor emphasizes the importance of BSI and standard precautions.*

35. Using protocols and standing orders is referred to as indirect medical control.
A) True **B)** False
[Reference text page 26]

36. Patients with serious medical problems often wear:
A) a Medic Alert® bracelet. **B)** an ankle bracelet.
C) a Vial of Life necklace. **D)** all of the above.
[Reference text page 29]

37. When assessing patients with medical emergencies, medical direction may instruct the EMT-Basic to administer:
A) oxygen for many types of emergencies.
B) activated charcoal for diabetics with low blood sugar.
C) oral glucose for ingestion of harmful substances.
D) all of the above.
[Reference text page 29]

38. Patient transport facility decisions are made based upon condition and extent of injuries.
A) True **B)** False
[Reference text page 30]

39. The EMT-Basic is an extension of the ________, who provides medical direction.
A) physician **B)** Medical Director
C) paramedic **D)** State EMS Director
[Reference text page 26]

40. Being a patient care advocate is not a part of the role of an EMT-Basic.
A) True **B)** False
[Reference text page 24]

CASE STUDIES

Use a separate piece of paper to answer the case study questions. Number your answers with the case study number and question letter (1A, 1B, etc.).

ACCESS TO THE EMS SYSTEM

1. As an EMT-Basic working for the local volunteer ambulance, you are dispatched to a non-emergency call for a patient with a non-life-threatening leg injury. Because the caller dialed the business number to the main ambulance offices, you are asked to advise the caller and patient on the proper methods for accessing the local EMS system.
   A) Describe the difference between the office numbers and a universal access number or emergency access number.
   B) How can you promote the use of the access number for your agency or locality?

LEVELS OF EMS TRAINING

2. You have just completed your EMT-Basic education and are employed with the local EMS agency. A college counselor has asked you to participate in a televised panel discussion on available jobs for college students. After explaining the four common levels of provider, the moderator presents you with several questions.
   A) Your descriptions of the EMT-Basic and First Responder were very similar. Are their roles actually similar? How do they differ?
   B) If most states allow an EMT-Basic to care for a patient in an ambulance, why do we need EMT-Intermediates and EMT-Paramedics? How are they different?
3. Your county has just hired an emergency manager. She has asked you to look at every phase of the EMS response and think of those who may be able to help during difficult responses or special rescue situations.
   A) Who else could be extended members of the EMS system in unusual situations?
4. As part of a new federal loan program, the EMS dispatch center is completing a renovation project. In addition to new hardware and a new communication system, several telecommunicators have just completed EMD training. The editor of the local newspaper, a personal friend, asks you to explain what EMD is and how it will benefit members of your community.
   A) What is EMD all about?
   B) What differences can a caller expect when talking with an operator trained in EMD?
   C) How will it improve patient care in your community?

ROLES AND RESPONSIBILITIES OF THE EMT-BASIC

5. The local vocational training program has requested that an EMT-Basic come over to the high school and describe "what it takes to be an EMT-Basic." Your battalion chief has given you this assignment and tells you to "make us look good."
   A) What type of personal and physical traits should all EMT-Basics possess?

B) What type of efforts must be made by every EMT-Basic to keep aware of changes in EMS?

C) What is the best strategy to ensure your patients always receive the best care you are capable of providing?

QUALITY IMPROVEMENT

6. The safety committee of a local manufacturing plant is discussing the benefits of quality improvement (QI) systems at the factory. As a veteran EMT-Basic, you have been actively involved in the QI system at the local volunteer EMS agency for many years. A fellow worker knows that you have experience with QI and has asked you for your opinion.

A) Explain the benefits that are realized by having a QI system in place with the EMS agency.

B) Describe how a QI system could be used in the EMS communications and human resources management standards of a high-quality EMS system.

C) What are a few ways the EMT-Basic can actively participate in a quality improvement system?

MEDICAL DIRECTION

7. Recent state legislation required a large lumber company to implement an emergency medical response team. As a member of the team, you are responsible for dealing with medical and trauma emergencies that occur at the mill. The local EMS agency has requested your team design specific communication policies for response, treatment, and off-line communications. The medical director for the local EMS agency has requested that you work together to create these policies, since your mill is located 15 miles from the agency's station.

A) Why is it important for the medical response team to work closely with medical direction in this case?

B) What mechanisms should exist when direct communication with a physician is impossible or disrupted?

C) Other than standing orders and written protocols, how might the physician be involved in the off-line medical direction of the medical emergency response team?

DUTIES OF THE EMT-BASIC

8. You are just completing your probationary period as an EMT-Basic with the local ambulance service. During your evaluation, your supervisor reprimands you for "neglecting your duties" as an EMT-Basic, but doesn't cite specific occurrences. You are concerned about how this will affect your career as an EMT-Basic.

A) What are the five most important duties of the EMT-Basic? Justify your selection of these top five.

KEY TERMS MATCHING

Assess your knowledge of the chapter key terms by matching the terms on the left to the definitions on the right.

_____ 1. Assessment

_____ 2. Emergency Medical Dispatchers (EMDs)

_____ 3. Emergency Medical Services Systems (EMSS) Act

_____ 4. EMT-Basic (EMT-B)

_____ 5. EMT-Intermediate (EMT-I)

_____ 6. EMT-Paramedic (EMT-P)

_____ 7. First Responder

_____ 8. Protocols

_____ 9. Quality Improvement (QI)

_____ 10. Standing Orders

_____ 11. Trauma Centers

(A) Specially trained personnel who answer calls for help; gather essential information, and when indicated, provide prearrival instructions over the phone until EMS personnel arrive.

(B) The most highly trained EMT personnel; perform invasive field care

(C) Evaluation of a situation or patient; the information is used to determine priorities for management

(D) Regional facilities having specialized physicians and equipment necessary for treating trauma injuries

(E) Preexisting written plans for treatment of specific complaints, interventions, or medications allowed by protocol without direct contact with medical direction.

(F) The 1973 Congressional Act that provided federal dollars to begin EMS systems throughout the United States

(G) Component of an EMS system that identifies the program's strengths and weaknesses and guarantees that the public receives the highest caliber of prehospital care

(H) One whose training emphasizes immediate care and scene control prior to the arrival of additional EMS services

(I) An advanced EMT trained in intravenous lines, airway techniques, manual defibrillation, and administration of some medications

(J) Medical orders designed by a physician for a given list of procedures or medications; will vary among localities

(K) Personnel trained in prehospital techniques including assessment and primary care for the ill or injured patient

D.O.T. OBJECTIVES CHECKLIST

Use the following list of knowledge objectives to check what you've learned. Check off only those objectives that you feel you completely understand and have mastered. For any objectives not checked, go back and review that section of the text chapter. Textbook page references have been provided to help you review the text material.

- [ ] Define Emergency Medical Services (EMS) systems. *(p. 6)*
- [ ] State the specific statutes and regulations in your state regarding the EMS system. *(p. 18)*
- [ ] Differentiate the roles and responsibilities of the EMT-Basic from other prehospital care providers. *(p. 21)*
- [ ] Describe the roles and responsibilities related to personal safety. *(p. 21)*
- [ ] Discuss the roles and responsibilities of the EMT-Basic for the safety of the crew, the patient, and bystanders. *(p. 22)*
- [ ] Define quality improvement and discuss the EMT-Basic's role in the process. *(p. 25)*
- [ ] Define medical direction and discuss the EMT-Basic's role in the process. *(p. 26)*

CHAPTER 2

The Well-Being of the EMT-Basic

CHAPTER 2 SUMMARY

Although there are many types of protective equipment and many safety procedures, you are ultimately responsible for your own well-being. When functioning as an EMT-Basic, you are also responsible for the safety of your crew, your patient, and bystanders (the general public).

Death is a normal occurrence. During your practice, you will encounter patients and family members in many stages of grief. Understanding the range of emotions they may be experiencing will enable you to help them, often simply by listening empathetically and offering calm, gentle reassurances.

One of the greatest long-term threats to the wellness of an EMT-Basic is stress. Stress is a normal side effect of performing emergency medical care. Certain situations will cause you greater stress than others. Develop healthy means of relieving the stress of your new duties. A healthy lifestyle is essential to dealing with stress effectively. A good diet, frequent exercise, and use of relaxation techniques will help. Seek a healthy balance between your duties as an EMT-Basic (which may also be your job), your family, recreational and religious activities, and your health.

CISD, or Critical Incident Stress Debriefings, are a relatively new tool to help emergency personnel deal with particularly stressful situations. A CISD allows providers to vent feelings in a nonthreatening, noncritical environment.

Body Substance Isolation (BSI) precautions, or standard precautions, and good handwashing technique are essential to protect you from exposure to an infectious disease. Assume any body substance is potentially infectious, and use barrier devices such as gloves, gowns, eye protection, and masks to prevent contact with a patient's body substances.

Although the EMT-Basic course prepares you to deal with many aspects of patient care, know your limitations. When faced with a Hazardous Material or Rescue situation, never enter the scene unless you are properly trained and equipped to do so. Law enforcement should control any scene involving a history of or potential for violence before you provide patient care.

REVIEW QUESTIONS

Please circle the best answer for each question.

1. The EMT-Basic needs to develop ways to cope with stressful situations in order to maintain his or her emotional health.
   A) True **B)** False
   [Reference text page 38]

2. In this chapter, you have learned what to expect and how to help yourself and others during and after stressful calls.
   A) True **B)** False
   [Reference text page 38]

3. Ungrateful, abusive, or violent patients can contribute to an EMT-Basic's stress level.
   A) True **B)** False
   [Reference text page 39]

4. The five stages that dying patients typically experience are denial, ________, bargaining, depression, and acceptance.
   A) resentment **B)** anger **C)** frustration **D)** anticipation
   [Reference text page 45]

5. Before accepting the loss of a loved one, the patient must move through the grieving process at his or her own pace.
   A) True **B)** False
   [Reference text page 45]

6. Irritability with coworkers, inability to concentrate, indecisiveness, loss of appetite, or isolation are all warning signs of:
   A) burnout. **B)** anxiety. **C)** stress. **D)** isolation.
   [Reference text page 39]

7. Exercising, eating a healthy diet, using relaxation techniques, and seeking professional counseling are all ways of managing:
   A) cancer. **B)** stress.
   C) anorexia. **D)** critical infections.
   [Reference text page 40]

8. Stress reducing techniques include:
   A) spouse and family support. **B)** community outreach programs.
   C) defusings. **D)** all of the above.
   [Reference text page 40]

9. The acronym BSI stands for body ________ isolation.
A) substance **B)** secretion **C)** segment **D)** stress
[Reference text page 48]

10. It is always necessary to wear gloves, protective eyewear, and a gown when working on a bleeding patient.
A) True **B)** False
[Reference text page 51]

11. Experts recommend an increase in sugar intake to help reduce the negative effects of stress.
A) True **B)** False
[Reference text page 41]

12. Experts recommend regular exercise and increasing carbohydrate intake to reduce the negative effects of stress.
A) True **B)** False
[Reference text page 41]

13. When you unexpectedly find yourself dispatched to a scene involving irrational individuals, individuals suspected of being intoxicated, dangerous pets, or weapons, you should immediately exit and:
A) request more EMT-Basic personnel. **B)** request law enforcement.
C) request fire department personnel. **D)** handle it yourself.
[Reference text page 55]

14. At a hazardous material scene, emergency care of the injured takes priority over the duties of the HAZ-MAT team.
A) True **B)** False
[Reference text page 54]

15. Anxiety is a/an:
A) disease process where the EMT-Basic feels badly after a particularly difficult call.
B) abnormal reaction to a traumatizing event experienced by the EMT-Basic.
C) normal reaction that occurs very infrequently during the career of an EMT-Basic.
D) natural emotional or physical reaction to threatening or challenging situations.
[Reference text page 39]

16. A CISD is a process that allows EMT-Basics to discuss their feelings after a difficult call. What does CISD stand for?
A) Critical Incident Stress Debriefing
B) Communicative Informational Stress Diagnosis
C) Conducted Informal Stress Debriefing
D) Critical Incident Stress Diagnosis
[Reference text page 42]

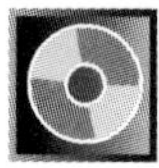

CD-ROM LINK: *Refer to the* EMT's Well-Being *video in Chapter 2 of the MedEMT CD-ROM where an EMS instructor discusses the importance of the CISD process.*

17. Which of the following is one of the reactions a family member may exhibit when confronted with death and dying?
A) betrayal
B) bargaining
C) sarcasm
D) support
[Reference text page 45]

18. What measures are designed to prevent the spread of communicable diseases from one individual to another?
A) body surface isolation
B) body substance infection
C) body source infection
D) body substance isolation
[Reference text page 48]

CD-ROM LINK: *Refer to the* BSI Precautions *video in Chapter 2 of the MedEMT CD-ROM where an instructor emphasizes the importance of BSI precautions.*

19. An EMT-Basic's family may experience responses such as:
A) anger at interruptions in normal life.
B) stress from the inability to plan activities.
C) frustration from not truly understanding your feelings.
D) all of the above.
[Reference text page 42]

20. During a stress debriefing, you may be judged for improperly managing the scene.
A) True
B) False
[Reference text page 42]

21. Defusing is a specialized process that can be done prior to an incident occurring.
A) True
B) False
[Reference text page 43]

22. The stages of the grieving process are: denial, bargaining, anger, ________, and depression.
A) renewal
B) acceptance
C) anticipation
D) removal
[Reference text page 45]

23. The first reaction to any loss is usually shock, disbelief, or:
A) anger.
B) denial.
C) depression.
D) bargaining.
[Reference text page 45]

24. One of the best techniques to use when working with death and dying is to just:
A) take a cold shower.
B) have a few cocktails.
C) avoid looking in people's eyes.
D) listen.
[Reference text page 47]

25. Without exception, the EMT-Basic must:
A) immediately assess all patients upon arrival at the scene.
B) assure that the scene is safe prior to entering.
C) wear gloves and an eye shield when dealing with patients.
D) do all of the above.
[Reference text page 48]

26. Ways of making the environment less disease-friendly are referred to as:
A) PPE.
B) work practices.
C) engineering controls.
D) none of the above.
[Reference text page 31]

27. A policy that prohibits recapping of needles is called a work practice control.
A) True **B)** False
[Reference text page 49]

28. When cleaning up after a call, it is a good practice to wear utility gloves.
A) True **B)** False
[Reference text page 50]

29. It is not necessary to change your gloves between calls.
A) True **B)** False
[Reference text page 50]

30. An example of an airborne disease of serious concern to EMT-Basics is tuberculosis.
A) True **B)** False
[Reference text page 51]

31. Roll-up flooring, which prevents pathogens from becoming trapped in the joints, is a type of:
A) engineering control.
B) PPE.
C) work practice control.
D) environmental impact control.
[Reference text page 49]

32. The most effective method of preventing the spread of pathogens is:
A) wearing rubber gloves.
B) handwashing.
C) wearing a mask.
D) patient isolation.
[Reference text page 49]

33. In instances where it is not practical to wash your hands after a patient contact, the CDC recommends the use of a 10% alcohol solution to rinse off with.
A) True **B)** False
[Reference text page 49]

34. To prevent bloodborne pathogen transmission, it is recommended that eye shields be worn whenever there is a potential for blood splash or body fluid splash.
A) True **B)** False
[Reference text page 52]

35. A mask should be worn by the EMT-Basic to help protect himself or herself from the spread of disease:
A) when the patient is elderly. **B)** during emergency childbirth.
C) when measuring the patient's BP. **D)** for minor bleeding control.
[Reference text page 51]

36. As an EMT-Basic, your role at a HAZ-MAT incident is to:
A) quickly identify potential hazards.
B) protect yourself, patients, and bystanders.
C) notify the appropriate authorities.
D) do all of the above.
[Reference text page 54]

37. At a HAZ-MAT scene, as a rule, EMS personnel:
A) do not treat patients until they have been decontaminated.
B) need to don self-contained breathing apparatus.
C) must treat all patients as quickly as possible.
D) must do none of the above.
[Reference text page 54]

38. EMT-Basics should work closely with law enforcement personnel to develop plans for answering calls in gang-controlled neighborhoods.
A) True **B)** False
[Reference text page 55]

39. When you arrive on the scene of a rescue, do not enter the scene unless you have been properly trained and equipped to reduce potential hazards such as electricity, fire or explosion.
A) True **B)** False
[Reference text pages 54-55]

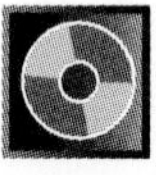

CD-ROM LINK: *Refer to the* Scene Safety *video in Chapter 2 of the MedEMT CD-ROM where an instructor discusses the importance of establishing scene safety for any emergency call.*

40. If, while on the scene, of a call you are threatened by the patient or his or her family, you should do all of the following EXCEPT:
A) quickly plan your route of escape.
B) notify law enforcement personnel.
C) stand up to the patient, as you do not have to take this abuse.
D) begin to retreat without confronting the patient.
[Reference text pages 55, 260-61]

CASE STUDIES

Use a separate piece of paper to answer the case study questions. Number your answers with the case study number and question letter (1A, 1B, etc.).

EMOTIONAL ASPECTS OF EMERGENCY CARE

1. The family of a frequent user of EMS has requested you to respond to their home. Upon arrival, you find the patient, Steven, yelling and screaming at everyone on scene. Steven's wife quietly explains that he has been diagnosed with terminal liver cancer and is expected to die rapidly. Steven's screaming blocks your attempts to talk with him.
A) How will you determine if Steven's reaction is normal under the circumstances?
B) What other emotions may Steven experience while dealing with the fact that he is dying?

2. After working for more than five years with the local rescue squad, you have seen many types of illness and injury. Recently, the new shift rotations have meant longer hours and greater call volumes for you and your partner. Your latest station assignment has also meant more trauma and abuse calls. You are aware of your own increased stress due to the changes.
A) What warning signs of stress should you and your partner be looking for?
B) What strategies can you use to help reduce or manage stress?
C) Describe the steps you would take to help control your own stress level.

3. Losing a fellow firefighter is never easy. You just cannot believe that Bill is gone. Last night's fire did not seem that bad, and everyone worked hard to contain it. All you can remember is finding Bill's lifeless body lying in the hallway. It appears that he may have had a heart attack during the initial stages of the fire. After discussion with the staff, the chief has decided that the entire department will participate in a CISD session this morning.
A) What is the purpose of a CISD session?
B) What makes up a comprehensive CISD stress management program?

4. The local volunteer rescue team is recruiting new members. You have just finished your EMT-Basic program and are excited about working with the team. During your first interview, the Captain of the team asks you to describe the principles of standard precautions and body substance isolation (BSI).
A) Define body substance isolation and how it relates to EMS.
B) What body substance isolation precautions are generally required during the measurement of a patient's blood pressure?

5. A significant number of residents in the area your EMS agency covers have been diagnosed with tuberculosis. The Health Department has notified your agency that it is currently treating a number of active cases of airborne diseases in your service area. The notification encourages responding crews to use appropriate precautions. Your department is concerned and has assigned you the responsibility to obtain the proper BSI equipment.
   A) What type of equipment will you need?
   B) What resources are available in your local area to gather information on BSI regulations?

SCENE SAFETY

6. The weather outside is unseasonably warm, which usually means busy shifts for EMS. Towards the middle of the shift, you and your partner are dispatched to a local high school for a head injury. The principal meets you at the door and informs you that the patient is lying in a bathroom, unconscious and bleeding severely. As you approach the scene, and while still several hundred feet away, you notice several dozen teenaged girls yelling, screaming, and threatening each other in the hallway. The girls seem to be split into two rival groups. A few faculty members appear to be losing control of the crowd.
   A) How would you handle this situation?

SAFETY PRECAUTIONS IN ADVANCE

7. The EMT-Basic Program Coordinator has advised the class that each student must obtain several immunizations prior to starting any clinical or field time. You are sure you were immunized as a child, but you have not taken the time to verify your status.
   A) What diseases can you be immunized against?
   B) What steps will you take to verify your immunization status?

KEY TERMS MATCHING

Assess your knowledge of the chapter key terms by matching the terms on the left to the definitions on the right.

_____ **1.** Body Substance Isolation Precautions (BSI)

_____ **2.** Critical Incident Stress Debriefing (CISD)

_____ **3.** High-efficiency particulate air (HEPA) respirator

_____ **4.** Pathogen (PATH-oh-jen)

(A) The first level of the Centers for Disease Control's revised set of guidelines regarding isolation precautions established in 1996. Replaces BSI and universal precautions.

(B) Microorganism that causes disease

(C) Equipment used by an emergency rescuer to protect against injury and infectious disease

(D) A meeting held after a critical incident that encourages emergency care workers to discuss their feelings openly with trained mental health professionals and peer counselors.

______ **5.** Personal Protective Equipment (PPE)	**(E)**	A specially filtered mask that is worn when caring for patients suspected or diagnosed with tuberculosis and other diseases caused by airborne pathogens
______ **6.** Standard Precautions	**(F)**	Natural emotional or physical reaction to threatening or challenging situations
______ **7.** Stress	**(G)**	Equipment and standards designed to prevent the spread of communicable diseases

LABELING DIAGRAM

Fill in the blanks in the "Protective Eyewear" column with *yes* or *no*, according to the situation presented on the left.

Guide to Preventing Bloodborne Pathogen Transmission

Situation	Disposable Gloves	Protective Eyewear	Mask	Gown
Bleeding control with spurting blood	Yes	**A.** ______	Yes	Yes
Bleeding control with minimal bleeding	Yes	**B.** ______	No	No
Emergency childbirth	Yes	**C.** ______	Yes	Yes
Endotracheal intubation	Yes	**D.** ______	Yes	No
Oral/nasal suctioning; manually clearing airway	Yes	**E.** ______	Yes	Yes
Handling/cleaning instruments with possible contamination	Yes	**F.** ______	Yes	Yes
Measuring blood pressure	Yes★	**G.** ______	No	No
Giving an injection	Yes	**H.** ______	No	No
Measuring temperature	Yes★	**I.** ______	No	No
Cleaning back of ambulance after a routine medical call	Yes	**J.** ______	No	No

★ Note: In your area, gloves may not be needed for measuring blood pressure and temperature. Check your local protocols.

SKILLS CHECKLIST

Check your knowledge of important EMT-B skills by marking off each step in the following skills sheet.

HANDWASHING

- [ ] Remove watch and rings. Roll up sleeves.
- [ ] Adjust water flow and temperature.
- [ ] Wet hands and distal forearms.
- [ ] Dispense soap onto hands.
- [ ] Scrub lower arms and hands. Clean around and under nails.
- [ ] Rinse thoroughly under running water to remove all soap. Do not touch sink!
- [ ] Use a paper towel to shut off faucet in order to avoid re-contaminating hands.

NOTE: Even though you wear protective gloves with your patients, handwashing must still be performed immediately after each call.

(reprinted from *Pocket Reference for The EMT-B and First Responder* by Bob Elling, Prentice Hall, 1999)

D.O.T. OBJECTIVES CHECKLIST

Use the following list of knowledge objectives to check what you've learned. Check off only those objectives that you feel you completely understand and have mastered. For any objectives not checked, go back and review that section of the text chapter. Textbook page references have been provided to help you review the text material.

- [ ] List possible emotional reactions that the EMT-Basic may experience when faced with trauma, illness, death, and dying. *(p. 44)*
- [ ] Discuss the possible reactions that a family member may exhibit when confronted with death and dying. *(p. 44)*
- [ ] State the steps in the EMT-Basic's approach to the family confronted with death and dying. *(p. 44)*
- [ ] State the possible reactions that the family of the EMT-Basic may exhibit due to their outside involvement in EMS. *(p. 41)*
- [ ] Recognize the signs and symptoms of critical incident stress. *(p. 39)*
- [ ] State possible steps that the EMT-Basic may take to help reduce/alleviate stress. *(p. 40)*
- [ ] Explain the need to determine scene safety. *(p. 48)*
- [ ] Discuss the importance of body substance isolation (BSI). *(p. 48)*
- [ ] Describe the steps the EMT-Basic should take for personal protection from airborne and bloodborne pathogens. *(p. 49)*
- [ ] List the personal protective equipment necessary for each of the following situations: *(p. 53)*
    - [ ] Hazardous materials
    - [ ] Rescue operations
    - [ ] Violent scenes

- [ ] Crime scenes
- [ ] Exposure to bloodborne pathogens
- [ ] Exposure to airborne pathogens

CHAPTER 3

Medical, Legal, and Ethical Issues

CHAPTER 3 SUMMARY

As an EMT-Basic, you have a legal and ethical responsibility to provide for the well-being of your patient. Some type of consent, or permission to treat, must be obtained from each patient. Expressed consent should be obtained from every conscious, mentally competent adult before you provide treatment. You must explain any procedures and their related risk. Implied consent exists when you treat a patient who is unable to give expressed consent (e.g., unconscious) and needs life-saving care. The consent of a parent or guardian is required prior for the treatment of minors. If the parent or guardian is unavailable, you should render care for life-threatening conditions based on implied consent.

A mentally competent adult can refuse treatment or withdraw from treatment at any time. Inform the patient of the risks and consequences of refusing care and obtain a release from liability. Good documentation is essential to provide any form of legal protection.

EMT-Basics may become involved in either the criminal and civil (tort) court systems. EMT-Basics may be called upon to offer testimony in criminal cases. Claims that an EMT-Basic was negligent or abandoned a patient are generally civil court issues. In order to prove negligence, the claimant must prove the following things: that the EMT-Basic had a duty to act, that the EMT-Basic breached his or her duty to act, that the patient suffered physical or psychological harm, and that the EMT-Basic's breach of duty caused the physical or psychological harm.

A duty to act is an obligation to provide medical care. Much like consent, it can be implied or expressed. An implied duty exists when you accept a call from dispatch. An expressed duty may exist as a result of a written contract with a government or business.

All patient information is confidential and should not be released except as allowed by law in your state or locality. Certain situations, such as sexual assault or suspected child abuse, may require you to report the incident to a specific agency. When working at a crime scene, your primary concern is patient care. Preserve evidence, if at all possible, and be sure to document carefully exactly what you observed.

REVIEW QUESTIONS

Please circle the best answer for each question.

1. Written protocols and standing orders define the EMT-Basic's authority to provide care. These are authorized by a combination of state laws and ________ direction.
   A) incident **B)** system **C)** medical **D)** state
   [Reference text page 63]

2. DNR orders are only for patients with terminal conditions.
   A) True **B)** False
   [Reference text page 65]

3. The patient's consent to treatment may occur in one of three ways: expressed, implied, or:
   A) parental. **B)** indirect. **C)** supervisory. **D)** none of the above.
   [Reference text pages 63, 67-68]

4. Consent for treatment that is assumed from an unconscious patient is called ________ consent.
   A) parental **B)** expressed **C)** implied **D)** applied
   [Reference text page 68]

5. An EMT-Basic can be charged with assault and battery if expressed consent is not obtained from a conscious, mentally competent patient.
   A) True **B)** False
   [Reference text page 68]

6. There are certain cases where an EMT-Basic should make the decision not to provide treatment or transport.
   A) True **B)** False
   [Reference text pages 73-74]

7. An implied obligation to provide care occurs when:
   A) a request for an ambulance has been confirmed.
   B) an EMT-Basic encounters an injury scene while off-duty.
   C) an ambulance service has contracted to provide emergency services.
   D) all of the above occur.
   [Reference text page 74]

8. As an EMT-Basic, if you decide to provide care to a patient while off-duty, you should treat the situation just as if you were on duty.
   A) True **B)** False
   [Reference text page 75]

9. When treating an organ donor patient, it is important to treat the patient like any other patient, but also to notify medical direction that you are treating a donor.
A) True **B)** False
[Reference text page 77]

10. It is not a problem if the EMT-Basic disturbs a potential crime scene.
A) True **B)** False
[Reference text page 78]

11. An example of an advanced directive would be:
A) implied orders. **B)** standing orders.
C) do not resuscitate orders. **D)** EMS protocols.
[Reference text page 65]

CD-ROM LINK: *Refer to the* Advance Directives *video in Chapter 3 of the MedEMT CD-ROM where an instructor points out how advance directives can sometimes relieve certain stresses of patient care.*

12. Expressed consent must be obtained from every:
A) patient prior to treatment.
B) conscious, mentally competent adult before rendering treatment.
C) Medical Director.
D) combative patient prior to treatment.
[Reference text page 68]

13. Implied consent is used when the patient is:
A) a minor. **B)** unconscious. **C)** uncooperative. **D)** emancipated.
[Reference text page 68]

14. Who may give parental consent?
A) The parent of an emancipated minor.
B) A physician.
C) The Medical Director.
D) A legal guardian of a minor.
[Reference text page 69]

15. Abandonment is acceptable only if the EMT-Basic is:
A) in fear of his or her own safety.
B) given permission by his or her supervisor.
C) assured the patient is faking illness.
D) turning over care to a bystander.
[Reference text page 73]

16. Organ donors may be identified by:
A) the back of a drivers license or a card in the patient's possession.
B) a friend.
C) the hospital admission clerk.
D) a national registry.
[Reference text page 77]

17. The primary responsibility of the EMT-Basic at a crime scene is the:
A) care of the patient. **B)** preservation of the crime scene.
C) investigation of the crime scene. **D)** care of the next of kin.
[Reference text page 78]

18. Which of the following is considered a special reporting situation in most states?
A) Alcohol abuse **B)** Child abuse **C)** Verbal abuse **D)** Homelessness
[Reference text page 76]

19. In order to prove negligence, the patient must prove that the EMT-Basic:
A) suffered a physical or psychological harm.
B) had no knowledge of the patient.
C) had a duty to act.
D) caused willful harm to the patient.
[Reference text page 74]

20. A tort is a:
A) civil wrong. **B)** criminal wrong.
C) criminal act. **D)** willful, unlawful act.
[Reference text page 70]

21. If you respond to the home of a patient who is unresponsive or too ill to respond, you may provide treatment; this is an example of ________ consent.
A) ethical **B)** implied **C)** parental **D)** expressed
[Reference text page 68]

22. A DNR order:
A) applies for only three days.
B) should not be followed until confirmed with Medical Director.
C) does not apply once the patient reaches the hospital.
D) requires a written physician's order in most states.
[Reference text page 65]

23. Expressed consent cannot be given by a patient who is:
A) terminally ill. **B)** mentally incompetent.
C) in extreme pain. **D)** conscious and alert.
[Reference text page 68]

24. An EMT-Basic's standard of care represents and defines:
A) the national curriculum of care taught by EMT-Basic instructors.
B) specific care provided to patients once they reach a hospital.
C) the minimum acceptable level of care provided in a community.
D) laws that define and govern the specific actions of EMT-Basics.
[Reference text page 63]

25. Which organization outlines the minimal standards for an EMT-Basic's scope of practice in the United States?
A) U.S. Department of Labor
B) World Health Organization
C) U.S. Department of Transportation
D) World Centers for Disease Control
[Reference text pages 62 & 4]

26. Documents signed by a patient that communicate his or her wishes regarding medical care are called:
A) automated care orders.
B) advance directives.
C) extended patient directives.
D) Physician orders.
[Reference text page 65]

27. A durable power of attorney for health care is an:
A) advance directive that identifies a person who can make decisions for the patient if he or she becomes incapacitated.
B) advance directive that identifies a relative who can sue an insurance company for health benefits if needed.
C) advance directive which, when presented, requires the EMT-Basic to not resuscitate a terminally ill patient.
D) attorney who specializes in health care issues for the elderly, terminally ill, and mentally ill patients.
[Reference text page 67]

28. Which of the following do the courts and juries NOT consider when evaluating negligence?
A) Whether the EMT-Basic had a duty to act
B) Whether the EMT-Basic asked permission to treat the patient
C) Whether the patient suffered injuries or damages
D) Whether the EMT-Basic's actions caused injuries or damage to the patient
[Reference text pages 73-74]

29. A mentally ill patient has the right to refuse emergency care or withdraw from treatment anytime.
A) True
B) False
[Reference text pages 68 & 71]

CD-ROM LINK: *Refer to the* Release Form *video in Chapter 3 of the MedEMT CD-ROM in which an EMS team explains the procedure for filling out a release form to a victim of a robbery attempt.*

30. Common skills within the EMT-Basic scope of practice include all of the following EXCEPT:
A) automated external defibrillation. **B)** spinal management.
C) triage. **D)** IV therapy.
[Reference text page 62]

31. In a legal action, the jury may determine if an EMT-Basic follows his or her standard of care, which is based upon:
A) textbooks. **B)** common practices.
C) professional journals. **D)** all of the above.
[Reference text pages 63-64]

32. Depending upon the state, ________ minors may be parents of their own children.
A) designated **B)** emancipated **C)** mentally ill **D)** graduated
[Reference text page 70]

33. An offensive physical contact or touching of another person without his or her consent is called assault.
A) True **B)** False
[Reference text page 71]

34. If a patient refuses medical assistance, the EMT-Basic should:
A) try to persuade the patient to accept treatment.
B) ask law enforcement personnel to speak with the patient.
C) ensure the patient can make rational informed decisions.
D) do all of the above.
[Reference text pages 72-73]

35. You should always describe the consequences of a refusal in a manner the patient understands.
A) True **B)** False
[Reference text page 73]

36. When determining negligence, the jury will consider what another ________ EMT-Basic would do in the same circumstances.
A) paid **B)** professional **C)** prudent **D)** experienced
[Reference text page 74]

37. Generally, the Good Samaritan Laws do NOT protect EMT-Basics from:
   A) being sued.
   B) gross negligence.
   C) acts that were not in good faith.
   D) all of the above.
   [Reference text page 75]

38. Examples of confidential information would be:
   A) patient history.
   B) assessment findings.
   C) treatment provided.
   D) all of the above.
   [Reference text page 75]

39. The EMT-Basic should avoid cutting through any knots or ties at a crime scene.
   A) True **B)** False
   [Reference text page 78]

40. The EMT-Basic should try to keep bystanders away from a potential crime scene to preserve evidence.
   A) True **B)** False
   [Reference text page 78]

CASE STUDIES

Use a separate piece of paper to answer the case study questions. Number your answers with the case study number and question letter (1A, 1B, etc.).

SCOPE OF PRACTICE

1. The local high school has sent a reporter to the station asking for a job description of an EMT-Basic. After explaining that your care is directed by a physician, the reporter asks you to explain the EMT-Basic's scope of practice.
   A) Explain the term "scope of practice."

ETHICS

Note: In each case below, you must make difficult choices in situations where there are no clear-cut answers. The suggested answers are based upon the EMT-Basic Code of Ethics; there is no absolute right or wrong answer for most ethical questions.

2. You observe another EMS crew bring a patient into the Emergency Department. The patient was involved in a motor vehicle collision and has obvious head and chest injuries, but is neither immobilized nor receiving supplemental oxygen.
   A) How would you act as an EMT-Basic in this situation?

3. Your partner is injured in a struggle to subdue a violent but critically injured patient. The patient has a life-threatening injury, but your partner's injury is also very serious.
   A) How would you act as an EMT-Basic in this situation?

4. You arrive on the scene of an injured child. One parent wants the child to be taken to the emergency department and the other does not. You suspect that one of the parents may have caused the injury through child abuse or neglect.
   A) How would you act as an EMT-Basic in this situation?

ADVANCE DIRECTIVES

5. You are dispatched for a man down at the local senior living center. When you arrive, the center's coordinator advises you that the man has been suffering a terminal illness for several months. Bystanders are performing CPR as you enter the room. The patient's daughter is sobbing in the corner and is too upset to speak to you. Someone hands you a bright orange envelope marked "Do Not Resuscitate." The orders inside the envelope appear to be valid.
   A) What type of document is in the envelope?
   B) Given the scenario, how will you proceed under your local protocols?
   C) What is a durable power of attorney for health care?
6. A recent television show highlighted the choices some terminally ill patients are making regarding their health care. During one section of the show, the host discussed the controversy of DNRs and living wills and their impact on emergency responders. Several of your friends have called you for clarification of how DNRs or advance directives are treated by EMS in your area and asked your opinion.
   A) How will you respond to their questions?
   B) What specific advice might you give them to help reduce the fear that EMS will disregard a family member's medical decision?

PATIENT CONSENT

7. You are dispatched to the local high school for an ill student. Upon arrival, you find a 14-year-old female unconscious on the bathroom floor. Her friends reveal she was sniffing glue before class and has a known history of chemical abuse, but they deny any narcotic use. There are no obvious signs of trauma and no track marks visible.
   A) What are your first actions in this case?
   B) Given this scenario, under what type of permission will you begin treatment?
   C) How will you obtain consent?
8. As the second unit on scene of an auto vs. train accident, you are directed toward a patient still trapped inside his small car. He is able to communicate with you even though you cannot see his face under the protective tarp. He is answering your questions appropriately and without difficulty. He has bilateral deformed, swollen, and painful thighs. He is also complaining of some facial trauma.
   A) What type of consent will you obtain from this patient?
9. A female passenger in the same car as above is unable to communicate clearly. She is confused and occasionally takes several seconds to respond to your questions. Given the mechanism of injury, you strongly believe the patient has suffered head trauma.
   A) What type of consent will you obtain from this patient?
   B) How does this patient differ from the first one?

ASSAULT AND BATTERY

10. A 40-year-old male who appears intoxicated has fallen down the stairs and is bleeding from the head. He doesn't want any help and says that if you touch him, he will charge you with assault and battery.

A) Explain the concept of assault.
B) Explain battery.
C) What is the major difference between these two definitions?

ABANDONMENT OR NEGLIGENCE

11. After a grueling 24-hour shift, the last call of the day is for an ill man. Tony is a 70-year-old regular caller who sometimes only seems interested in having some company during the night. Your crew has often been dispatched to take him to the county hospital. This time Tony cannot remember why he called you. He complains that his ankle pain is no different than the last few weeks. He forgot to take his medications today, and he doesn't seem as sharp as usual. You believe that Tony is just nervous and advise him not to go to the hospital.

A) If you leave, what could you be charged with?
B) What is medical abandonment?
C) If Tony refused treatment, what steps could you take to avoid a later claim of abandonment of your patient?
D) What is negligence?

DUTY TO ACT

12. One bright Sunday morning you are rushing to church with your family, late as usual. As you reach the church parking lot, you see that two cars have collided in the intersection in front of you. Bystanders are just exiting their vehicles. It appears that at least two people are injured. No EMS has arrived, and as a new EMT-Basic, you know the volunteer fire service is at least ten minutes away.

A) Do you have a legal duty to act?
B) Do you have an ethical duty to act?
C) What is the difference between a legal duty to act and an ethical duty to act?
D) What is a contractual duty to act?

POTENTIAL CRIME SCENE/EVIDENCE

13. You just graduated from your EMT-Basic program and are volunteering at the local fire department when you are dispatched to an injured female. En route to the call, fire dispatch advises that the patient is a victim of domestic violence and that her assailant has left the scene. As you arrive, law enforcement officers and family members wave you up to the house. As you enter the home, you notice the officer is handling a small handgun found next to the wounded woman. Just as she loses consciousness, she tells you who shot her.

A) Describe the steps you will use to control the scene as you begin patient care.

B) During your rapid physical exam of the patient, you observe that she has been shot once in the back and twice in the abdomen. What special precautions should you take while quickly removing the patient's clothing?

SPECIAL REPORTING SITUATIONS

14. As you enter the home of a patient with shortness of breath, you notice the smell of human and animal wastes and see several small animals running around inside. The elderly couple appears to be bedridden. Both are nearly blind and deaf. The woman is moderately short of breath and must be transported to the local hospital. A neighbor agrees to watch the husband until a family member can be contacted.

A) What action might you take on behalf of your patient's husband once you arrive at the hospital?

15. You recently transported a young male from a homeless shelter to the hospital. He was complaining of chest pain and a fever. Later, the emergency department called to advise you the patient tested positive for an infectious airborne disease.

A) Describe your actions after learning of the patient's status.

KEY TERMS MATCHING

Assess your knowledge of the chapter key terms by matching the terms on the left to the definitions on the right.

______ **1.** Abandonment

______ **2.** Advance Directive

______ **3.** Assault

______ **4.** Battery

______ **5.** Confidentiality

(A) Failure to act as a reasonable, prudent, similarly trained person would act under similar circumstances

(B) A description of the specific care and actions expected and allowed by law

(C) The minimum acceptable level of care provided in an EMS system

(D) Physician experienced and knowledgeable in all aspects of emergency care who delegates emergency medical practice to non-physician providers, such as EMT-Basics and other EMS personnel

(E) Used for unconscious or mentally incompetent patients requiring emergency intervention; based on the assumption that the patient would give permission to treat life-threatening conditions

______ **6.** Do Not Resuscitate (DNR) Orders

______ **7.** Durable Power of Attorney for Health Care (DPAC)

______ **8.** Duty to Act

______ **9.** Expressed Consent

______ **10.** Implied Consent

______ **11.** Medical Director

______ **12.** Negligence

______ **13.** Scope of Practice

______ **14.** Standard of Care

(F) Permission for treatment from a patient who is of legal age and is able to make rational decisions; expressed consent is given after the patient is informed of procedures involved in a treatment in a language he or she understands

(G) A contractual or legal obligation to care for any patient who requests services; does not apply if caring for the patient endangers the EMT-Basic's life

(H) A type of advance directive that assigns another person to make medical decisions on the patient's behalf; used only if an individual becomes unable to make decisions

(I) Written physician's order directing health care providers to withhold lifesaving care from a patient in cardiac or respiratory arrest.

(J) An obligation to protect the patient's privacy by not disclosing information to unauthorized individuals

(K) Actual offensive physical contact or touching of another person without his or her consent; usually combined with a charge of assault, particularly if threatening words were exchanged between the parties

(L) Termination of care without the patient's consent and without making any provisions for continuing care at the same or higher level

(M) A legal statement of a patient's wishes regarding his or her health care; used in the event the patient becomes unable to make decisions

(N) Threatening or attempting to inflict offensive physical contact; physical contact is not necessary

SKILLS CHECKLIST

Check your knowledge of important EMT-B skills by marking off each step in the following skills sheet.

REFUSAL OF EMERGENCY CARE

- [ ] Spend time effectively communicating with patient (includes reasoning, persistence, and strategies to convince patient to go to hospital).
- [ ] Clearly inform patient of consequences of not going to hospital.
- [ ] Consult with medical direction.
- [ ] Contact family to help convince patient.
- [ ] Call law enforcement who may be able to order or "arrest" serious patient in order to force patient to go to hospital.
- [ ] Try to determine why patient is refusing care.
- [ ] Complete thorough documentation of refusal, have patient sign refusal release, and have witness sign the release (e.g., bystander, police, family).

NOTE: Procedure may differ by state and jurisdiction. Always follow your medical director's advice.

(reprinted from *Pocket Reference for The EMT-B and First Responder* by Bob Elling, Prentice Hall, 1999)

D.O.T. OBJECTIVES CHECKLIST

Use the following list of knowledge objectives to check what you've learned. Check off only those objectives that you feel you completely understand and have mastered. For any objectives not checked, go back and review that section of the text chapter. Textbook page references have been provided to help you review the text material.

- [ ] Define the EMT-Basic scope of practice. *(p. 62)*
- [ ] Discuss the importance of Do Not Resuscitate (DNR) advance directives and local or state provisions regarding EMS application. *(p. 65)*
- [ ] Define consent and discuss the methods of obtaining consent. *(p. 67)*
- [ ] Differentiate between expressed and implied consent. *(p. 68)*
- [ ] Explain the role of consent of minors in providing care. *(p. 69)*
- [ ] Discuss the implications for the EMT-Basic in patient refusal of transport. *(p. 71)*
- [ ] Discuss the issues of abandonment, negligence, and battery and their implications to the EMT-Basic. *(p. 71)*
- [ ] State the conditions necessary for the EMT-Basic to have a duty to act. *(p. 74)*
- [ ] Explain the importance, necessity, and legality of patient confidentiality. *(p. 75)*
- [ ] Discuss the considerations of the EMT-Basic in issues of organ retrieval. *(p. 77)*
- [ ] Differentiate the actions that an EMT-Basic should take to assist in the preservation of a crime scene. *(p. 78)*
- [ ] State the conditions that require an EMT-Basic to notify local law enforcement officials. *(p. 77)*

CHAPTER 4

The Human Body

CHAPTER 4 SUMMARY

Knowledge of the human body and how it works is important to you as an EMT-Basic. It enables you to communicate with other health care professionals effectively and allows you to perform a competent assessment. In order for you to recognize things that are wrong with the patient, you must know what "normal" is.

Each system has specific purposes, although they all work together to keep us healthy. The musculoskeletal system gives the body shape, allows movement, and protects internal organs. The respiratory system provides oxygen to the bloodstream and removes waste gases. The circulatory system is responsible for transport of blood cells, plasma, and platelets throughout the body. The control of the voluntary and involuntary activities of the body is the function of the nervous system. The skin (integumentary system) protects the body from the environment, bacteria, and other organisms. The endocrine system secretes chemicals responsible for regulating body activities and functions.

REVIEW QUESTIONS

Please circle the best answer for each question.

1. As a broad base for EMT-Basic assessment skills, it is important to have an understanding of the basic ________ of the human body.
   A) position **B)** anatomy **C)** purpose **D)** precautions
   [Reference text page 88]

2. The heart is ________ or anterior to the spinal column.
   A) posterior **B)** caudad **C)** ventral **D)** cephalad
   [Reference text page 91]

3. A patient in the supine position is:
   A) standing facing forward. **B)** lying face down.
   C) sitting with the back straight. **D)** lying flat on the back.
   [Reference text page 89]

4. The abdominal region lies ________ to the pelvic region.
   A) superior **B)** posterior **C)** anterior **D)** inferior
   [Reference text page 91]

5. The eyes are protected by the:
   A) cranial cavity. **B)** bony orbit. **C)** frontal sinus. **D)** hard palate.
   [Reference text page 96]

6. The vertebrae are largest in the ________ region.
   A) cervical **B)** thoracic **C)** lumbar **D)** frontal
   [Reference text page 98]

7. The rib ________, or thoracic cavity, protects the organs of the chest and assists in breathing.
   A) muscles **B)** cage **C)** column **D)** structure
   [Reference text pages 98-99]

8. Ribs are attached to the sternum with:
   A) cartilage. **B)** bone. **C)** tendons. **D)** ligaments.
   [Reference text page 99]

9. The _______ is the anterior portion of the pelvis which lies in front of the bladder.
   A) fusion **B)** intersection **C)** pubis **D)** fontenelle
   [Reference text page 98]

10. The hip bones, ________, and coccyx form the bowl called the pelvis.
A) symphysis **B)** sacrum **C)** lumbar **D)** acetabulum
[Reference text pages 98-99]

11. The rim of the pelvis that can be felt when you put your hands on your hips is the:
A) iliac crest. **B)** symphysis pubis.
C) greater trochanter. **D)** pelvic tuberosity.
[Reference text pages 99, 302]

12. The palpable wing of the pelvis is called the:
A) iliac crest.
B) ischium.
C) pubis.
D) none of the above.
[Reference text page 99]

13. The ________ malleolus, a prominent knobby surface landmark, can be palpated on the inner side of the ankle joint.
A) lateral **B)** medial **C)** left **D)** central
[Reference text page 101]

14. The ________, or heel bone, is the largest bone in the foot.
A) talus **B)** tarsal **C)** calcaneus **D)** metatarsal
[Reference text page 101]

15. The bone that runs between the hip and the knee is called the:
A) pelvis. **B)** tibia. **C)** femur. **D)** fibula.
[Reference text page 101]

16. The two bones of the lower leg are the:
A) radius and fibula. **B)** femur and fibula.
C) tibia and femur. **D)** tibia and fibula.
[Reference text page 101]

17. The kneecap is called the:
A) femur. **B)** patella. **C)** tibia. **D)** calcaneus.
[Reference text page 101]

18. The tip of the scapula, where it is attached to the clavicle is called the:
A) supraclavicular joint.
B) acromion process.
C) acromion palpation.
D) costal joint.

[Reference text pages 102-103]

19. The ________ is often broken by a fall on an outstretched arm, and is the most frequently broken bone in the body.
A) femur **B)** clavicle **C)** tibia **D)** radius
[Reference text page 102]

20. The carpal bones of the wrist are connected to each other by:
A) ligaments. **B)** articulations. **C)** metacarpals. **D)** cartilage.
[Reference text page 103]

21. The collarbone is also known as the:
A) scapula. **B)** clavicle. **C)** trochanter. **D)** talus.
[Reference text page 102]

22. The long bone of the upper arm, between the shoulder and the elbow, is the:
A) humerus. **B)** femur. **C)** radius. **D)** ulna.
[Reference text page 103]

23. Which two bones are found in the forearm?
A) Humerus and ulna
B) Ulna and radius
C) Tibia and fibula
D) Radius and fibula
[Reference text page 103]

24. The bones of the finger and toes are called:
A) tarsals. **B)** phalanges. **C)** carpals. **D)** metacarpals.
[Reference text pages 102 & 104]

25. The bones of the hand are called:
A) tarsals. **B)** metatarsals. **C)** carpals. **D)** metacarpals.
[Reference text page 104]

26. The bones of the wrist are called:
A) metacarpals. **B)** phalanges. **C)** carpals. **D)** metatarsals.
[Reference text pages 103-104]

27. Ligaments connect:
A) muscles to bones.
B) muscles to muscles.
C) bones to bones.
D) cartilage to bones.
[Reference text page 95]

28. Abduction is:
A) movement of a limb closer to the midline.
B) lateral movement of a limb away from the midline.
C) a bone rotating upon its own axis.
D) none of the above.
[Reference text page 105]

29. The articulations of the metacarpal bones of the hand with the phalanges of the fingers (the knuckles) are hinge joints.
A) True **B)** False
[Reference text page 106]

30. The articulation between the acetabulum and the head of the femur is a ________ joint.
A) gliding **B)** condyloid **C)** ball-and-socket **D)** pivot
[Reference text pages 104-106]

31. Functions of the muscular system include voluntary movement, generation of ________, maintenance of posture, and protection of internal organs.
A) heat **B)** energy
C) light **D)** electrical impulses
[Reference text pages 106-107]

32. Around the bronchi in the respiratory tree, you would expect to find ________ muscle tissue.
A) cardiac **B)** striated **C)** smooth **D)** dry
[Reference text page 109]

33. Contraction of the smooth muscles controls the flow through tubular structures.
A) True **B)** False
[Reference text page 109]

34. The skeletal muscles that provide for movement are under ________ control.
A) voluntary **B)** manual **C)** involuntary **D)** cardiac
[Reference text page 108]

35. Cardiac muscle is supplied with oxygen by the blood flowing through the heart's chambers.
A) True **B)** False
[Reference text page 110]

36. Skeletal muscles are attached to bones by:
A) cartilage. **B)** ligaments.
C) tendons. **D)** none of the above.
[Reference text page 94]

37. The trachea divides into the:
A) bronchi. **B)** bronchioles. **C)** carina. **D)** alveoli.
[Reference text page 113]

38. The bronchi divide into the:
A) pulmonary capillaries. **B)** bronchioles.
C) carina. **D)** alveoli.
[Reference text pages 113-114]

39. The nasopharynx lies above the oropharynx.
A) True **B)** False
[Reference text page 111]

40. The larynx is constructed mainly of ________ and muscles.
A) skin **B)** bone **C)** cartilage **D)** tendons
[Reference text page 112]

41. During swallowing, the epiglottis is pushed over the top of the larynx, preventing food from entering the respiratory tract.
A) True **B)** False
[Reference text page 112]

42. The part of the airway that can create the greatest resistance to air flow is the:
A) nasal cavity. **B)** trachea. **C)** bronchi. **D)** bronchioles.
[Reference text page 114]

43. The ________ are the functional units of the lungs, where gas exchange takes place.
A) alveoli **B)** bronchi **C)** mast cells **D)** carina
[Reference text page 115]

44. Carbon dioxide is:
A) an end product of normal cell metabolism.
B) the result of abnormal metabolism.
C) required for normal cell metabolism.
D) a cellular nutrient.
[Reference text page 118]

45. Oxygen is:
A) an end product of normal cell metabolism.
B) an end product of abnormal cell metabolism.
C) required for normal cell metabolism.
D) carried in the blood as a dissolved ion.
[Reference text pages 110, 118]

46. A network of capillaries covers each alveolus for the purpose of gas exchange between blood and air.
A) True B) False
[Reference text page 115]

47. What occurs during normal expiration?
A) The intercostals and diaphragm relax.
B) The intercostals and diaphragm contract.
C) The intercostals relax and diaphragm contracts.
D) The intercostals contract and diaphragm relaxes.
[Reference text page 117]

48. When the diaphragm contracts, the thoracic cavity becomes:
A) injured. B) smaller. C) collapsed. D) larger.
[Reference text page 117]

49. The movement of air into and out of the lungs occurs because pressure gradients are created.
A) True B) False
[Reference text page 117]

50. The volume of air that moves in and out of the airways in a normal breath (inspiration, followed by expiration) is called the:
A) residual volume. B) tidal volume.
C) vital capacity. D) expiratory reserve volume.
[Reference text page 119]

51. Inadequate respirations may cause:
A) hypoxia B) pale, bluish color C) breathing D) orientation
[Reference text page 119]

52. Breathing by using the accessory muscles would generally be considered to be:
A) adequate. B) inadequate. C) prolonged. D) appropriate.
[Reference text page 119]

53. A person with breath sounds that are present and equal in both lungs is most likely breathing:
A) adequately. B) rapidly. C) inadequately. D) slowly.
[Reference text page 119]

54. The respiratory rate of a person experiencing respiratory distress is:
A) normal. **B)** faster than normal.
C) slower than normal. **D)** any of the above.
[Reference text page 119]

55. Oxygen-poor blood is pumped to the lungs from the right atrium through which vessel?
A) Aorta **B)** Pulmonary artery
C) Vena cava **D)** Pulmonary vein
[Reference text page 124]

56. The ________ pumps blood through the aorta to the rest of the body.
A) left atrium **B)** left ventricle **C)** right ventricle **D)** right atrium
[Reference text pages 121-122]

57. The pulmonary veins are the only veins that carry ________ blood.
A) oxygen poor **B)** capillary **C)** oxygen-rich **D)** cardiac
[Reference text pages 121 & 124]

58. The upper chambers of the heart are known as the:
A) septum. **B)** ventricles. **C)** atria. **D)** sinus nodes.
[Reference text page 121]

59. The right atrium pumps blood to the:
A) left atrium. **B)** left ventricle.
C) right ventricle. **D)** pulmonary artery.
[Reference text page 121]

60. The right ventricle pumps blood to the:
A) pulmonary vein. **B)** pulmonary artery.
C) aorta. **D)** left ventricle.
[Reference text page 121]

61. Blood returns to the heart from the lungs by way of the:
A) venae cavae. **B)** aorta.
C) right heart. **D)** pulmonary vein.
[Reference text page 121]

62. Unoxygenated blood first enters the heart's:
A) right atrium. **B)** left atrium. **C)** right ventricle. **D)** left ventricle.
[Reference text page 121]

63. There are two main circulatory routes of the blood: the systemic circulation and the pulmonic circulation.
A) True **B)** False
[Reference text page 120]

64. Systemic circulation moves blood from the heart's ________ through blood vessels to all parts of the body.
A) left ventricle **B)** right ventricle
C) left atrium **D)** right atrium
[Reference text page 122]

65. The vessels that pass blood from the tissues back to the heart are called:
A) arteries. **B)** veins. **C)** capillaries. **D)** nodes.
[Reference text pages 123 & 127]

66. The heart is located in an area called the mediastinum.
A) True **B)** False
[Reference text page 120]

67. The two AV valves regulate the passageways between the ventricles and lungs.
A) True **B)** False
[Reference text pages 121-122]

68. One complete heartbeat, called the cardiac cycle, includes a contraction phase called systole, and a relaxation phase called diastole.
A) True **B)** False
[Reference text pages 121-122]

69. The blood supply for the heart itself is provided by the ________ arteries.
A) pulmonary **B)** carotid **C)** coronary **D)** cardiac
[Reference text page 124]

70. The major artery leaving the heart to supply the systemic circulation is the:
A) coronary artery. **B)** vena cava.
C) pulmonary artery. **D)** aorta.
[Reference text page 124]

71. The major artery of the thigh is the:
A) femoral. **B)** tibial. **C)** popliteal. **D)** brachial.
[Reference text page 126]

72. The left and right brachial arteries supply blood to the:
A) skull. **B)** arms. **C)** legs. **D)** kidneys.
[Reference text page 125]

73. The ________ aorta divides into the left and right iliac arteries that feed the legs.
A) ascending **B)** arch of the **C)** thoracic **D)** abdominal
[Reference text page 125]

74. Pulsations of the ________ arteries can be palpated on the lateral anterior surface of each wrist.
A) brachial **B)** radial **C)** ulnar **D)** medial
[Reference text page 125]

75. The left and right pulmonary veins drain:
A) the heart. **B)** the lungs. **C)** the brain. **D)** all of the above.
[Reference text page 127]

76. The vessels that pass blood through the tissues for exchange of materials are called:
A) arteries. **B)** veins.
C) capillaries. **D)** none of the above.
[Reference text page 126]

77. What is the job of the white blood cell?
A) Transport carbon dioxide **B)** Transport oxygen
C) Fight infection **D)** Regulate temperature
[Reference text page 129]

78. What is the job of the platelet?
A) Produce antibodies **B)** Excrete hormones
C) Form blood clots **D)** Produce red blood cells
[Reference text page 129]

79. Oxygenated hemoglobin gives erythrocytes their red color.
A) True **B)** False
[Reference text page 128]

80. White blood cells carry oxygen and carbon dioxide in the blood.
A) True **B)** False
[Reference text pages 128-129]

81. Besides transporting cells, the plasma carries dissolved nutrients and metabolic wastes.
A) True **B)** False
[Reference text page 129]

82. Perfusion occurs in the:
A) arteries. **B)** veins.
C) organs and tissues. **D)** capillary bed.
[Reference text page 130]

83. What happens during perfusion?
A) Oxygen and nutrients are delivered; carbon dioxide and wastes are picked up.
B) Vessels constrict to maintain the blood pressure.
C) The diaphragm descends and the rib cage lifts to create a relative vacuum, causing air to rush into the lungs.
D) Blood from the left ventricle exerts pressure on arterial walls.
[Reference text page 130]

84. In adults, assessment of the circulation can be performed by measuring the ________ and blood pressure.
A) respiratory rate **B)** pulse
C) skin temperature **D)** capillary refill
[Reference text page 130]

85. The pulse can be palpated in places where an artery lying near the skin surface also runs over a bone.
A) True **B)** False
[Reference text page 130]

86. Blood pressure reaches its maximum after the left ventricle contracts. This reading is known as the ________ pressure.
A) systolic **B)** diastolic **C)** constant **D)** venous
[Reference text page 130]

87. In the face of injury, the body will adjust cardiac output and blood vessel diameter to maintain a normal blood pressure.
A) True **B)** False
[Reference text page 130]

88. The condition of shock results if inadequate circulation prevents the tissues from receiving enough ________ to meet their energy needs.
A) sugar **B)** oxygen
C) carbon dioxide **D)** leukocytes
[Reference text page 130]

89. Symptoms of shock can include pale, cool skin; shallow breathing; a weak, rapid pulse; and restless behavior.
A) True **B)** False
[Reference text page 130]

90. The functions of the nervous system are sensation of changes, integration of information, and control of body processes.
A) True **B)** False
[Reference text page 131]

91. The ________ are specialized nerve cells, capable of transmitting electrical impuslses over distances as short as one millimeter or as long a meter or more:
A) protons. **B)** synapses. **C)** networks. **D)** neurons.
[Reference text page 131]

92. The liquid that bathes the brain and spinal cord is called cerebro________ fluid.
A) vascular **B)** neuro
C) spinal **D)** none of the above
[Reference text page 132]

93. The portion of the head housing the brain is the:
A) cerebrum. **B)** cranium. **C)** cerebellum. **D)** brain stem.
[Reference text page 133]

94. The central nervous system (CNS) consists of the brain:
A) and spinal cord. **B)** and brain stem.
C) stem and spinal nerves. **D)** and peripheral nerves.
[Reference text pages 132-133]

95. The largest part of the brain is the:
A) cerebellum. **B)** cerebrum. **C)** pons. **D)** brain stem.
[Reference text page 132]

96. The peripheral nervous system, consisting of 12 pairs of cranial nerves, 31 pairs of spinal nerves, and all other branches, carries impulses between the CNS and ________:
A) various receptors. **B)** glands. **C)** internal organs **D)** all of the above
[Reference text page 133]

97. The peripheral nervous system carries information between muscles in the extremities and the:
A) autonomic nervous system. **B)** adrenal glands.
C) muscles in the arms. **D)** brain.
[Reference text page 133]

98. During stress, the fight-or-flight response of the sympathetic nervous system institutes characteristic physiological changes, including:
A) dilation of blood vessels in organs. **B)** release of epinephrine.
C) rise in blood glucose levels. **D)** all of the above.
[Reference text pages 134 & 138]

99. The division of the nervous system that regulates the activities of many internal organs is the:
A) somatic nervous system. **B)** autonomic nervous system.

C) peripheral nervous system. **D)** cranial nerves.
[Reference text page 134]

100. The sympathetic and ________ divisions make up the motor portion of the autonomic nervous system.
A) automatic **B)** parasympathetic
C) sensory **D)** spinal
[Reference text page 134]

101. Which of the following is NOT a sign of sympathetic activation?
A) Increased heart rate **B)** Dilation of the pupils
C) Increased digestive functions **D)** Rapid and deep breathing
[Reference text page 134]

102. The autonomic nervous system usually operates without conscious awareness.
A) True **B)** False
[Reference text page 134]

103. Blood vessels and sweat glands in the skin play an important role in regulation of body temperature.
A) True **B)** False
[Reference text page 135]

104. Which of the following is NOT a function of the skin?
A) Protection from infection **B)** Production of white blood cells
C) Temperature regulation **D)** Excretion of wastes
[Reference text pages 135-136]

105. The layer of skin located between the epidermis and the subcutaneous layer is the:
A) dermis. **B)** subdermal. **C)** muscle layer. **D)** sebaceous.
[Reference text page 136]

106. All of the cells of the epidermis are dead.
A) True **B)** False
[Reference text page 136]

107. The dermis is generally thinner than the epidermis.
A) True **B)** False
[Reference text page 136]

108. The outer layer of the skin is called the:
A) subcutaneous tissue. **B)** dermis.
C) merkel cells. **D)** epidermis.
[Reference text page 136]

109. The layer of fat and soft tissue beneath the skin is called the:
A) subcutaneous layer.
B) dermis.
C) connective tissue.
D) hypodermis.
[Reference text page 136]

110. The layer of skin containing the blood vessels, nerves, and hair follicles is called the:
A) epidermal ridge.
B) sebaceous layer.
C) dermis.
D) epidermis.
[Reference text page 136]

CASE STUDY

Use a separate piece of paper to answer the case study questions. Number your answers with the case study number and question letter (1A, 1B, etc.).

1) Your EMS crew is on standby at the local high school for a regional football game. During halftime, a fan loses her balance on the bleachers and falls to the ground from a height of five feet. Although alert and oriented, she is in severe pain. She landed on her right hip and knee, and there is no indication of cervical spine injury. Her leg is in an awkward position.
A) You straighten the leg and position the patient for transport. You notice that the right leg appears shorter than the left and that the patient's right foot is turned outward. Describe the nature and site of the injury in anatomical terms.
B) What internal structures may have been damaged by the injury?

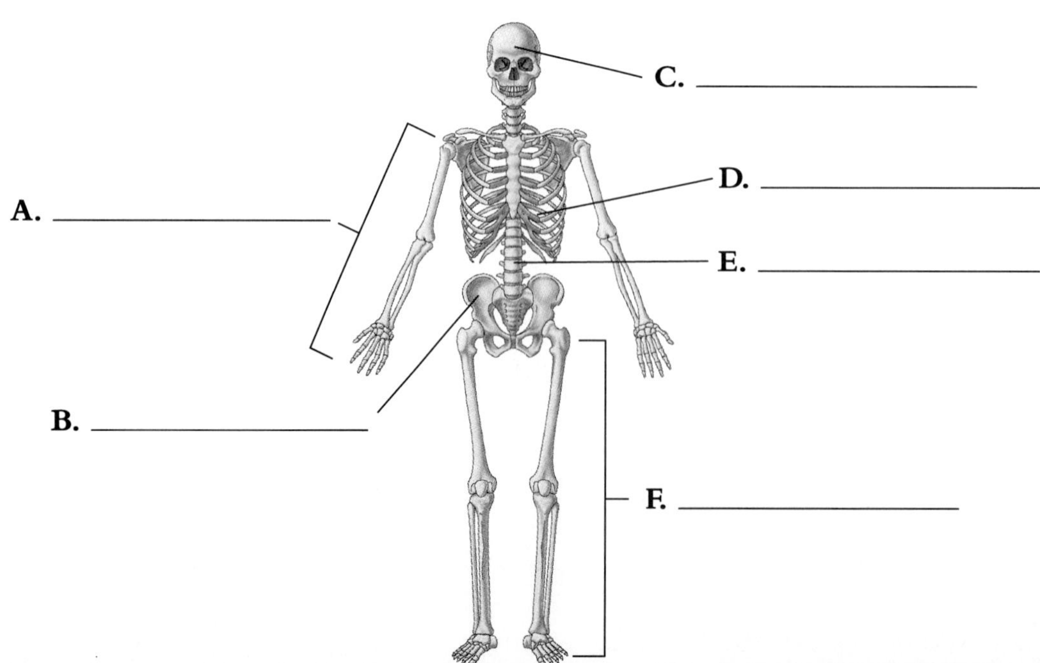

LABELING DIAGRAMS

Fill in the blanks on the following diagrams with the correct anatomical term.

REGIONS OF THE HUMAN SKELETON

THE HUMAN SKULL

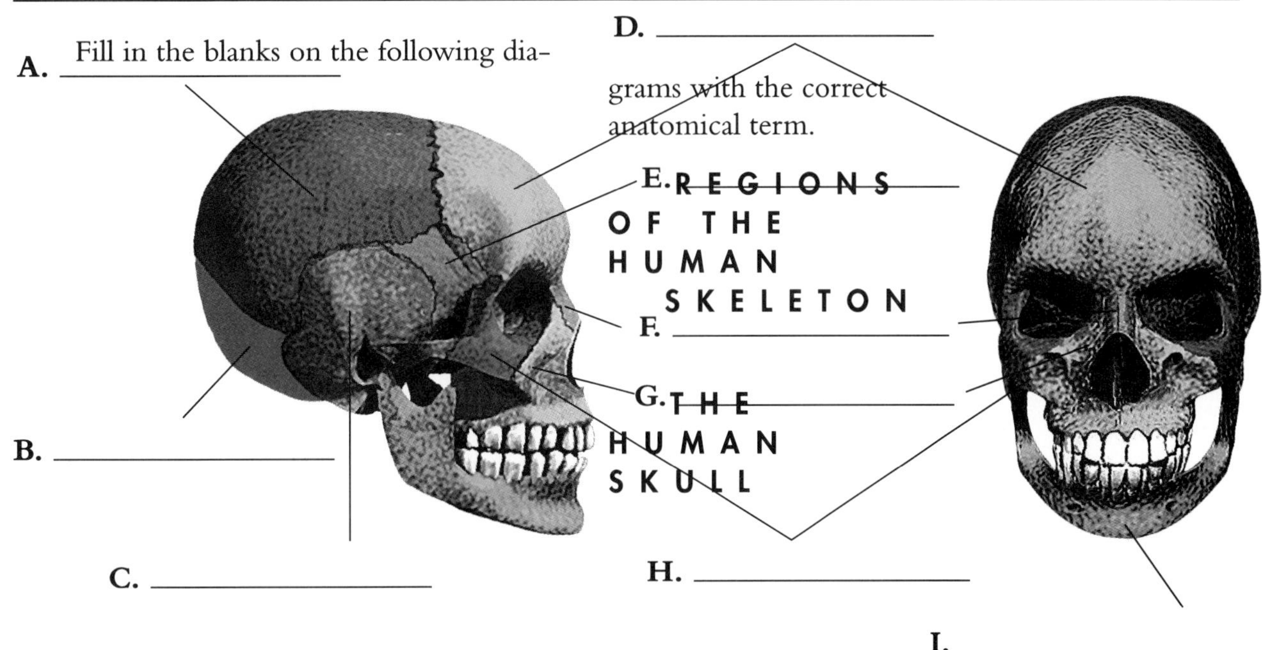

THE UPPER RESPIRATORY TRACT

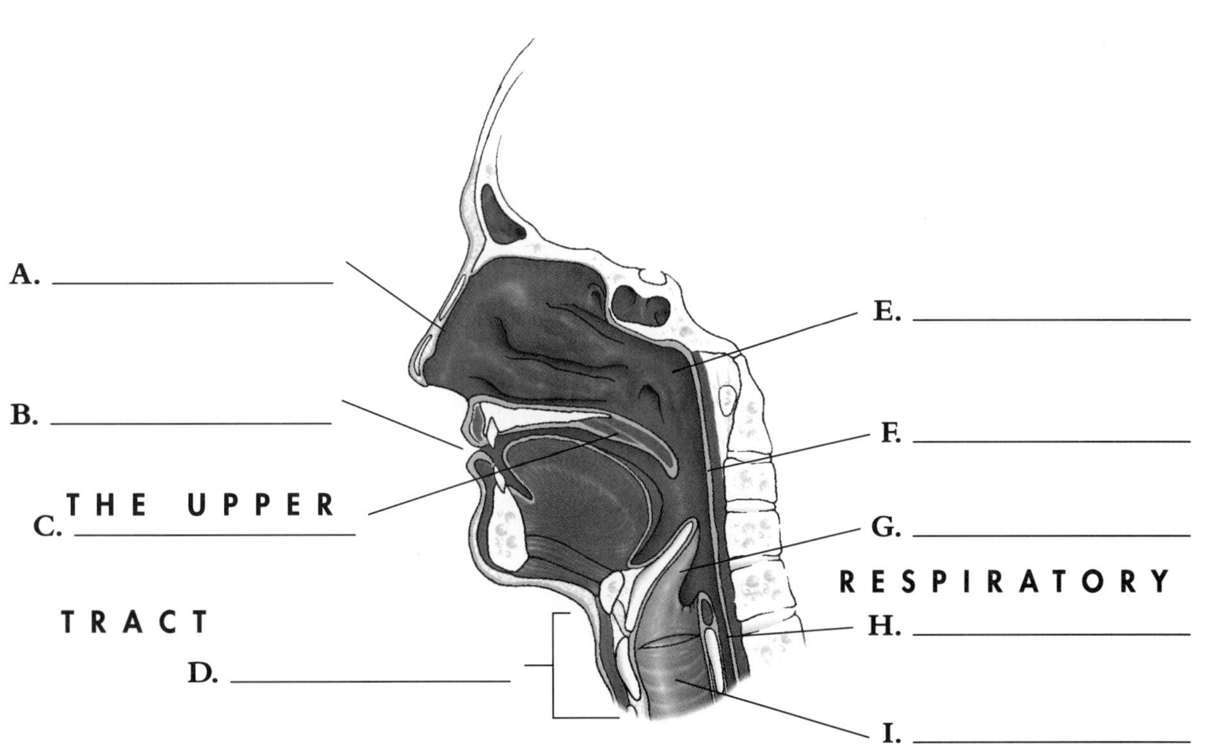

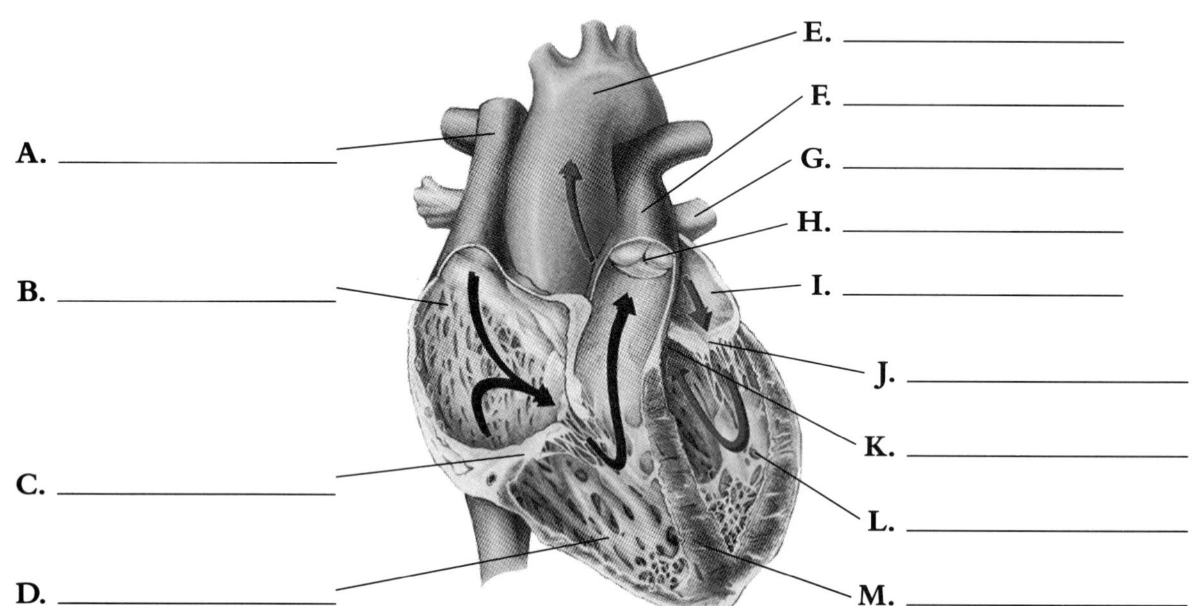
E.
F.
G.
H.
I.
J.
K.
L.
M.
A.
B.
C.
D.

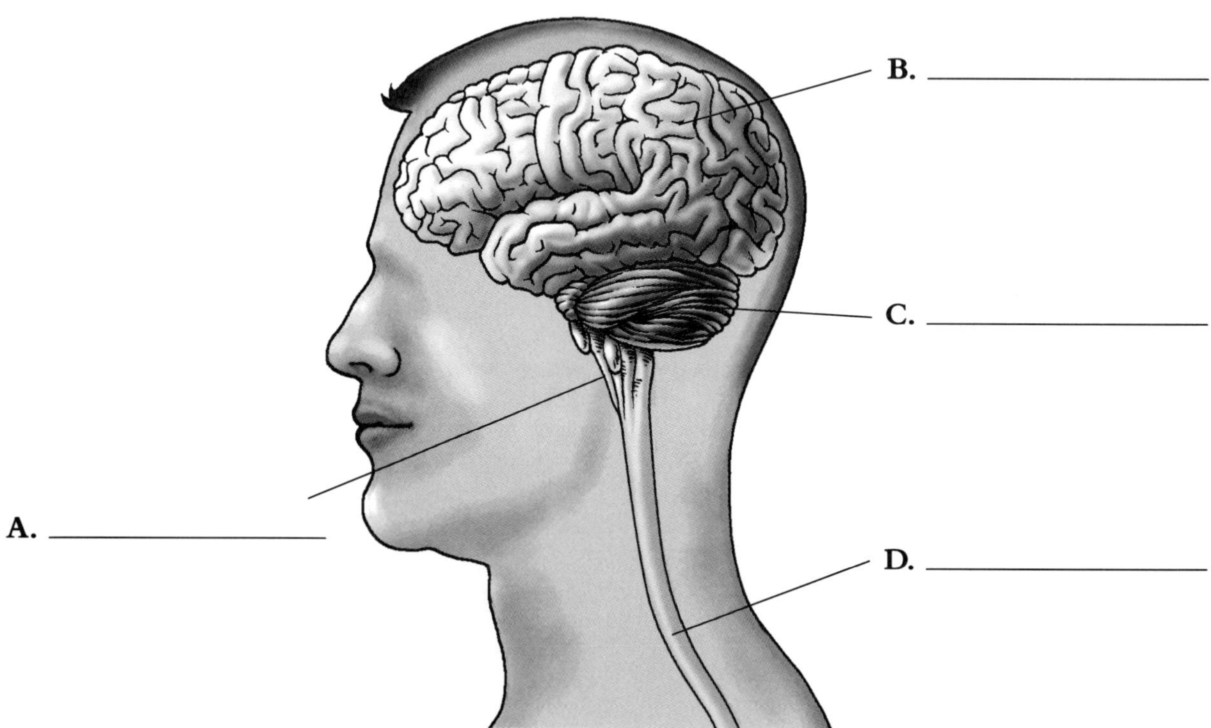
B.
C.
A.
D.

THE BLOOD FLOW THROUGH THE HEART

THE BRAIN

(A) The inferior tip of the sternum; it is prominent and easy to palpate

(B) The cheek bones

(C) Cells in the blood responsible for controlling disease conditions, such as infections caused by microorganisms

(D) Muscles that are under conscious control

(E) Block-like bones that stack upon one another to form the spinal column

(F) The smallest branches of the veins

(G) Inferior and superior; the final vein of the systemic circulation; it empties into the right atrium of the heart

(H) Front of the body; also called anterior

(I) Exchange of air between lungs and ambient air

(J) The two lower chambers of the heart

(K) Vessels carrying blood back to the heart

(L) Structures within the heart and circulatory system that prevent backflow of blood

(M) The small structure that hangs from the roof of the mouth just in front of the oropharynx; made of connective tissue

(N) The trunk of a body, not including the head or limbs

(O) Bone forming the medial side of the forearm

(P) The supine position inclined with the feet elevated about a foot above the head level

(Q) The windpipe; main air passage, arising from larynx and dividing into bronchi

(R) On one side of the body

KEY TERMS MATCHING

Assess your knowledge of the chapter key terms by matching the terms on the left to the definitions on the right.

_____ **1.** Abdominal cavity

_____ **2.** Acromion (ah-KRO-me-un)

_____ **3.** Anatomy

_____ **4.** Anterior

_____ **5.** Aorta (ay-OR-tuh)

_____ **6.** Arteries

_____ **7.** Arterioles (ar-TEAR-ee-olz)

_____ **8.** Atrium (AY-tree-um)

_____ **9.** Ball-and-Socket Joint

_____ **10.** Bilateral

_____ **11.** Blood Pressure

_____ **12.** Brachial (BRAY-kee-ul) Artery

_____ **13.** Bronchi (BRONG-kee)

_____ **14.** Bronchioles

_____ **15.** Calcaneus (kal-KAY-ne-us)

_____ **16.** Capillaries (KA-pul-air-eez)

_____ **17.** Cardiac Muscle

_____ **18.** Carina (kah-REE-nuh)

(S) The shin bone

(T) Part of the body between the neck and abdomen

(U) The ankle bone

(V) The third layer of skin located under the dermis; attaches the skin to underlying structures

(W) Above another structure

(X) Lying on the back

(Y) Flat bone in the center of the anterior chest; the breastbone

(Z) Reference position in which the body is standing upright, facing the EMT with feet flat, arms at the side, palms forward

(AA) The five fused vertebrae that form the rigid part of the posterior side of the pelvis

(BB) Cranium; the bones that comprise and protect the head

(CC) The shoulder blade

(DD) Vertebral column; consists of the cervical, thoracic, and lumbar vertebrae

(EE) Breathing rate; measured in breaths per minute

(FF) Component of blood that contains hemoglobin; transport oxygen to the body's cells and remove carbon dioxide

(GG) Originates in the right ventricle and enters the lungs where it branches off and follows the bronchi of the lungs

(HH) Major artery of the forearm

(II) Bone forming the lateral side of the forearm

(JJ) Bony structure forming anterior part of hip bone

______ **19.** Carotid (kah-RAH-tid) Artery

______ **20.** Carpals (KAR-pulz)

______ **21.** Central Nervous System

______ **22.** Cerebellum (seh-reh-BEL-em)

______ **23.** Cerebrum (seh-REE-brem)

______ **24.** Cervical (SUR-vi-kul), Cervical Vertebrae

______ **25.** Circulation

______ **26.** Clavicle (KLA-vi-kul)

______ **27.** Coccyx (KOK-siks), Coccygeal Bones

______ **28.** Contralateral

______ **29.** Coronary artery

______ **30.** Cranium (KRAY-nee-em)

______ **31.** Cricoid (KRY-koyd) Cartilage

______ **32.** Dermis (DER-mus)

______ **33.** Distal

______ **34.** Dorsal

______ **35.** Dorsalis Pedis (dor-SAL-is PEE-dis) Artery

______ **36.** Endocrine System

______ **37.** Epidermis (ep-i-DER-mus)

______ **38.** Epiglottis (ep-i-GLOT-us)

(KK) Nearer to the head, trunk, or point of origin

(LL) Lying on the stomach, face down

(MM) The serum, or fluid component, of blood

(NN) Component of blood essential for clotting

(OO) Toward the back of the body; also called dorsal

(PP) Pertaining to the sole of the foot

(QQ) The study of the normal functions of the human body

(RR) The throat

(SS) Small bones of the fingers and toes

(TT) The kneecap

(UU) Microcirculation of blood within the organs and tissues, when oxygen and nutrients are delivered to the cells and their waste products are removed

(VV) The massive cup-shaped ring of bone at the lower end of the trunk; formed by the hip bones

(WW) The sensory and motor nerves that extend from the spinal cord throughout the body

(XX) Ventral surface of the hand; the palm of the hand

(YY) Part of pharynx above the level of the soft palate

(ZZ) Eye socket

(AAA) Elbow bone; tip of the elbow

(BBB) Part of pharynx between the soft palate and upper end of epiglottis

(CCC) Bone of the nose

_____ **39.** Esophagus (eh-SOF-eh-gus)

_____ **40.** Face

_____ **41.** Femur (FEE-mer)

_____ **42.** Femoral (FEM-or-ul) Artery

_____ **43.** Fibula (FIB-yuh-luh)

_____ **44.** Fowler's Position

_____ **45.** Glottis (GLOT-is)

_____ **46.** Heart

_____ **47.** Hemoglobin (HEE-muh-glow-ben)

_____ **48.** Hinge joint

_____ **49.** Hormones

_____ **50.** Humerus (HYU-me-rus)

_____ **51.** Hypoperfusion (HY-po-per-few-zhun)

_____ **52.** Iliac (ILL-e-ak) Crest

_____ **53.** Inferior

_____ **54.** Involuntary Muscles

_____ **55.** Ischium (ISH-e-em)

_____ **56.** Joint

_____ **57.** Larynx (LAIR-inks)

_____ **58.** Lateral

_____ **59.** Lateral Recumbent Position

(DDD) Imaginary line drawn through the middle of the clavicle (or collar bone), dividing the body into unequal right and left sides

(EEE) An imaginary vertical line that divides the body into equal right and left sides

(FFF) Consists of the muscular system and the skeletal system. A human body functions through the actions and interactions of these systems

(GGG) Imaginary line drawn vertically through the side of the body, extending from the middle of the armpit to the ankle, dividing the body into front and back sides

(HHH) Foot bones

(III) The hand bones

(JJJ) Toward the middle of a body or region

(KKK) The two fused bones that form the upper jaw

(LLL) Lying on one side

(MMM) The five vertebrae forming the lower back

(NNN) The surface landmark of the ankle

(OOO) Respiratory organs that exchange oxygen, carbon dioxide, and water between the blood and the outside atmosphere

(PPP) The lower jaw bone

(QQQ) Superior portion of the sternum

(RRR) Away from the midline, to the sides

(SSS) Part of respiratory tract between the pharynx and the trachea, responsible for the production of voice; also called the voice box

(TTT) A place where bones connect

(UUU) One of the bones forming the pelvis

_______ **60.** Lumbar (LUM-bar), Lumbar Vertebrae

_______ **61.** Lungs

_______ **62.** Malleolus (ma-LEE-oh-lus)

_______ **63.** Mandible (MAN-di-bul)

_______ **64.** Manubrium (ma-NEW-bre-um)

_______ **65.** Maxillae (mak-SIL-ee)

_______ **66.** Medial

_______ **67.** Metacarpals (me-tuh-KAR-pulz)

_______ **68.** Metatarsals (me-tuh-TAR-sulz)

_______ **69.** Mid-axillary (mid-AKS-ul-eh-ree) Line

_______ **70.** Mid-clavicular (mid-kluh-VIK-yu-ler) Line

_______ **71.** Midline

_______ **72.** Musculoskeletal system

_______ **73.** Nasal bone

_______ **74.** Nasopharynx (nay-zo-FAIR-inks)

_______ **75.** Olecranon (oh-LEK-re-non)

_______ **76.** Orbit

_______ **77.** Oropharynx (or-oh-FAIR-inks)

(VVV) Muscles that carry out the automatic muscular functions of the body

(WWW) Shock; inadequate cardiac output causing a decrease in the delivery of oxygen and clearance of carbon dioxide

(XXX) Upper part of the pelvis

(YYY) Below or beneath another structure

(ZZZ) The upper arm bone

(A1) Biologically active substances secreted by an endocrine gland; travel through the bloodstream to exert an influence on distant organs or body tissues

(A2) Joint that allows movement in one plane, forward and backward

(A3) Supine position with the upper body elevated by a 45°–60° bend at the hips

(A4) Organ located in the thoracic cavity that receives blood from the veins and pumps it to the arteries

(A5) Space between the vocal cords; sound is produced when air passes through opening, causing vocal cords to vibrate

(A6) Protein in red blood cells responsible for oxygen transport

(A7) The lateral and smaller bone of the lower leg

(A8) The major artery in the thigh

(A9) The thigh bone

(A10) Consists of orbits, nasal bone, maxilla, mandible, and zygomatic bones

(A11) Outermost layer of skin

(A12) A leaf-shaped, lid-like structure attached to the top of the larynx; closes during swallowing, preventing food or liquid from entering the respiratory tract

(A13) Part of the gastrointestinal tract that joins the pharynx to the stomach

______ **78.** Palmar

______ **79.** Patella (pa-TELL-uh)

______ **80.** Pelvis

______ **81.** Perfusion (per-FEW-zhun)

______ **82.** Peripheral Nervous System

______ **83.** Phalanges (fuh-LAN-jeez)

______ **84.** Pharynx (FAIR-inks)

______ **85.** Physiology

______ **86.** Plantar

______ **87.** Plasma

______ **88.** Platelets

______ **89.** Posterior

______ **90.** Prone (Position)

______ **91.** Proximal

______ **92.** Pubis (PEW-bis)

______ **93.** Pulmonary Artery

______ **94.** Radial Artery

______ **95.** Radius

______ **96.** Red Blood Cells

______ **97.** Respiratory (RES-pruh-tor-ee) Rate

______ **98.** Sacrum, Sacral Vertebrae

(A14) Farthest from head or source; opposite of proxima

(A15) Artery located on the upper surface of the foot; can be used to assess blood supply distal to a leg injury

(A16) Pertaining to the back of the body; also called posterior

(A17) Collection of ductless glands that internally secrete hormones into the bloodstream

(A18) Layer of skin located beneath the epidermis that supplies the skin with nutrients

(A19) Ring of cartilage that forms the bottom of the larynx and is an anatomical landmark

(A20) The skull

(A21) Blood vessels that supply the heart with blood

(A22) The largest part of the brain; consists of two hemispheres

(A23) The last four vertebrae; the tailbone

(A24) Bone of the shoulder girdle that joins the sternum to the scapula; collarbone

(A25) Flow of blood from the heart through arteries to capillaries and returning to the heart through veins

(A26) First seven vertebrae; the neck

(A27) On the opposite side of the body

(A28) Portion of the brain that coordinates voluntary muscular movements

(A29) The brain and spinal cord

(A30) The eight bones of the wrist

(A31) Major artery in the neck

(A32) A triangular projection of the lowest tracheal cartilage; forms the division of the primary bronchi

_____ **99.** Scapula (SKA-pyu-luh)

_____ **100.** Skull

_____ **101.** Spinal Column

_____ **102.** Standard Anatomical Position

_____ **103.** Sternum

_____ **104.** Subcutaneous (sub-kew-TAY-ne-is) Layer

_____ **105.** Superior

_____ **106.** Supine (Position)

_____ **107.** Tarsal (TAR-sul)

_____ **108.** Thorax

_____ **109.** Tibia (TIB-e-uh)

_____ **110.** Torso

_____ **111.** Trachea (TRAY-kee-uh)

_____ **112.** Trendelenburg Position

_____ **113.** Ulna

_____ **114.** Unilateral

_____ **115.** Uvula (YEW-vyu-luh)

_____ **116.** Valves

_____ **117.** Veins

(A33) The heel bone

(A34) Tiny vessels that carry blood through the tissues; the network of capillaries in the tissues and organs is called the capillary bed

(A35) Involuntary muscle tissue of the heart that is usually not under conscious control

(A36) Subdivisions of the bronchi; terminate in the alveoli

(A37) The two major subdivisions of the trachea

(A38) Major artery of the upper arm

(A39) Force of the blood on the vessels; systolic pressure is the working pressure; diastolic pressure is the resting pressure

(A40) Cup-shaped surface of a bone that joins with the ball-shaped head of a long bone

(A41) On both sides of the midline (right and left sides)

(A42) One of two upper chambers of the heart

(A43) Smaller vessels that branch off the arteries and lead to the capillaries

(A44) Blood vessels that carry blood away from the heart

(A45) The highest point of the shoulder

(A46) Toward the front; front of the body; also called ventral

(A47) The study of the structures of the body and how they relate to one another

(A48) The main trunk of the arterial system of the body; it leaves the heart from the upper surface of the left ventricle

(A49) The portion of the torso beneath the thorax and above the pelvis; contains the liver, gallbladder, stomach, pancreas, intestines, spleen, kidneys, and ureters

______ **118.** Vena Cava (VEE-nuh KAY-vuh)

______ **119.** Ventilation

______ **120.** Ventral

______ **121.** Ventricles

______ **122.** Venules

______ **123.** Vertebrae (VER-te-bray)

______ **124.** Voluntary muscles

______ **125.** White Blood Cells

______ **126.** Xiphoid Process (ZY-foyd)

______ **127.** Zygomatic (ZI-go-MA-tik) Bones

CHAPTER 5

Vital Signs and SAMPLE History

CHAPTER 5 SUMMARY

Obtaining baseline vital signs and a SAMPLE history is an important part of the assessment process you will learn in Chapter 8. Vital signs include an evaluation and measurement of the patient's breathing, pulse, blood pressure, pupils, and skin. The assessment process is a very organized, systematic approach that ensures you obtain all pertinent information about the patient.

Obtain the chief complaint, age and sex of every patient. Obtain the respiratory rate and evaluate quality as normal, shallow, labored, or noisy. Check for the presence of a peripheral pulse (radial in adults, brachial for patients less than one year old). If there is no peripheral pulse, check for a carotid pulse. Obtain the pulse rate and evaluate the pulse as either strong or weak and regular or irregular.

Evaluate the skin color in the nail beds, oral mucosa, and conjunctiva and characterize as pale, cyanotic, flushed, or jaundiced. Evaluate the skin temperature as normal, hot, cool, or cold. Also note whether the skin is wet, moist, or dry. Assess the pupils by briefly shining a light into the patient's eyes and determine pupil size and reactivity. Note whether pupils are equal in size; whether they react equally to light; and whether they are dilated, constricted, or normal. Obtain a blood pressure by either palpation or auscultation.

Obtain a SAMPLE history by asking the patient short, simple questions. If the patient is incapacitated, you can obtain much of the information by talking with family members. Ask about the signs or symptoms the patient is experiencing. Find out if the patient has any known allergies or takes any medications. Ask if the patient has any previous medical history, and ask when the patient's last oral intake (food or liquid) was. It is also very important to ask about the events or circumstances that led up to the call for assistance.

REVIEW QUESTIONS

Please circle the best answer for each question.

1. Recording vital signs several times during the call aids in determining a trend in the patient's condition.
   A) True **B)** False
   [Reference text page 148]

2. It is important to only address the chief complaint while on a call.
   A) True **B)** False
   [Reference text pages 146-47]

3. When assessing a patient's vital signs, which of the following do you want to record?
   A) Pulse **B)** Blood pressure **C)** Respiration **D)** All of the above
   [Reference text page 147]

4. A patient with chronic high blood pressure, a mild cough, and allergies was working in the yard when she suddenly felt a severe pain radiating up her neck and down her arm. Her husband called the EMS. What is her chief complaint?
   A) Allergies
   B) Cough
   C) High blood pressure
   D) Pain radiating up the neck and down one arm.
   [Reference text page 146]

5. The main components of an adult's vital signs include assessment of breathing, skin, pupils, blood pressure, and:
   A) respiratory distress. **B)** pulse.
   C) capillary refill. **D)** all of the above.
   [Reference text page 147]

6. The initial set of readings for a patient are called the ________ vital signs.
   A) historical **B)** serial **C)** ongoing **D)** baseline
   [Reference text page 148]

7. The convention for reporting breathing rate is in respirations per:
   A) second. **B)** minute. **C)** hour. **D)** heartbeat.
   [Reference text page 148]

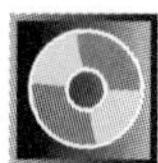

CD-ROM LINK: *Review the* Assessment of Breathing *video in Chapter 5 of the MedEMT CD-ROM.*

8. Which artery should be checked first for a pulse in the unresponsive infant?
A) Carotid **B)** Brachial
C) Apical **D)** Femoral
[Reference text pages 151 & 153]

9. On an older child, which is the primary site for evaluating a peripheral pulse?
A) Carotid **B)** Brachial
C) Radial **D)** Femoral
[Reference text pages 151 & 53]

10. The skin should be assessed for:
A) temperature, rigidity, and moisture. **B)** color, temperature, and condition.
C) temperature, strength, and color **D)** strength, wetness, and condition.
[Reference text pages 148, 154-56]

11. The pink color of oxygenated skin can be masked by a person's natural skin color.
A) True **B)** False
[Reference text page 154]

12. Cool, moist skin may indicate anxiety or:
A) shock. **B)** hypothermia. **C)** brain injury. **D)** heat stress.
[Reference text page 155]

13. In a dark room, the normal pupil should:
A) constrict. **B)** dilate.
C) not react. **D)** blink frequently
[Reference text page 158]

14. If you shine a light in one eye of an unconscious patient, the normal reaction is constriction of both pupils.
A) True **B)** False
[Reference text page 158]

15. Drug use can cause the pupils to become:
A) dilated. **B)** constricted.
C) either dilated or constricted. **D)** unequally sized.
[Reference text page 158]

16. Arterial pressure exerted by the blood when the left ventricle contracts is detected:
A) as the first sound heard when pressure in the BP cuff is released.
B) when sounds of the pulse disappear during deflation of the BP cuff.
C) by a stethoscope as the diastolic reading.
D) by none of the above.
[Reference text page 159]

17. One size of sphygmomanometer cuff fits all patients.
A) True **B)** False
[Reference text page 163]

18. When measuring the blood pressure, inflate the cuff to ________ mmHg above the point where the pulse disappears.
A) 10 **B)** 30 **C)** 50 **D)** 70
[Reference text page 162]

19. When measuring blood pressure, the cuff is deflated until two consecutive beats are heard through the stethoscope. This measures the ________ pressure.
A) diastolic **B)** residual **C)** systolic **D)** venous
[Reference text page 162]

CD-ROM LINK: *Review the* Vital Signs—Blood Pressure *video in Chapter 5 of the MedEMT CD-ROM.*

20. When a blood pressure is written as 100/80, the diastolic pressure is 110.
A) True **B)** False
[Reference text page 162]

21. A symptom can be objectively measured by the EMT-Basic.
A) True **B)** False
[Reference text page 167]

22. You are treating a patient complaining of chest pressure. You completed your assessment, applied oxygen, and are transporting him to the hospital now that the pain has subsided. His vital signs are BP134/70, HR 78, RR 22. How often should you reassess this patient's vital signs?
A) every minute **B)** every 5 minutes
C) every 10 minutes **D)** every 15 minutes
[Reference text page 165]

23. Sally has an open fracture of the right femur after colliding with a tree while skiing. The wound is bleeding and painful. How often should you reassess her vital signs en route to the hospital?
A) every minute **B)** every 5 minutes
C) every 10 minutes **D)** every 15 minutes
[Reference text page 165]

24. You are treating Mr. Harris for a possible stroke. During transport, he becomes unable to speak, and then becomes unresponsive. How will you best assess the nature and seriousness of his condition?

A) Repeat vital signs.
B) Call medical control.
C) Ask his wife about any other medical history.
D) Continue to try to arouse him.
[Reference text page 165]

25. Which of the following is a sign that your patient is in respiratory distress?

A) He complains of shortness of breath.
B) He complains of chest pain.
C) He has numbness and tingling in his fingers.
D) He has a rapid respiratory rate.
[Reference text pages 167 & 366]

26. Your patient fell from a roof. He has a laceration to the forehead, which is bleeding profusely. His vital signs are: BP140/100, HR 60, RR12. Which symptom may indicate this patient has a head injury?

A) bleeding
B) laceration
C) nausea
D) altered mental status
[Reference text page 167]

27. Which piece of information about your chest pain patient could NOT be obtained by a SAMPLE history alone?

A) He complains of shortness of breath.
B) He had a sudden onset of this episode.
C) He has a family history of high blood pressure.
D) He takes nitroglycerin pills.
[Reference text pages 167-69]

28. Noisy breathing is characterized by:

A) a rapid respiratory rate.
B) an increase in audible sounds.
C) a decrease in audible sounds.
D) none of the above.
[Reference text page 149]

29. The average range for an adult's pulse would be:

A) 60 to 100.
B) 55 to 105.
C) 70 to 110.
D) 80 to 120.
Reference text page 147]

30. The average range for an adult's respirations would be:

A) 10 to16.
B) 12 to 20.
C) 20 to 30.
D) 24 to 32.
[Reference text page 147]

31. The average range for systolic blood pressure for an adult would be:
A) 80 to 110. **B)** 80 to 120. **C)** 90 to 150. **D)** 100 to 120.
[Reference text page147]

32. Impaired blood flow to the skin may be caused by:
A) anemia. **B)** hemorrhage.
C) low cardiac output. **D)** all of the above.
[Reference text page 154]

33. The four categories of respiration characteristics are normal, shallow, labored, and noisy breathing.
A) True **B)** False
[Reference text page 148]

34. Examples of accessory muscles of breathing are the ________ muscle(s).
A) sternocleidomastoid **B)** diaphragm
C) lumbar **D)** bicep
[Reference text page 149]

35. A turbulent breathing sound that may be present during inspiration is called:
A) wheezing. **B)** grunting. **C)** crowing. **D)** all of the above.
[Reference text page 149]

36. The pulse that is palpated posterior to the medial malleolus is called the ________ pulse.
A) femoral **B)** brachial **C)** posterier tibial **D)** pedal
[Reference text page 151]

37. Applying excessive pressure to the corotid artery when checking a pulse can cause the patient's heart rate to slow dramatically.
A) True **B)** False
[Reference text page 152]

38. A true picture of the patient's oxygenation can be found by checking the skin color in:
A) the conjunctiva. **B)** the oral mucosa. **C)** the nail beds. **D)** all of the above.
[Reference text page 154]

39. A very bright, cherry red complexion is a late sign of:
A) carbon monoxide poisoning. **B)** shock.
C) hypothermia. **D)** cardiac arrest.
[Reference text page 155]

40. A nonreactive pupil is suggestive of:
A) stroke. **B)** head injury. **C)** a glass eye. **D)** all of the above.
[Reference text page 158]

41. Changes in the blood pressure can be caused by:
A) heart disease. **B)** valve disease.
C) ruptured aneurysm. **D)** all of the above.
[Reference text page 163]

42. Sustained hypertension can result in all of the following EXCEPT:
A) stroke. **B)** myocardial infarction.
C) shock. **D)** blood clots.
[Reference text page 164]

43. Kidney disease, which causes fluid retention, can lead to hypotension.
A) True **B)** False
[Reference text page 164]

44. Vital signs should be reassessed every ________ minutes in a stable patient.
A) 5 **B)** 10 **C)** 15 **D)** 20
[Reference text page 165]

45. Examples of medications that patients may be allergic to include:
A) penicillin and MRI contrast fluid. **B)** eggs and ragweed.
C) pollen and bee venom. **D)** all of the above.
[Reference text page 167]

CASE STUDIES

Use a separate piece of paper to answer the case study questions. Number your answers with the case study number and question letter (1A, 1B, etc.).

CHIEF COMPLAINT

1. As the newest member of the company emergency response team, your responsibility for the next ten shifts is to complete an initial assessment and report the patient's chief complaint to the responding EMS crews. The mining facility is rather small, so you will have only a few minutes to complete your assessment before the EMS crew arrives. As you complete your equipment check-out, the supervisor asks you to explain the term "chief complaint."
A) What does chief complaint mean?
B) What kinds of questions can you quickly ask your patient to help determine the chief complaint?

THE VITAL SIGNS

2. You are dispatched to a man down. Upon arrival, you find several bystanders kneeling beside an elderly man who has collapsed outside a grocery store. The patient is alert and oriented and complains of hip pain and a small abrasion on his left elbow. He states he "must have tripped on the curb." Your partner asks you to obtain a set of baseline vital signs.

A) What are the primary components included in a set of vital signs?
B) Why is it important that you take a set of baseline vitals?
C) When reporting the baseline vital signs, what is important to report besides the numbers?

3. As a member of the high school staff, you knew tonight's championship basketball game could spell trouble. After your school won, students gathered in the parking lot to celebrate. Unfortunately, several students from the opposing high school decided to make trouble. As the two groups began arguing, someone sprayed pepper spray into the crowd. Instantly, six students dropped to their knees and began coughing and crying.

A) What will you do first?
B) Describe normal breathing in an adult.
C) How do you determine the breathing rate of a patient?
D) What are the four categories of breathing effort?

4. As a competitive bicyclist and EMT, you have volunteered to provide medical care along a particularly dangerous section of the mountain trail. Your first patient took a bad spill and appears to have a fractured right arm. You complete your initial assessment and begin taking vital signs. The patient is alert and oriented. He is very upset about losing the race and complains loudly about the splint your partner is applying.

A) Where will you try to take a baseline pulse on this patient?
B) Besides the rate, what other characteristics or information about the patient's pulse will you report?

5. As the on-site EMT-Basic, you spend a lot of time responding to requests for minor soft tissue wounds, foreign objects in the eye, and muscle aches. However, the weather has been changing drastically and unexpectedly during the last two weeks. Several field employees are working in very hot or very cold environments, or both temperature conditions on the same shift. The job superintendent, concerned about worker safety, wants you to give a brief presentation to the crews about skin signs (colors) and skin temperature and what they mean.

A) Describe the normal and abnormal skin colors and the conditions each color typically represents.
B) What is a typical relative skin temperature?
C) How do you assess a patient's skin temperature?

6. Around 7:30 A.M., Dispatch requests that you respond to an automobile vs. bicycle crash. While en route, the First Responder crew advises you that the 5-year-old bicycle rider has an altered level of consciousness. When you arrive, you notice the boy is pale and cool to the touch. You ask your partner to measure vital signs as you begin your rapid trauma assessment.

A) Explain the steps necessary to check capillary refill time.
B) What is the meaning behind abnormal capillary refill findings?

7. The local soccer club has hired you, an EMT-Basic, to provide EMS duties at their soccer games every weekend. During your first game, a 10-year-old girl is kicked in the head.

She has not lost consciousness. She is complaining of dizziness, feeling nauseous, and a severe headache.

A) What steps are required to assess this patient's pupils?

B) List and describe the classifications of pupil size and reactivity to ambient light.

8. The chief of EMS has asked you to prepare a brief presentation on blood pressure for the volunteer First Responder agency. He specifically wants you to describe what happens inside the body to cause the blood pressure sounds we hear.

A) What is blood pressure?

B) What are the two phases of blood pressure we measure called?

C) What is the physiological cause behind the sound we hear while measuring blood pressure?

D) What are some conditions that can be caused by high blood pressure?

9. As you approach a housing complex, you notice several bystanders standing around an adult lying on the ground. The call was for a woman down. While assessing the scene, you see the woman's walker fallen on its side. The patient is an elderly female who, according to witnesses, tripped and fell. She denies losing consciousness or hitting her head. Her only complaint is severe hip pain. She feels cool to the touch with slightly moist skin.

A) Describe the steps you would take to measure the patient's blood pressure, using a blood pressure cuff and stethoscope.

B) Describe the steps in taking a blood pressure with only a cuff and no stethoscope.

C) What are average blood pressure ranges for infants, children, and adults?

SAMPLE HISTORY

10. The large senior center at the golf course is a common location for difficult EMS calls. Frequently, the patients are unable to communicate clearly due to various significant medical problems. Today's response is no exception. Bill appears to have suffered another stroke while playing golf with his wife. After appropriately managing the ABCs, your partner begins a physical exam while you gather information about Bill's medical history.

A) What is a medical history?

B) Describe what the letters stand for in the SAMPLE acronym.

C) How can the OPQRST questions fit into the gathering of a SAMPLE history?

11. The fog is so bad tonight you wonder how anyone could safely drive along this stretch of freeway. The shift battalion chief gets on the radio and requests that several backup units respond to a crash scene just outside the city limits. You and your partner are in the fourth ambulance to arrive. The Paramedic on scene asks you to manage a low-priority patient complaining of right leg pain and minor lacerations on his face. Your patient denies any loss of consciousness. He was wearing his seat belt. You glance at the vehicle he was driving and notice major front end damage. The air bag appears to have deployed.

A) Describe the questions you would ask to determine the severity of the patient's leg pain.

B) What two questions are important to ask during the "M" phase of the SAMPLE history assessment?

LABELING DIAGRAMS

Label the diagrams below by filling in the proper term(s) that corresponds to the letters in the acronym:

SAMPLE HISTORY

S	________	**A)**	Last oral intake
A	________	**B)**	Pertinent past medical history
M	________	**C)**	Events leading up to
P	________	**D)**	Allergies
L	________	**E)**	Medications
E	________	**F)**	Signs and symptoms

OPQRST HISTORY

O	________	**A)**	Radiation
P	________	**B)**	Severity
Q	________	**C)**	Time
R	________	**D)**	Onset
S	________	**E)**	Provocation
T	________	**F)**	Quality

PULSE LOCATIONS

Write the correct pulse location in the blanks in the diagram.

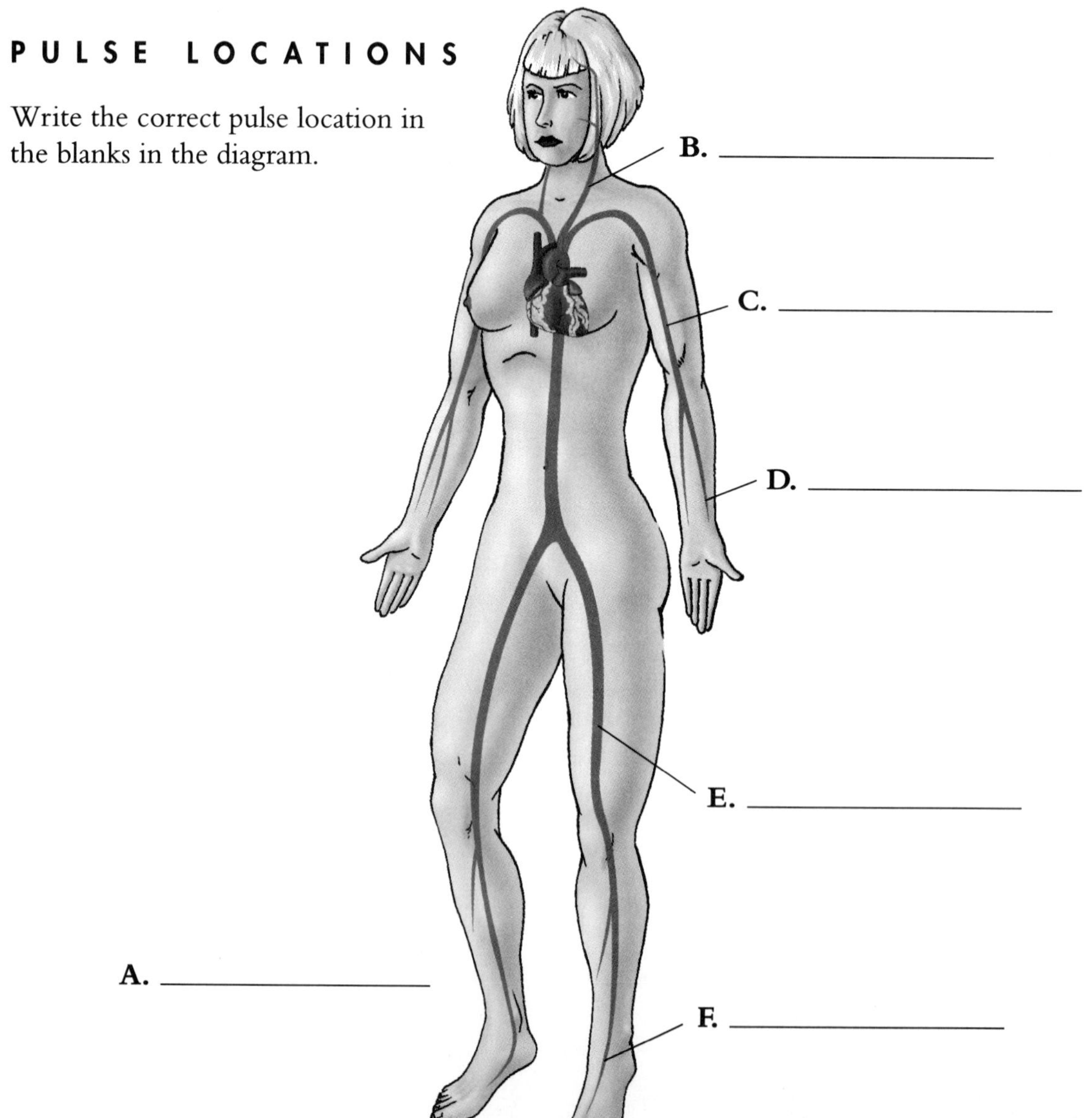

KEY TERMS MATCHING

Assess your knowledge of the chapter key terms by matching the terms on the left to the definitions on the right.

______ 1.	Auscultation	(A)	Condition described by the patient that can't be observed
______ 2.	Brachial Pulse	(B)	An unusually rapid heart rate
______ 3.	Bradycardia (bray-deh-KAR-de-uh)	(C)	The pressure in the arterial system when the left ventricle contracts; first sound heard when assessing blood pressure by auscultation
______ 4.	Chief Complaint	(D)	Pulse rate and quality, breathing rate and quality, blood pressure, skin color, skin temperature, skin condition, pupil size and quality, and capillary refill in children
______ 5.	Conjunctiva (kon-junk-TIE-vuh)	(E)	Harsh, high-pitched sound during inspiration
______ 6.	Cyanosis (Sy-uh-NO-sis)	(F)	Blood pressure cuff
______ 7.	Diastolic Pressure (di-uh-STALL-ik)	(G)	An observable indication of illness or injury
______ 8.	Expiration	(H)	Outermost layer of the eyeball; whites of the eyes
______ 9.	Femoral (FEM-or-ul) Pulse	(I)	Mnemonic used to summarize a patient's relevant medical history (Signs/Symptoms, Allergies, Medications, Past history, Last oral intake, Events leading to injury or illness)
______ 10.	Hypertension	(J)	The flow of blood through the radial artery; palpated on the anterior lateral surface of the wrist, proximal to the thumb
______ 11.	Inspiration	(K)	Breathing; process through which air enters and leaves the lungs
______ 12.	Jaundice (JAWN-dis)	(L)	Circular opening in the iris that allows passage of light into the eye
______ 13.	Lens		

_____ **14.** Oral Mucosa

_____ **15.** Palpation

_____ **16.** Pulse

_____ **17.** Pupil

_____ **18.** Radial Pulse

_____ **19.** Respiration (res-per-AY-shun)

_____ **20.** SAMPLE History

_____ **21.** Sclera

_____ **22.** Sign

_____ **23.** Sphygmomanometer (sfig-mo-mah-NOM-eh-ter)

_____ **24.** Stridor

_____ **25.** Symptom

_____ **26.** Systolic (sis-TALL-ik) Pressure

_____ **27.** Tachycardia (tak-eh-KAR-de-uh)

_____ **28.** Vital Signs

(M) Yellow deposits in skin and whites of the eyes caused by increased bilirubin in the blood; indication of liver abnormality

(N) Assessment by touch or feel

(O) Pink membrane lining the inside of the mouth

(P) Refracting structure of the eye located directly behind the pupil

(Q) Pressure caused by contraction of the heart; can be palpated where an artery lies close to underlying bone; an indication of cardiac output

(R) Taking air into the lungs (inhalation)

(S) Abnormally high blood pressure

(T) The flow of blood through the femoral artery in the upper thigh

(U) Expelling air from the lungs (exhalation)

(V) The pressure exerted on the walls of the arteries when the heart is at rest; when assessing blood pressure by auscultation, measured at point when the sound stops

(W) Patient's self-described worst or most serious concern

(X) Membrane lining the eyelids and the surface of the sclera of the eye

(Y) Blue coloring of the skin; may indicate poor oxygen uptake or reduced perfusion

(Z) Slow heart rate

(AA) The flow of blood through the brachial artery, in the medial aspect of the upper arm

(BB) Listening for sounds with a stethoscope

SKILLS CHECKLISTS

Check your knowledge of important EMT-B skills by marking off each step in the following skills sheets.

BLOOD PRESSURE BY AUSCULTATION

- [ ] Place stethoscope around your neck.
- [ ] Patient should be seated or lying down.
- [ ] If patient has not been injured, support his or her arm at heart level.
- [ ] Place cuff snugly around upper arm so that bottom of cuff is about one inch above crease of elbow.
- [ ] With your fingertips, palpate brachial artery at crease of elbow.
- [ ] Place the tips of stethoscope in your ears.
- [ ] Position the diaphragm of the stethoscope directly over the brachial pulse or over medial anterior elbow if no brachial pulse can be felt.
- [ ] Inflate cuff with bulb valve closed.
- [ ] Once you no longer hear brachial pulse, continue to inflate cuff until gauge reads 30 mm Hg higher than the point where pulse sound disappeared.
- [ ] Slowly release air from cuff by opening bulb valve, allowing pressure to fall smoothly at rate of approximately 10 mm per second.
- [ ] When you hear the first clicking or tapping sounds, note the reading on the gauge. This is the systolic pressure.
- [ ] Continue to deflate cuff and listen for point at which these distinctive sounds fade. When sounds turn to dull, muffled thuds, the reading on gauge is the diastolic pressure.
- [ ] After obtaining diastolic pressure, let cuff deflate rapidly.

BLOOD PRESSURE BY PALPATION

- [ ] Find radial pulse on the arm to which blood pressure cuff is applied.
- [ ] With bulb valve closed, inflate cuff to a point where you can no longer feel the radial pulse.
- [ ] Note this point on gauge and continue to inflate cuff until gauge reads 30 mm Hg higher than point where pulse disappeared.
- [ ] Slowly deflate cuff, noting reading at which the radial pulse returns. This reading is the systolic pressure.
- [ ] After obtaining systolic reading, let cuff deflate.

NOTE: You cannot determine diastolic reading by palpation.

(reprinted from *Pocket Reference for The EMT-B and First Responder* by Bob Elling, Prentice Hall, 1999)

D.O.T. OBJECTIVES CHECKLIST

Use the following list of knowledge objectives to check what you've learned. Check off only those objectives that you feel you completely understand and have mastered. For any objectives not checked, go back and review that section of the text chapter. Textbook page references have been provided to help you review the text material.

- [ ] Identify the components of vital signs. *(p. 147)*
- [ ] Describe the methods to obtain a breathing rate. *(p. 148)*
- [ ] Identify the attributes that should be obtained when assessing breathing. *(p. 148)*
- [ ] Differentiate between shallow, labored, and noisy breathing. *(p. 148)*
- [ ] Describe the methods to obtain a pulse rate. *(149)*
- [ ] Identify the information obtained when assessing a patient's pulse. *(p. 153)*
- [ ] Differentiate between a strong, weak, regular, and irregular pulse. *(p. 153)*
- [ ] Describe the methods to assess the skin color, temperature, condition (capillary refills in infants and children). *(p. 154)*
- [ ] Identify the normal and abnormal skin colors. *(p. 154)*

- [ ] Differentiate between pale, blue, red, and yellow skin color. *(p. 154)*
- [ ] Identify the normal and abnormal skin temperature. *(p. 155)*
- [ ] Differentiate between hot, cool, and cold skin temperature. *(p. 155)*
- [ ] Identify normal and abnormal skin conditions. *(p. 155)*
- [ ] Identify normal and abnormal capillary refill in infants and children. *(p. 156)*
- [ ] Describe the methods to assess the pupils. *(p. 157)*
- [ ] Identify normal and abnormal pupil size. *(p. 157)*
- [ ] Differentiate between dilated (big) and constricted (small) pupil size. *(p. 157)*
- [ ] Differentiate between reactive and nonreactive pupils and equal and unequal pupils. *(p. 157)*
- [ ] Describe the methods to assess blood pressure. *(p. 160)*
- [ ] Define systolic pressure. *(p. 159)*
- [ ] Define diastolic pressure. *(p. 159)*
- [ ] Explain the difference between auscultation and palpation for obtaining a blood pressure. *(p. 160)*
- [ ] Identify the components of a SAMPLE history. *(p. 165)*
- [ ] Differentiate between a sign and a symptom. *(p. 167)*
- [ ] State the importance of accurately reporting and recording the baseline vital signs. *(p. 165)*
- [ ] Discuss the need to search for additional medical identification. *(p. 167)*

CHAPTER 6

Lifting and Moving Patients

CHAPTER 6 SUMMARY

Safely moving your patient to the stretcher and the ambulance is an important part of patient care. How you move the patient and the speed with which you do so can have a dramatic impact on his or her condition. Proper movement techniques are also important to your well-being. Lifting, reaching, carrying, pushing, and pulling are frequent sources of injury in EMT-Basics. Always use proper body mechanics when moving patients, stretchers, or other devices.

Moves can be qualified as emergency, urgent, and nonurgent (routine). Emergency moves are used when there is an immediate threat to the patient, such as fire, explosion, an inability to protect the patient from other hazards, or the inability to access other patients in need of care. There is a danger of aggravating spinal injuries in these moves, so they are only used when absolutely needed. Urgent moves are used when there is an immediate threat to the patient's life. An altered mental status or compromise of the patient's airway, breathing, or circulation indicate the need for an urgent move.

Your positioning of the patient may affect the patient's injury or illness. When providing care and deciding on the most appropriate device in which to move the patient, always be aware of any special positioning needs of the patient.

REVIEW QUESTIONS

Please circle the best answer to each question.

1. What is the key to reducing your chance for back injury?
   A) Practice **B)** Positioning **C)** Prevention **D)** Posture
   [Reference text page 178]

2. What are body mechanics?
   A) Principals and applications that focus on safe and efficient methods for using your body
   B) Methods developed for the proper positioning of the patient during lift and move operations
   C) Concepts developed by physical therapists to rehabilitate injuries
   D) The practice of developing upper body strength to compensate for lower back injuries
   [Reference text page 179]

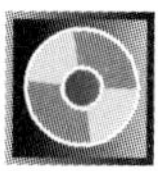

CD-ROM LINK: *Review the* Lifting and Moving *video in Chapter 6 of the MedEMT CD-ROM.*

3. A key element of body mechanics is to use the muscles of your legs instead of your back.
   A) True **B)** False
   [Reference text page 179]

4. It is not necessary to keep the weight of an object you are lifting close to your body when safely lifting.
   A) True **B)** False
   [Reference text page 179]

5. General guidelines for lifting include all of the following EXCEPT:
   A) know your own physical limitations.
   B) consider the size and weight of the patient.
   C) communicate clearly and frequently.
   D) position your feet approximately six inches apart.
   [Reference text page 179]

6. Wearing a support belt when lifting helps the EMT-Basic lift heavier patients.
   A) True **B)** False
   [Reference text page 180]

7. A specialized lifting and moving technique that uses the large muscles of the legs is called a:
A) leg lift. **B)** power lift. **C)** back grip. **D)** power grip.
[Reference text page 180]

8. When preparing to lift, the EMT-Basic should assess the ground for obstructions, slippery conditions, or other potential hazards
A) True **B)** False
[Reference text page 180]

9. Bending all fingers at the same angle and placing the hands ten inches apart are two key elements to:
A) the stretcher operation. **B)** the power grip.
C) the power lift. **D)** none of the above.
[Reference text page 180]

10. A specialized device used for the transportation of patients down stairs or through narrow spaces is called a:
A) wheeled ambulance cot. **B)** KED.
C) stairchair. **D)** blanket roll.
[Reference text page 182]

11. To minimize the risk of injury, avoid reaching:
A) overhead. **B)** more than 15 to 20 inches.
C) while bending backwards. **D)** in all of the above ways.
[Reference text page 183]

12. When carrying with one hand, the EMT-Basic should lean to the opposite side to compensate for the unbalanced weight.
A) True **B)** False
[Reference text page 182]

13. Techniques for moving a patient whose condition is life threatening are called:
A) urgent. **B)** emergency.
C) nonurgent. **D)** none of the above.
[Reference text page 184]

14. Lifting and moving patients when there is no immediate threat to life is called:
A) an emergency move. **B)** an urgent move.
C) a nonurgent move. **D)** none of the above.
[Reference text page 184]

15. The greatest threat to a patient requiring an emergency move is aggravating the spine.
A) True **B)** False
[Reference text page 184]

16. It is not necessary for the EMT-Basic to rule out the possibility of a spinal injury before performing a nonurgent move.
A) True **B)** False
[Reference text pages 185-87]

17. Which of the following moves are NOT considered emergency moves?
A) Blanket drag **B)** Rapid extrication
C) Clothing drag **D)** Foot drag
[Reference text pages 185-87]

18. Emergency moves may be necessary if:
A) the patient is really screaming.
B) additional calls are holding.
C) the patient has to go to the bathroom.
D) there is an imminent building collapse.
[Reference text page 185]

19. Rolling a patient onto a blanket to provide a move is called a/n:
A) foot drag **B)** blanket roll
C) blanket drag **D)** armpit forearm drag
[Reference text page 186]

20. If a patient is very critical and found wedged between a toilet and the wall, the move you should use will be:
A) an emergency move. **B)** a routine move.
C) an urgent move. **D)** none of the above.
[Reference text page 185]

21. Situations in which urgent moves are necessary include:
A) major bleeding. **B)** airway compromise.
C) altered mental status. **D)** all of the above.
[Reference text page 187]

22. A specialized technique for quickly removing a patient from a vehicle without compromising the spine is called:
A) KED application. **B)** rapid extrication.
C) a two-rescuer spinal assist. **D)** rapid takedown.
[Reference text page 187]

23. Ensuring that the patient's spine is not compromised is the key to rapid extrication.
A) True **B)** False
[Reference text page 187]

24. Throughout the rapid extrication procedure, the EMT-Basic should not let go and move position until another rescuer's hands take over.
A) True **B)** False
[Reference text page 187]

25. Nonurgent techniques for moving patients without spine injury include:
A) direct extremity lift. **B)** draw sheet method.
C) direct carry. **D)** all of the above.
[Reference text page 188]

26. When moving a patient who has no suspected trauma from the ground, the EMT-Basic should use either a direct ground lift or:
A) straddle slide. **B)** extremity lift.
C) blanket drag. **D)** draw sheet method.
[Reference text page 189]

27. Two techniques commonly used to move supine patients from a bed to a stretcher are the draw sheet method and:
A) the extremity lift. **B)** the blanket drag.
C) the direct carry. **D)** none of the above.
[Reference text page 191]

28. To do a direct carry properly takes a minimum of two rescuers.
A) True **B)** False
[Reference text page 191]

29. If the terrain is unstable or uneven, it may help to roll the stretcher in its lowest position.
A) True **B)** False
[Reference text page 194]

30. A flexible device used to help immobilize the spine in confined spaces such as a bucket seat is a:
A) KED. **B)** Reeves stretcher.
C) short backboard. **D)** scoop stretcher.
[Reference text page 197]

31. A stretcher that has two halves that actually assemble right around the patient is called a:
A) Reeves stretcher. **B)** scoop stretcher.
C) KED. **D)** vest-type device.
[Reference text page 197]

32. A device designed for moving patients over rough or irregular terrain is called a:
A) scoop stretcher. **B)** stokes stretcher.
C) stair chair. **D)** flexible stretcher.
[Reference text page 198]

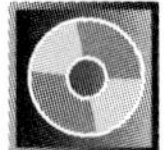
CD-ROM LINK: *Review the video* Climber's Descent *in Chapter 6 of the MedEMT CD-ROM.*

33. The seated position on a wheeled stretcher is called which of the following?
A) Recovery position **B)** Fowler's position
C) Trendelenberg position **D)** Supine
[Reference text page 200]

34. When a patient is unable to protect his or her airway, the patient should be placed in the ________ position.
A) Trendelenberg **B)** Fowler's **C)** recovery **D)** prone
[Reference text page 199]

35. A carrying device that is assembled directly around the patient in a confined space, not used in suspected spinal injury cases, is called which of the following?
A) Scoop stretcher **B)** Long spinal board
C) Extrication device **D)** Short board
[Reference text page 197]

CASE STUDIES

Use a separate piece of paper to answer the case study questions. Number your answers with the case study number and question letter (1A, 1B, etc.).

LIFTING TECHNIQUES

1. A set of new EMT-Basics is just finishing the week-long employee orientation. As a field training officer, you have been assigned to educate them about the company's back safety program and proper lifting and moving techniques.
A) Define the term "body mechanics."
B) Describe standard guidelines and safety precautions necessary when lifting any patient.
C) Describe the standard guidelines and safety precautions necessary when carrying a patient or equipment.

2. A sheriff's officer is first on scene at the old farmhouse, located 50 minutes away from the nearest hospital. When you arrive, the officer advises you that the patient is wedged face down between two large bookcases. The patient is disoriented to time and place, and you are unable to properly complete your assessment while he remains in his current position.

You are able to observe that the patient has some right-sided facial drooping and significant drooling.

A) Should you consider an urgent move for this patient? Justify your answer.

3. You have been running calls all day. Just as you lie down for a quick nap, the alarm sounds again. The call is for a woman who has fallen out of bed. As you arrive, you find a 22-year-old female lying on the floor. She is a paraplegic and unable to move. She denies any injury.

A) List the lifting techniques used in nonurgent moves.

B) Describe the steps required to complete a nonurgent move.

4. The large convalescent center has been shut down because of a long-term loss of electricity to the area. Your shift is preparing to quickly transport all the patients to different facilities in the region. The day shift supervisor has asked you to review with the crews the proper steps for reaching, pushing, and pulling.

A) Describe the steps for reaching correctly.

B) Describe special considerations for reaching during a log roll.

C) List the guidelines for proper pushing and pulling.

PATIENT TRANSPORT EQUIPMENT

5. Dispatch advises of a single vehicle rollover. Someone drove over the side of the new levee just outside of town. As you arrive on scene, you see your patient upside down in his overturned sport utility vehicle. The vehicle is 150 feet down the embankment and has come to rest against two very large rocks. The embankment is made of soft dirt and small brush.

A) What type of stretcher or cot would you choose for the rescue of this patient?

B) What immobilization device is necessary in addition to the stretcher or cot?

6. This old midtown hotel was built with long, narrow hallways and no elevators. The only access to the upper floors of this building is through a large central staircase structure. The 65-year-old patient you are about to transport complains of general weakness and is unable to walk. After several attempts, it is obvious that the wheeled stretcher is too large to make it around some of the corners.

A) List the stretchers or cots that would be acceptable to use in this situation.

B) Which device seems most appropriate? Justify your answer.

7. You receive a call for a man down at the base of the stairs. When you arrive, you find an obese patient (approximately 400 lbs.) who managed to crawl across the living room floor and is lying in a large stuffed chair. His vital signs are stable, his mental status is alert, but he is now complaining of low back pain.

A) What type of move does he need?

B) From your safety point of view, what should you consider right away?

C) How could you and your team properly immobilize this patient to remove from the chair if the KED definitely will not fit?

KEY TERMS MATCHING

Assess your knowledge of the chapter key terms by matching the terms on the left to the definitions on the right.

_____ **1.** Body Mechanics

_____ **2.** Emergency Moves

_____ **3.** Flexible Stretcher

_____ **4.** Hyperextension

_____ **5.** Long Backboard

_____ **6.** Nonurgent (routine) Moves

_____ **7.** Portable Stretcher

_____ **8.** Power grip

_____ **9.** Power lift

_____ **10.** Rapid Extrication

_____ **11.** Recovery Position

_____ **12.** Scoop Stretcher

_____ **13.** Short Backboard

(A) Carrying device used for patient transport over rough or irregular terrain

(B) Specialized device used for transportation of patients down stairs or through narrow spaces; may have wheels

(C) A flexible device used to help immobilize the spine in confined spaces

(D) Techniques for moving a patient whose condition is life threatening; cervical spine procedures are taken

(E) Most commonly used ambulance stretcher; may be rolled on smooth surfaces; adjustable height

(F) Device for immobilizing the upper part of the spine when a long board cannot be used

(G) Device used to move patients with no suspected spinal injuries from confined areas

(H) Light, collapsible stretcher useful in small spaces

(I) Standard transportation position for a patient without spinal injury; patient is rolled onto one side, usually the left

(J) Carrying device made of flexible materials with large carrying handles; used for moving patients in narrow or confined spaces

(K) A specialized lifting and moving technique that uses the large muscles of the legs to lift and carry the weight

(L) Gripping items with palms and fingers in complete contact with the object; fingers bent at the same angle and hands ten inches apart

______ 14. Stair Chair	(M)	Lifting and moving patients when there is no immediate threat to life
______ 15. Urgent Moves	(N)	Device used for full spinal immobilization
	(O)	Extension of a joint beyond its normal limit during movement
______ 16. Vest-Type Extrication Device	(P)	Specialized techniques for quickly removing a patient from a vehicle without compromising the cervical spine
______ 17. Wheeled Stretcher	(Q)	Specific extrication or lifting and moving techniques used when immediate danger threatens the EMT or the patient
______ 18. Wire Basket Stretcher (Stokes Litter)	(R)	Moving your body correctly while lifting and moving to prevent injury

SKILLS CHECKLIST

Check your knowledge of important EMT-B skills by marking off each step in the following skills sheets.

ONE-RESCUER ASSIST

- [ ] Place patient's arm around your neck.
- [ ] Grasp patient's hand in your hand.
- [ ] Place your other arm around patient's waist.
- [ ] Help patient walk to safety, communicating with him or her about obstacles or uneven terrain.

TWO-RESCUER ASSIST

- [ ] Each rescuer stands at a side of patient.
- [ ] Each places a patient's arm around his or her shoulder and grips the patient's hand.
- [ ] Each rescuer then places own free arm around patient's waist.
- [ ] They both then help patient walk to safety.

EXTREMITY CARRY

- [ ] Rescuer A: Place patient on his or her back with knees flexed.
- [ ] Rescuer A: Kneel at patient's head and place your hands under patient's shoulders.

- [ ] Rescuer B: Kneel at patient's feet and grasp his or her wrists.
- [ ] Rescuer B: Then lift patient forward, while Rescuer A slips arms under patient's armpits and grasps patient's wrist.
- [ ] Rescuer B: Grasp patient's knees while facing patient, or turn and grasp patient's knees while facing away from patient.
- [ ] Rescuers A and B: Crouch, then stand at same time and move as a unit when carrying patient.

DIRECT CARRY

- [ ] Rescuers A and B: Get in position along one side of patient. Rescuer A is at head-end; Rescuer B at foot-end.
- [ ] Rescuer A: Cradle patient's head and neck by sliding one arm under patient's neck to grasp shoulder.
- [ ] Rescuer B: Slide hand under patient's hip and lift slightly.
- [ ] Rescuer A: Slide your other arm under patient's back.
- [ ] Rescuer B: Place your arms under patient's hips and calves.
- [ ] Rescuers A and B: Slide patient to edge of bed and bend toward him or her with your knees slightly bent.
- [ ] Then lift and curl patient to your chests and return to standing position.
- [ ] Rotate, and then slide patient gently onto stretcher.

LOADING WHEELED STRETCHER

- [ ] Lift rear step of ambulance.
- [ ] Move stretcher as close to ambulance as possible.
- [ ] Make sure stretcher is locked in its lowest level before lifting (depends on local procedure and type of stretcher).
- [ ] Rescuers A and B: Get in position on opposite sides of stretcher, bend at knees, and grasp lower bar of stretcher frame.
- [ ] Come to a full standing position with backs straight.
- [ ] Use oblique stepping movements to move stretcher to ambulance.
- [ ] Secure stretcher into ambulance using the appropriate securing device.
- [ ] Engage both forward and rear catches to hold stretcher in place.

BLANKET DRAG

- [ ] Gather half of blanket up against patient's side.
- [ ] Roll patient toward your knees.
- [ ] Gently roll patient onto blanket.
- [ ] Roll up blanket by patient's head, neck, and shoulders and drag this rolled material, keeping patient's head as low to ground as possible.

RAPID EXTRICATION

Step 1: Perform an initial assessment.

- [ ] Rescuer A: Maintain manual stabilization of patient's head and neck.
- [ ] Rescuer B: Conduct initial assessment of patient and determine need for rapid extrication based on patient status. Assess pulses, motor ability, and sensory response (PMS) in four extremities.

Step 2: Apply a cervical collar.

- [ ] Rescuer B: Apply a properly sized cervical collar.
- [ ] Rescuer A: Continue to maintain manual stabilization before, during, and after application of collar.

Step 3: Lift patient and position the long backboard.

- [ ] Rescuer B: Hold patient's armpit, and join hands with Rescuer C under patient's thighs.
- [ ] Rescuer A: Call for a lift, while maintaining manual stabilization.
- [ ] Rescuers B: Lift patient approx. two inches off seat with Rescuer C.
- [ ] Bystander (or 4th Rescuer): Insert long backboard under patient on seat.

(reprinted from *Pocket Reference for The EMT-B and First Responder* by Bob Elling, Prentice Hall, 1999)

D.O.T. OBJECTIVES CHECKLIST

Use the following list of knowledge objectives to check what you've learned. Check off only those objectives that you feel you completely understand and have mastered. For any objectives not checked, go back and review that section of the text chapter. Textbook page references have been provided to help you review the text material.

- [ ] Define body mechanics. *(p. 179)*

- [ ] Discuss the guidelines and safety precautions that need to be followed when lifting a patient. *(p. 179)*
- [ ] Describe the safe lifting of cots and stretchers. *(p. 187)*
- [ ] Describe the guidelines and safety precautions for carrying patients and/or equipment. *(p. 181)*
- [ ] Discuss one-handed carrying techniques. *(p. 182)*
- [ ] Describe correct and safe carrying procedures on stairs. *(p. 182)*
- [ ] State the guidelines for reaching and their application. *(p. 183)*
- [ ] Describe correct reaching for log rolls. *(p. 183)*
- [ ] State the guidelines for pushing and pulling. *(p. 184)*
- [ ] Discuss the general considerations of moving patients. *(p. 184)*
- [ ] State three situations that may require the use of an emergency move. *(p. 185)*
- [ ] Identify the following patient carrying devices: *(p. 194)*
    - [ ] Wheeled ambulance stretcher
    - [ ] Portable ambulance stretcher
    - [ ] Stair chair
    - [ ] Scoop stretcher
    - [ ] Long spine board
    - [ ] Basket stretcher
    - [ ] Flexible stretcher

CHAPTER 7

Airway Management

CHAPTER 7 SUMMARY

Airway management is a critical intervention that the EMT-Basic must master. Without an airway, your patient cannot breathe. If your patient cannot breathe, he or she will die.

Open the airway, by using either the jaw-thrust or head-tilt/chin-lift maneuver, depending on the probability of a cervical spine injury. Suction the patient if necessary. Consider placing an oropharyngeal airway (OPA) or a nasopharyngeal airway (NPA) to help maintain patency. Your evaluation of the patient's airway and breathing is crucial and can be summarized as adequate or inadequate.

If breathing is inadequate, immediate intervention is necessary. Assist the patient's ventilations, using the mouth-to-mask technique, two-person bag-valve-mask device technique, flow-restricted, oxygen powered ventilation device (FROPVD), or one-person bag-valve-mask device technique. Regardless of device or technique, supplement with high-flow oxygen. For all patients who are breathing adequately, consider applying oxygen via non-rebreather mask at high-flow rates. The only indication for a nasal cannula is that the patient will not tolerate the non-rebreather mask.

Always use BSI precautions when performing airway management skills. There is often a chance that blood, vomitus, or other materials obstructing the airway will be expelled with force, so do not forget to wear goggles to protect your eyes.

REVIEW QUESTIONS

Please circle the best answer for each question.

1. The EMT-Basic must assure that every patient has a patent airway, has adequate ________, and is receiving sufficient oxygen.
   A) breathing. **B)** capillary refill.
   C) skin color. **D)** brachial pulse.
   [Reference text page 208]

2. The term "patent" refers to an open and clear airway.
   A) True **B)** False
   [Reference text page 208]

3. The term "alveoli" refers to microscopic sacs of the lungs where the exchange of gases occurs.
   A) True **B)** False
   [Reference text page 210]

4. The parts of the lower airway are the:
   A) trachea, pharynx, and alveoli.
   B) larynx, bronchioles, and nasopharynx.
   C) trachea, bronchi, bronchioles, and alveoli.
   D) esophagus, larynx, and bronchi.
   [Reference text page 208]

5. The epiglottis protects the lower airway by preventing food from entering it.
   A) True **B)** False
   [Reference text page 209]

6. The trachea is also called the voice box.
   A) True **B)** False
   [Reference text page 209]

7. The passage of oxygen and carbon dioxide between the ________, and the ________, of the lung is called gas exchange.
   A) alveoli, venules **B)** alveoli, arterioles **C)** alveoli, capillaries **D)** arteries, veins
   [Reference text page 210]

8. The movement of air into and out of the lungs is called:
   A) exhalation. **B)** ventilation.
   C) respiration. **D)** inhalation.
   [Reference text page 210]

9. As the thoracic cavity increases in size during inhalation, a negative pressure is created within the chest cavity causing air to flow into the lungs.

A) True **B)** False
[Reference text pages 117 & 210]

10. An adult's breathing is said to be labored when additional thoracic muscles are required for ventilation.
A) True **B)** False
[Reference text page 211]

11. During exhalation, the size of the thoracic cavity:
A) increases. **B)** decreases.
C) stays the same. **D)** expands rapidly.
[Reference text pages 99 & 211]

12. Retractions refer to noisy breathing.
A) True **B)** False
[Reference text page 211]

13. A large amount of swelling is required before there is airway obstruction in children.
A) True **B)** False
[Reference text page 239]

14. When opening a child's airway, you must avoid hyperextension or flexion of the neck.
A) True **B)** False
[Reference text page 240]

15. You should use the crossed-finger technique to open an unconscious patient's mouth.
A) True **B)** False
[Reference text page 213]

16. When performing a head-tilt/chin-lift maneuver on an infant, tilt the head back gently to a ________, or "sniffing," position.
A) hyperextended **B)** flexed **C)** neutral **D)** reversed
[Reference text pages 240-41]

CD-ROM LINK: *Review the* Head-Tilt/Chin-Lift *and* Jaw Thrust *videos in Chapter 7 of the MedEMT CD-ROM.*

17. Immediate suctioning may be required if the patient presents with gurgling sounds.
A) True **B)** False
[Reference text pages 213, 216, 232 & 331]

18. Rigid suction catheters ("tonsil tip" catheters) should NOT be:
A) used to suction the oropharynx.
B) inserted as far as the EMT-Basic can see.
C) used in responsive patients.
D) used on children.
[Reference text page 217]

19. The nasopharynx is suctioned with a soft catheter or a French catheter.
A) True **B)** False
[Reference text page 217]

20. When suctioning, you must always use gloves, gown, protective eyewear, and a respirator.
A) True **B)** False
[Reference text page 217]

21. When suctioning an endotracheal tube, use a soft catheter or a French catheter.
A) True **B)** False
[Reference text page 217]

22. An oropharyngeal airway adjunct can be used in an unresponsive patient without a gag reflex.
A) True **B)** False
[Reference text page 219]

CD-ROM LINK: *Review the* Suctioning *video in Chapter 7 of the MedEMT CD-ROM.*

23. If a patient has stopped breathing or has inadequate breathing, perform:
A) suctioning. **B)** assisted artificial ventilation.
C) triage. **D)** CPR.
[Reference text page 225]

24. Mouth-to-mask ventilation protects the EMT-Basic from direct patient contact.
A) True **B)** False
[Reference text page 228]

25. The bag-valve-mask maneuver is most effective when used by:
A) one EMT-Basic. **B)** two EMT-Basics.
C) someone trained in CPR. **D)** a physician.
[Reference text pages 225 & 228]

26. The flow-restricted, oxygen-powered ventilation device is used on infants and children.
A) True **B)** False
[Reference text page 232]

27. Which statement is false?
A) Oxygen is required for life.
B) Hypoxic means "without any oxygen."
C) Oxygen therapy can supplement the body's need for oxygen.
D) Anoxia means "without oxygen."
[Reference text page 225]

28. A person with a tracheostomy tube:
A) can be ventilated by attaching a bag-valve directly to the tube.
B) may require frequent suctioning.
C) may have air escape from the mouth or nose.
D) all of the above.
[Reference text pages 243-44]

29. Blunt injuries to the face may result in severe swelling or bleeding.
A) True **B)** False
[Reference text page 245]

30. For complete airway obstruction by a foreign body, all of the following are correct EXCEPT:
A) use abdominal thrusts and finger sweeps for adults.
B) in infants, use back blows and chest thrusts.
C) administer oxygen by non-rebreather mask, without moving the patient.
D) obese patients may require chest thrusts.
[Reference text pages 112, 797-800]

31. Bag-valve masks are available in infant, child, and adult sizes.
A) True **B)** False
[Reference text page 244]

32. You are ventilating a patient in respiratory arrest with a bag-valve mask. He has a tracheostomy due to throat cancer. You are not getting adequate chest rise and fall. What should you do?
A) Ventilate through the mouth and plug the stoma.
B) Switch to a positive pressure ventilatory device.
C) Seal the stoma and attempt to ventilate through the mouth and nose.
D) Increase the oxygen flow to compensate for poor tidal volume.
[Reference text page 244]

33. You should suction an infant for no more than how many seconds?
A) 25 **B)** 30 **C)** 15 **D)** 5
[Reference text page 217]

34. All oi the following are signs and symptoms of inadequate breathing in infants and children EXCEPT:
A) nasal flaring
B) shallow breathing
C) cyanosis in the nail beds
D) unequal pupils
[Reference text page 242]

35. The vocal cords are found in the:
A) alveoli.
B) epiglottis.
C) larynx.
D) bronchi.
[Reference text page 209]

36. The ________ separates the chest cavity from the abdominal cavity.
A) trachea
B) larynx
C) diaphragm
D) epiglottis
[Reference text page 210]

37. What gases are exchanged during the process of respiration?
A) Oxygen and nitrogen
B) Nitrogen and carbon dioxide
C) Oxygen and carbon dioxide
D) Nitrogen and carbon monoxide
[Reference text page 211]

38. The most common cause of airway obstruction in the unconscious adult is:
A) incompletely chewed food.
B) facial trauma.
C) small foreign objects.
D) the tongue.
[Reference text page 212]

39. Stridor is a:
A) low-pitched sound resulting from a partial airway obstruction.
B) dull, hoarse cough that accompanies shortness of breath.
C) serious condition that causes secretions to build up in the airway.
D) high-pitched sound resulting from partial airway obstruction.
[Reference text page 213]

40. Which airway maneuver should be used during suctioning?
A) crossed-finger technique
B) chest thrust, back blow
C) head tilt/chin lift
D) jaw thrust
[Reference text page 213]

41. Which body substance isolation precautions should be used during suctioning?
A) gloves, mask, and skin precautions
B) gloves, gown, and respirator
C) gloves, skin precautions, and respirator
D) gloves, mask, and eye protection
[Reference text page 217]

42. Causes of pharynx obstruction include:
A) accumulation of vomitus.
B) tissue swelling from trauma.
C) destruction of the airway.
D) all of the above.
[Reference text page 209]

43. Extreme use of accessory muscles to breathe is called retractions.
A) True **B)** False
[Reference text page 211]

44. All of the following are methods of assessing breathing EXCEPT:
A) listening to breath sounds.
B) auscultating the diastolic pressure.
C) measuring the respiratory rate.
D) evaluating the depth of respirations.
[Reference text page 223]

45. Artificial ventilation may be indicated if the patient has:
A) been hyperventilating.
B) a respiratory rate that is too slow or fast.
C) a normal mental status.
D) none of the above.
[Reference text page 225]

46. When ventilating a patient, if the abdomen is distended, you may be allowing air to get into the esophagus
A) True **B)** False
[Reference text page 231]

47. It is acceptable to use a water-soluble lubricant prior to using a nasal airway.
A) True **B)** False
[Reference text page 222]

48. A full tank of oxygen usually contains:
A) 500 psi.
B) 1000 psi.
C) 2000 psi.
D) 2500 psi.
[Reference text page 235]

49. An "E" cylinder usually holds ________ liters.
A) 350
B) 625
C) 1250
D) 2000
[Reference text page 235]

50. The flow requirements for a nasal cannula are:
A) 1 to 4 lpm.
B) 2 to 6 lpm.
C) 8 to 12 lpm.
D) none of the above.
[Reference text page 237]

51. The preferred ventilation device for prehospital care is:
A) the simple face mask.
B) the non-rebreather mask.
C) the nasal cannula.
D) none of the above.
[Reference text page 237]

52. With the correct mask seal, the non-rebreather mask delivers about ________ percent oxygen to the patient.
A) 75
B) 90
C) 100
D) none of the above
[Reference text page 237]

53. A punctured oxygen tank or broken valve assembly can act like a missile.
A) True
B) False
[Reference text page 237]

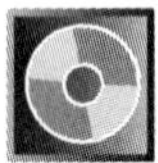

CD-ROM LINK: *Review the* Nasal Cannula *video in Chapter 7 of the MedEMT CD-ROM.*

54. Differences between adult, child, and infant airways include:
A) infants are often nose breathers.
B) children have a smaller, narrower trachea.
C) the cricoid of a child is less rigid than an adult's.
D) all of the above.
[Reference text page 240]

55. All of the following are signs and symptoms of inadequate breathing in a child EXCEPT:
A) retraction above the clavicles and between the ribs.
B) breathing through the nose.
C) seesaw breathing pattern.
D) shallow breathing.
[Reference text page 242]

CASE STUDIES

Use a separate piece of paper to answer the case study questions. Number your answers with the case study number and question letter (1A, 1B, etc.).

THE RESPIRATORY SYSTEM

1. Your EMT-Basic education has been exciting and rewarding. The instructor team placed a lot of emphasis on learning basic anatomical structures. Your first call as a certified Emergency Medical Technician-Basic is for a patient who has been assaulted. Upon your arrival, you find a 25-year-old male who was struck in the face and neck with a baseball bat. There is significant facial trauma with bleeding into the oropharynx.
A) What respiratory structures might the blows have injured?

B) Where might the blood in the oropharynx drain if not suctioned? What complications can this cause?

AIRWAY MANAGEMENT

2. Family members were worried about their grandfather and decided to call 911. As you arrive, you notice oxygen tanks and oxygen tubing throughout the house. According to the family, the patient has not been out of bed for three days. You find the 72-year-old male lying in bed with moderate respiratory distress. He is using three pillows to prop himself up and the window is open, despite the cold weather. He looks fatigued and you hear audible wheezes during his inhalations. He denies any productive cough, seems slightly agitated, and has cyanosis around the fingertips. The patient has a long history of chronic obstructive pulmonary disease and heart failure. His physician recently increased his home oxygen to two liters via cannula 24 hours a day.

A) Given this patient's signs of "air hunger," what treatment would you suggest?

3. The motorcycle appears to have struck the vehicle just behind the driver's door. The motorcy-cle driver, an 18-year-old male, is alert and oriented. He feels cold to the touch and complains of severe neck and back pain. He is wearing a helmet and denies any significant medical history. You notice an open fracture in the lower left leg with minor blood loss. The patient cannot feel or move his toes on either side. He states it is "a little hard to breathe." You count his respirations at 28 per minute, observing that each breath is slightly labored. A highway patrol officer, who believes the driver of the car is under the influence of alcohol, estimates the impact at approximately 45 mph.

A) What is the patient's airway status? Justify your answer.

B) What interventions are indicated for this patient?

C) As you load the motorcycle driver into the ambulance, you suddenly hear snoring respi-rations. The patient's mental status is deteriorating, and the respiratory rate has increased to 34. What is the most likely cause of the snoring respirations?

D) What should you do now?

4. Based on your request, the department has just purchased ten new suction units to replace the outdated ones currently in use. The manufacturer's representative has given you an orientation on the benefits, maintenance, and use of these units. Knowing that you have this knowledge, the supervisor asks you to give the day shift a quick lesson on the new devices.

A) Describe the basic components of all suction devices.

B) Describe the different types of suction units available.

C) What special considerations are necessary when using the rigid suction catheter?

D) What special considerations are necessary for the use of rigid suction catheters in infants and children?

5. Your latest patient collapsed just after eating a large dinner. During resuscitation efforts, the patient begins to vomit large quantities of stomach contents. Much of the material is large and chunky. Your job is to maintain the airway of the patient.

A) What safety considerations should you be aware of when clearing a patient's airway?

B) As you attempt to suction the airway with a tonsil-tip (rigid) catheter, very little material is actually being cleared. What steps can you take to improve airway patency and suction efforts?

6. The early-morning crash scene is full of twisted metal, broken glass, and the muffled sounds of several people moaning. As a new EMT-Basic, you are almost overwhelmed by it all. Your partner asks you to suction the nasal airway of her patient. The patient's teeth are clenched and your partner has not been able to open the airway manually.
   A) What adjunct could you use to manage the airway of this patient?
   B) Describe the equipment and technique you would use to suction the patient.
7. Katarina is a 70-year-old female who has been a regular patient of Ambulance 7 for more than two years. She calls 911 often because of complaints associated with her chronic respiratory disease. This evening she cannot catch her breath and believes she is having another "anxiety attack." You listen to her lung sounds and cannot hear any air movement. While en route to the hospital, you notice the patient has become exhausted and her respirations have dropped to eight per minute. She is now unresponsive to painful stimulus but maintains a strong gag reflex.
   A) What airway adjunct is preferred in this case? Why?
   B) How does inserting a nasopharyngeal airway differ from inserting an oropharyngeal airway?
8. You are driving to the ball game with some friends from work. As you enter the highway, you witness a high-speed single-vehicle rollover. Since everyone in your car is involved in EMS, you stop to render assistance. The single occupant of the vehicle was ejected and has sustained massive head injuries. She is female, approximately 25 years old, and is breathing at eight to ten breaths per minute. You are only carrying a basic first aid kit including a pocket mask. Your friend advises you that EMS is ten minutes out.
   A) How will you open this patient's airway?
9. As a lead lifeguard for over five years, you are glad when the department finally decides to outfit each station with a bag-valve mask and small oxygen tank. You are sure these will be very useful during the upcoming summer season. As both a lifeguard and a new EMT-Basic, you have been asked to evaluate equipment for adoption.
   A) What features will you look for when deciding which bag-valve-mask device to purchase?
   B) Within a week after placing the devices at each station and completing staff training on the use of BVM's, a non-breathing patient is pulled from the surf. Your staff is ventilating
   using the bag-valve mask and oxygen. How do they know they are ventilating the patient effectively?
10. You are dispatched to pick up the local EMS medical director who has asked to ride along with your crew for the next few hours. She wants to observe how artificial ventilation procedures are being used in the field. After several minor calls, you are dispatched to a man down at the bus station. As you arrive, you see that bystanders and a security guard have started CPR. You are assigned to airway management while your partner takes over chest compressions. You quickly attach the demand-valve to the flow-restricted, oxygen-powered ventilation device mask and begin hyperventilating the patient.
   A) Describe the basic features of a flow-restricted, oxygen-powered ventilation device.
   B) After you have placed the face mask over the patient's mouth and nose, list the steps necessary to properly use the flow-restricted, oxygen-powered ventilation device.

C) What is the most significant complication to avoid during artificial ventilation when using a flow-restricted, oxygen-powered ventilation device?

11. Mr. Van has waited several days to call 911. As you enter his one-bedroom apartment, you notice that Mr. Van is using all his neck and chest muscles to breathe. He can only speak one or two words at a time. You immediately place a non-rebreather mask on the patient, but within seconds, you notice that oxygen is not filling the reservoir bag. You find that the portable D cylinder is empty.

A) What measures could have prevented this situation?

B) What safety measures should you observe as you quickly change cylinders?

C) What is the approximate regulator reading for a full D tank?

12. The allergy season is in full swing, and it seems like during every shift, someone at the plant experiences shortness of breath. A seasoned supervisor places an urgent call for a man down at the far end of the facility. Something about the supervisor's voice tells you to respond immedi-ately. As you arrive, a 42-year-old male is complaining of severe chest pain and shortness of breath. He is conscious, very anxious, and says he feels like he cannot catch his breath. He is cool, pale, and moist to the touch. His respiratory effort is severely labored at 28 breaths per minute.

A) What type of oxygen delivery device is most appropriate at this time?

B) List other common indications for the use of this oxygen delivery device.

C) What low-flow device is available to deliver oxygen to a conscious and alert patient?

D) After applying the non-rebreather mask, your patient becomes irritated, repeatedly stat-ing "I can't breathe" and trying to remove the mask. He is becoming anxious and agi-tated. What is an appropriate course of action?

SPECIAL CONSIDERATIONS

13. You are taking a break from your studies when you hear a terrible collision just down the street. You can see that the car is severely damaged. As you arrive with your jump kit, you see that bystanders have already removed a teenaged female from the vehicle. An off-duty firefighter is attending to the driver in the car and he asks you to take care of the passenger. The teenager was not restrained and was ejected from the car through a side window. In your initial assessment, you notice that the patient is breathing through a tracheostomy tube. Her respiratory rate is eight breaths per minute.

A) How does the tracheostomy tube change your assessment of the patient?

B) A quick evaluation of respiratory status after discovery of the stoma leads you to conclude that the patient needs ventilatory assistance. Can you ventilate directly into the tra-cheostomy tube?

C) After several minutes of ventilation, it becomes harder to squeeze the bag-valve device. You check the port of the tube and see a pink mucous mixture there. How do you clear the airway?

D) How would this process change if the patient had a stoma instead of a tube?

14. As you finish fueling your vehicle, dispatch requests an emergency response for an unrespon-sive male at the high school. You are nearby and arrive in less than two minutes. In the principal's office, you find a 57-year-old male who is pulseless and apneic. The principal's secretary states that she heard a loud thump behind his door and could not get an answer. He was complaining of not feeling well when he arrived for work.

You immediately open the patient's airway and attempt to ventilate. For some reason, you are unable to get a good seal around his mouth. It appears that his dental appliance has partially dislodged.

A) What should you do to correct the situation and maintain a tight seal?

KEY TERMS MATCHING

Assess your knowledge of the chapter key terms by matching the terms on the left to the definitions on the right.

______ **1.** Agonal (AY-gun-ul) Respirations

______ **2.** Airway Adjunct

______ **3.** Alveoli (al-VEE-o-li)

______ **4.** Aspiration

______ **5.** Bag-Valve Mask Device

______ **6.** Diaphragm

______ **7.** Head-Tilt/Chin-Lift Maneuver

______ **8.** Hypoxia (high-POKS-e-uh)

______ **9.** Intercostal Muscles

______ **10.** Jaw-Thrust Maneuver

______ **11.** Laryngectomy (lair-en-JEK-tuh-mee)

______ **12.** Nasal Cannula (NAY-zul KAN-yuh-luh)

______ **13.** Nasopharyngeal (NAY-zoh-fair-en-GEE-ul) Airway

(A) A surgically created opening into a body cavity

(B) Surgical opening of the trachea

(C) The amount of air inhaled and exhaled in a single breath

(D) Body cavity enclosed by the sternum, ribs, and vertebral column

(E) A specialized airway device for surgical placement into a tracheal stoma; used to maintain an airway passage

(F) A soft catheter used for suctioning the nasopharynx and in other situations where a rigid catheter cannot be used

(G) Nonflexible catheter used to suction an unresponsive patient

(H) Open; accessible

(I) Muscles located between the ribs; involved in breathing

(J) High-flow oxygen delivery device characterized by an inflatable oxygen reservoir bag and a one-way valve that prevents exhaled air from being reinhaled

(K) A soft rubber airway device inserted through the nose; designed to maintain an open airway by displacing the tongue off the pharynx

(L) A curved plastic device with a flange inserted in the patient's mouth; used to keep the tongue from blocking the pharynx

(M) Removal of the larynx

(N) The preferred method for opening and maintaining an airway in a patient with suspected spinal injury

_______ 14.	Non-Rebreather Mask	(O)	A tube inserted into the nose to deliver low-flow oxygen
_______ 15.	Oropharyngeal (or-oh-FAIR-en-GEE-ul) Airway	(P)	Deficiency of oxygen
_______ 16.	Patent (PAY-tent)	(Q)	Depressions in the neck, above the shoulder blades, between and below the ribs; indicates extensive muscle use during breathing due to respiratory distress
_______ 17.	Retraction	(R)	The preferred method for opening and maintaining an airway in a patient without suspected neck injury
_______ 18.	Rigid Suction Catheter	(S)	Primary muscle of breathing; forms the bottom portion of the thoracic cavity
_______ 19.	Soft Suction Catheter	(T)	Device that helps keep the airway open by keeping the tongue away from the back of the throat
_______ 20.	Stoma	(U)	To draw foreign material, a foreign body, or fluid into the respiratory tract while inhaling
_______ 21.	Thoracic (tho-RAS-ik) Cavity	(V)	Termination of the respiratory passages; the functional units of the lungs, across whose walls gas exchange occurs
_______ 22.	Tidal Volume	(W)	An oxygen delivery device comprised of a self-inflating bag face mask, one-way valve, and oxygen reservoir
_______ 23.	Tracheostomy (tray-kee-AHS-tuh-mee)	(X)	Occasional gasping breaths that may occur in the final stage of death
_______ 24.	Tracheostomy Tube		

LABELING DIAGRAMS

Fill in the correct anatomical terms corresponsing to the labels on the diagram.

THE RESPIRATORY SYSTEM

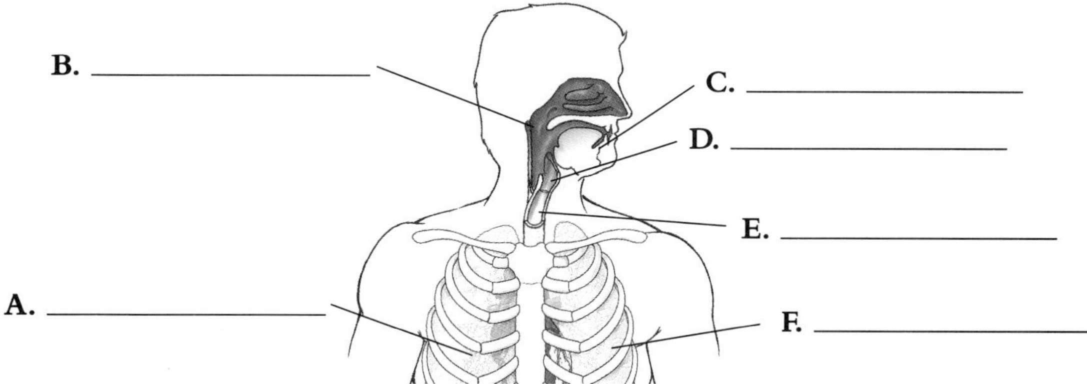

RESPIRATORY SIGNS

Fill in the correct characteristic of adequate and inadequate respiraiton in the table below.

Characteristic	Adequate Respiration	Inadequate Respiration
Rate	**A.**	**E.**
Effort of Breathing	Easy, effortless	Labored
Breath Sounds	**B.**	**F.**
Grunting	Absent	Present on exhalation
Chest Expansion	**C.**	**G.**
Nasal Flaring	Absent	Present (especially in children)
Retractions	**D.**	**H.**
Body Position	Relaxed	Sitting upright or leaning forward

SKILLS CHECKLISTS

Check your knowledge of important EMT-B skills by marking off each step in the following skills sheets.

JAW-THRUST MANUVER

☐ Take BSI precautions.

☐ Carefully keep the patient's head, neck, and spine aligned, moving him as a unit as you place him in a supine position.

☐ Then kneel approximately 18 inches above the head of the supine patient.

☐ Reach forward and gently place one hand on each side of patient's lower jaw. Run your fingers along jaw until you just pass the angle of the jaw.

☐ Stabilize the patient's head with your palms and forearms.

☐ Using your index fingers, push the angles of patient's lower jaw forward.

☐ To keep the mouth open, use an oropharyngeal airway on a patient with no gag reflex.

☐ Do not tilt or rotate the patient's head.

NOTE: Remember the purpose of jaw-thrust maneuver is to open the airway without moving the head or neck from a neutral position.

HEAD-TILT/CHIN-LIFT MANEUVER

☐ Take BSI precautions.

☐ Once the patient is supine, place one hand on the forehead. Place the fingertips of your other hand under the bony area at the center of patient's lower jaw.

☐ Tilt the head by applying gentle pressure to patient's forehead.

☐ Use your fingertips to lift chin and to support lower jaw. Move jaw forward to a point where lower teeth are almost touching upper teeth. Do not compress soft tissues under lower jaw.

☐ Do not close the patient's mouth. It is best to insert an oropharyngeal airway if the patient has no gag reflex.

OROPHARYNGEAL SUCTIONING

☐ Take BSI precautions.

☐ Position yourself at patient's head and turn patient onto his side.

☐ A rigid tip (Yankauer) is preferred. While it does not need to be measured, never lose sight of the tip.

☐ Measure a flexible suction catheter (distance between patient's ear lobe and corner of mouth, or center of mouth to angle of jaw).

☐ Turn suction unit on. Attach the catheter and test for suction.

☐ Open and clear the patient's mouth.

☐ Place the rigid pharyngeal tip so that the convex (bulging-out) side is against roof of patient's mouth. Insert tip just to the base of the tongue. Do not push tip down into the throat or larynx.

☐ Apply suction only after the tip of the catheter or rigid tip is in place, suctioning on the way out, moving tip from side to side. Suction for no longer than 15 seconds. (As per U.S. Department of Transportation, suction toddlers for no longer than 10 seconds and infants for no longer than 5 seconds.)

☐ Hyperventilate the patient with 100 percent oxygen.

MOUTH-TO-MASK WITH OXYGEN

☐ Take BSI precautions.

☐ Connect one-way valve to mask.

- [ ] Connect oxygen to inlet on face mask. Oxygen should be run at 15 lpm.
- [ ] Kneel about 18 inches above the head of the supine patient.
- [ ] Open the airway (manually or with adjunct).
- [ ] Position mask on patient's face so that the apex is over bridge of nose and the base is between lower lip and prominence of chin.
- [ ] Establish and maintain a proper mask-to-face seal (jaw-thrust maneuver) by placing both thumbs on top sides of mask and with index, third, and fourth fingers of each hand grasp lower jaw on each side, between angle of jaw and ear lobe, to jut the jaw forward.
- [ ] Ventilate patient at proper volume and rate. That is, 800 to 1200 ml per breath, 10 to 20 breaths per minute, 1.5 to 2 seconds for each adult breath.
- [ ] Remove your mouth from port to allow for passive exhalation.

NOTE: Do not delay mouth-to-mask ventilation if oxygen is not immediately available.

OROPHARYNGEAL (ORAL) AIRWAY INSERTION

- [ ] Take BSI precautions.
- [ ] Select appropriate size airway.
- [ ] Measure airway (center of mouth to angle of jaw, or corner of mouth to tip of ear lobe).
- [ ] Insert airway without pushing tongue back into throat. Insert upside down and flip 180 degrees over tongue, or insert straight in with a tongue blade holding tongue forward.
- [ ] Remove oropharyngeal airway quickly if patient gags.

NASOPHARYNGEAL (NASAL) AIRWAY INSERTION

- [ ] Take BSI precautions.
- [ ] Select appropriate size airway (diameter of patient's little finger). An alternative method is to measure from patient's nostril to earlobe or to angle of jaw.
- [ ] Measure airway (nostril to ear lobe).
- [ ] Lubricate nasopharyngeal airway with water-soluble gel.
- [ ] Fully insert airway with bevel facing nasal septum.

TWO-RESCUER BVM VENTILATION

- [ ] Take BSI precautions.
- [ ] Open the medical patient's airway using head-tilt/chin-lift maneuver.
- [ ] Suction and insert an oropharyngeal airway.
- [ ] Select correct bag-valve-mask size (adult, child, or infant). A pop-off valve is not acceptable!
- [ ] Kneel approximately 18 inches above the head of the supine patient.
- [ ] Position mask on patient's face so that the apex is over bridge of nose and the base is between the lower lip and prominence of chin.
- [ ] Position thumbs over top half of mask, index and middle fingers over bottom half.
- [ ] Use ring and middle fingers to bring patient's jaw up to mask and maintain head-tilt, chin-lift. *Tilt the head back as if you were trying to stand patient on his or her head!*
- [ ] The second rescuer should connect bag to mask, if not already done. While you maintain mask seal, second rescuer should squeeze the bag with two hands until patient's chest rises.
- [ ] The second rescuer should release pressure on the bag and let the patient exhale passively. While this occurs, the oxygen reservoir is refilling.
- [ ] Patient can be hyperventilated if his or her condition warrants it.

NOTE: This technique may be used for a trauma patient by combining a jaw-thrust maneuver with manual stabilization of the head and neck.

PREPARING OXYGEN DELIVERY SYSTEM

- [ ] Select desired cylinder. Check label and hydrostat date.
- [ ] Place cylinder in an upright position and stand to one side.
- [ ] Remove plastic wrapper or cap protecting cylinder outlet.
- [ ] Keep plastic washer (some set-ups).
- [ ] Crack main valve for one second to clean it out.
- [ ] Select correct pressure regulator and flowmeter.
- [ ] Place cylinder valve gasket on regulator oxygen port.
- [ ] Make certain that pressure regulator is closed.

- [ ] Align pins, or thread by hand.
- [ ] Tighten T-screw for pin yoke.
- [ ] Tighten with a wrench for a threaded outlet.
- [ ] Attach tubing and delivery device.

OXYGEN ADMINISTRATION VIA NONREBREATHER

- [ ] Take BSI precautions.
- [ ] Assemble regulator onto tank.
- [ ] Open main valve on tank.
- [ ] Check for leaks.
- [ ] Check tank pressure.
- [ ] Attach nonrebreather mask.
- [ ] Adjust liter flow to 12 to 15 liters per minute.
- [ ] Pre-fill reservoir.
- [ ] Apply and adjust mask to patient's face, explaining need for oxygen.
- [ ] Secure tank during transport.

OXYGEN ADMINISTRATION VIA NASAL CANNUAL

- [ ] Take BSI precautions.
- [ ] Assemble regulator onto tank.
- [ ] Open main valve on tank.
- [ ] Check for leaks.
- [ ] Check tank pressure.
- [ ] Attach nasal cannula to regulator.
- [ ] Place nasal prongs into the patient's nose, and adjust tubing for patient comfort.
- [ ] Adjust liter flow to 1–6 lpm.
- [ ] Secure tank during transport.

DISCONTINUING OXYGEN ADMINISTRATION

- [ ] Remove delivery device from patient.
- [ ] Turn off the liter flow rate.
- [ ] Close the main valve.
- [ ] Remove the delivery tubing.
- [ ] Bleed the flowmeter.
- [ ] Change the tank if volume is 200 psi or less.

INSERTION OF THE NASOGASTRIC TUBE

- [ ] Take BSI precautions.
- [ ] Prepare and assemble the equipment.
- [ ] Oxygenate the patient.
- [ ] Measure tube from tip of nose, over ear, to below xiphoid process.
- [ ] Lubricate end of tube, and pass tube gently downward along nasal floor to stomach.
- [ ] To confirm correct placement, auscultate over epigastrium. Listen for bubbling while injecting 10 to 20 cc air into tube.
- [ ] Use suction to aspirate stomach contents.
- [ ] Secure tube in place.

(reprinted from *Pocket Reference for The EMT-B and First Responder by Bob Elling,* Prentice Hall, 1999)

D.O.T. OBJECTIVES CHECKLIST

Use the following list of knowledge objectives to check what you've learned. Check off only those objectives that you feel you completely understand and have mastered. For any objectives not checked, go back and review that section of the text chapter. Textbook page references have been provided to help you review the text material.

- [ ] Name and label the major structures of the respiratory system on a diagram. *(p. 208)*
- [ ] List the signs of adequate breathing. *(p. 222)*
- [ ] List the signs of inadequate breathing. *(p. 222)*

- [ ] Describe the steps in performing the head-tilt/chin-lift maneuver. *(p. 214)*
- [ ] Relate mechanism of injury to opening the airway. *(p. 214)*
- [ ] Describe the steps in performing the jaw thrust maneuver. *(p. 214)*
- [ ] State the importance of having a suction unit ready for immediate use when providing emergency care. *(p. 215)*
- [ ] Describe the techniques of suctioning. *(p. 217)*
- [ ] Describe how to artificially ventilate a patient with a pocket mask. *(p. 226)*
- [ ] Describe the steps in performing the skill of artificially ventilating a patient with a bag-valve mask while using the jaw thrust maneuver. *(p. 230)*
- [ ] List the parts of a bag-valve-mask system. *(p. 228)*
- [ ] Describe the steps in performing the skill of artificially ventilating a patient with a bag-valve mask for one and two rescuers. *(p. 228)*
- [ ] Describe the signs of adequate artificial ventilation using the bag-valve mask. *(p. 231)*
- [ ] Describe the signs of inadequate artificial ventilation using the bag-valve mask. *(p. 231)*
- [ ] Describe the steps in artificially ventilating a patient with a flow-restricted, oxygen-powered ventilation device. *(p. 232)*
- [ ] List the steps in performing the actions taken when providing mouth-to-mouth and mouth-to-stoma artificial ventilation. *(p. 243)*
- [ ] Describe how to measure and insert an oropharyngeal (oral) airway. *(p. 219)*
- [ ] Describe how to measure and insert a nasopharyngeal (nasal) airway. *(p. 222)*
- [ ] Define the components of an oxygen delivery system. *(p. 234)*
- [ ] Identify a non-rebreather mask and state the oxygen flow requirements needed for its use. *(p. 237)*
- [ ] Describe the indications for using a nasal cannula versus a non-rebreather mask. *(p. 237)*
- [ ] Identify a nasal cannula and state the flow requirements needed for its use. *(p. 237)*

CHAPTER 8

Scene Size-Up and Initial Assessment

CHAPTER 8 SUMMARY

A thorough, organized patient assessment is the key to providing good patient care. All care that you give should be based on assessment. The scene size-up is an evaluation for threats to the EMT-Basic's safety and that of the crew and patient as well. The need for additional resources is identified during this phase. The EMT-Basic will also determine the mechanism or nature of the injury or illness during this phase of assessment.

Scene assessment does not stop after the EMT-Basic approaches the patient. Continuous evaluation of the scene, while caring for the patient, needs to be done to maintain a safe scene. The EMT-Basic should monitor for changes that may threaten his or her safety and the safety of the crew, the patient, or bystanders.

Body substance isolation (BSI) precaution measures are initiated before approaching the patient. BSI and standard precautions are an important protective measure at an emergency scene.

The initial assessment focuses on identification and treatment of life-threatening problems related to the mental status, airway, breathing, or circulation.

The EMT-Basic's general impression is an important tool that, when refined by experience, will help to manage a patient correctly. The impression includes basic information on the mechanism of injury or illness, the patient's sex, age, and chief complaint.

If a traumatic injury is suspected, the EMT-Basic should always remember to control the cervical spine while assessing the patient's mental status and airway patency.

REVIEW QUESTIONS

Please circle the best answer for each question.

1. Patient assessment is designed to:
   A) guide you in setting priorities.
   B) identify signs and symptoms.
   C) guide your treatment decisions.
   D) do all of the above.
   [Reference text page 255]

2. Upon arrival at the scene, you should immediately evaluate each of the following EXCEPT:
   A) the patient's chief complaint.
   B) the need for additional help.
   C) the patient's breath sounds.
   D) the mechanism of injury.
   [Reference text page 256]

3. Scene safety assessment protects:
   A) all EMS personnel.
   B) the patient (s).
   C) bystanders.
   D) all of the above.
   [Reference text page 256]

4. Which of the following statements about body substance isolation precautions is true?
   A) Wear gloves, mask, gown, and eye protection as necessary to prevent contact.
   B) A HEPA mask helps protect against toxic fumes.
   C) Gloves need only be worn when blood is present.
   D) A mask should be worn at all times.
   [Reference text page 257]

5. An example of a scene that may have a particular hazard or concern is a low-oxygen area.
   A) True
   B) False
   [Reference text page 259]

6. Loud, boisterous conduct at the scene of a call is a ________ sensory clue.
   A) sight
   B) smell
   C) hearing
   D) tactile
   [Reference text page 257]

7. The presence of a concealed weapon on a patient is an example of a ________ clue.
   A) sight
   B) smell
   C) hearing
   D) tactile
   [Reference text page 257]

8. Potential hazards at the scene of a crash or rescue include:
   A) vehicle instability.
   B) smoke or fire.
   C) leaking fuel.
   D) all of the above.
   [Reference text page 258]

9. If upon arrival at the scene, there are multiple patients with respiratory complaints, you should suspect:

A) the collision was a rollover.
B) the presence of toxic substances.
C) the patients have a history of asthma.
D) none of the above.

[Reference text page 259]

CD-ROM LINK: *Review the* Fallen Climber *and* Rescuers Descent *videos in Chapter 8 of the MedEMT CD-ROM.*

10. Which of the following statements about the mechanism of injury is NOT true?

A) It will influence the specific type of injury sustained.
B) It is unrelated to patient care.
C) It is helpful when assessing and treating a patient's traumatic injuries.
D) It may help predict the type of injuries found.

[Reference text page 263]

11. If you are working in an area with snow and ice, you should take safety precautions to stabilize your footing.

A) True
B) False

[Reference text page 259]

12. Requiring rescuers to wear PFDs while around a body of water is not necessary

A) True
B) False

[Reference text page 260]

13. The area approximately 150 yards and 120 degrees in front of the suspected site of firearms is called:

A) the inner circle.
B) the kill zone.
C) the hot zone.
D) none of the above.

[Reference text page 260]

14. Situating yourself behind an object so a hostile person can't see you is called:

A) camouflage.
B) concealment.
C) cover.
D) none of the above.

[Reference text page 261]

15. Hiding behind an object that will protect you from gunfire is called:

A) camouflage.
B) concealment.
C) cover.
D) kill zone.

[Reference text page 261]

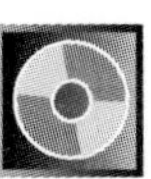

CD-ROM LINK: *Review the* Stabbing *video in Chapter 8 of the MedEMT CD-ROM.*

16. When approaching a patient at a crime scene, walk single file and the lead person should hold a flashlight by his or her side.
A) True **B)** False
[Reference text page 261]

17. The EMT-Basic should try to protect the patient from:
A) extremes of cold or heat. **B)** danger from traffic.
C) the news media. **D)** all of the above.
[Reference text page 262]

18. The final step in scene size-up is to determine the number of patients and the need for additional help or specialized rescue services.
A) True **B)** False
[Reference text page 270]

19. Hospital personnel rely heavily upon the information the EMT-Basic provides about the accident scene and the mechanism of injury.
A) True **B)** False
[Reference text page 263]

20. All patients require an initial assessment to identify and treat life-threatening injuries, regardless of the mechanism of injury.
A) True **B)** False
[Reference text page 254]

21. The outcome of a fall can be affected by all of the following EXCEPT the:
A) distance fallen.
B) type of surface impacted.
C) patient's sex.
D) part of the body that hits first.
[Reference text page 266]

22. Tissue compression caused by the pressure wave of a projectile is called:
A) compression. **B)** cavitation.
C) profile. **D)** insertion.
[Reference text page 267]

23. When a motorcyclist is thrown over the handlebars, it is common to break both tibias.
A) True **B)** False
[Reference text page 266]

24. Cavitation is the compression of tissue caused by the pressure wave of a projectile.
A) True **B)** False
[Reference text page 267]

25. The severity of injuries from firearms is determined by:
A) type of bullet. **B)** bullet caliber.
C) distance fired. **D)** all of the above.
[Reference text page 268]

26. In a blast injury, there is (are) ________ distinct pattern(s) of explosive injury.
A) 1 **B)** 2 **C)** 3 **D)** 4
[Reference text page 269]

27. The process of prioritizing patients to receive the appropriate level of care or transportation is called:
A) ordering. **B)** triage. **C)** flagging. **D)** coding.
[Reference text page 271]

28. Of the following, which is not a step in the initial assessment?
A) Assess mental status. **B)** Form a general impression.
C) Assess circulation. **D)** Obtain SAMPLE history.
[Reference text page 272]

29. Part of the general impression includes:
A) the patient's age and gender.
B) an evaluation of the scene safety.
C) calling for additional resources.
D) evaluation of the back and buttocks.
[Reference text page 273]

30. When a patient responds only to the EMT-Basic's commands, his mental status is called:
A) A **B)** V **C)** P **D)** U
[Reference text page 274]

31. When a patient fails to respond to a painful stimuli, her mental status is called:
A) A **B)** V **C)** P **D)** U
[Reference text page 274]

CD-ROM LINK: *Review the* Mental Status—AVPU *video in Chapter 8 of the MedEMT CD-ROM.*

32. The mechanism of injury as well as the patient's age determines the method of opening the airway.
A) True **B)** False
[Reference text page 275]

33. Conditions that suggest a high priority for immediate transport are:
A) unresponsive patient.
B) poor general impression.
C) uncontrolled bleeding.
D) all of the above.
[Reference text pages 279-80]

34. If breathing is adequate and the patient is responsive, oxygen may be indicated.
A) True **B)** False
[Reference text page 276]

35. Capillary refill should only be checked in children under 6 years of age.
A) True **B)** False
[Reference text page 279]

CASE STUDIES

Use a separate piece of paper to answer the case study questions. Number your answers with the case study number and question letter (1A, 1B, etc.).

SCENE SIZE-UP AND ASSESSMENT

1. The captain has just finished the afternoon drill when dispatch requests an emergency response for a laceration. Dusk makes it hard to see the details of the scene. As you approach the address, you notice bystanders watching a young man throwing clothes into the street. The young man looks up, notices the ambulance, and waves you forward. Your partner sees what looks like blood on the man's pants and on the pavement. The man is becoming more agitated and holds his arms up, questioning why you have not moved up the street. The bystanders begin moving back as the man starts to yell.
A) What is your primary responsibility when arriving on every EMS call?
B) As the EMT-Basic in charge, what is your major concern at this exact moment? How do you address this concern?

2. A tractor is almost completely upside down. Several people are attempting to dig around a 20-year-old male who is trapped inside the cab. You notice the patient bleeding from a laceration on his scalp. The tractor is spilling fuel and is beginning to lean heavily to one side. You are not familiar with tractor rollovers, and the patient is pinned.
A) What are some of the threats to safety at rescue or accident scenes?
B) Describe the concept of mechanism of injury and its importance.
C) What other types of scenes can present special hazards or concerns?
D) Is there a significant mechanism of injury in this case? What are other mechanisms that can be considered significant?

INITIAL ASSESSMENT

3. The mine safety office recently purchased two new First Responder vehicles. As you are checking out your squad's equipment, the central dispatch center advises of a medical aid call in Tunnel 18. You find a small crowd of miners gathered around someone lying motionless on a flatbed cart. As you get closer, it looks like the patient may be the victim of a crushing injury. Some of the men are holding pressure on a severe bleed on the patient's left forearm. Another miner is holding pressure against the patient's right thigh. The patient is slow to respond to questions and looks like he may be losing consciousness. You begin an initial assessment on the patient.

A) What is the function of the initial assessment?
B) What are the components of the initial assessment?
C) What type of body substance isolation would you suggest for the above scenario? (Assume the bleeding is quite severe.)

4. You are dispatched to a motorcycle collision in an intersection where the bike crashed into the rear of a parked car. The motorcyclist is lying unconscious on the ground.

A) If he went over the handlebars, what type of injury would you expect?
B) If the patient's helmet is cracked, what type of injuries should you suspect?
C) If the patient is verbally responsive and was thrown approximately 75 feet, what should his priority be?

KEY TERMS MATCHING

Assess your knowledge of the chapter key terms by matching the terms on the left to the definitions on the right.

______ **1.** AVPU

______ **2.** Blunt Trauma

______ **3.** Cavitation

______ **4.** General Impression

______ **5.** Initial Assessment

______ **6.** Interventions

______ **7.** Mechanism of Injury (MOI)

______ **8.** Nature of Illness

______ **9.** Penetrating Trauma

(A) The process of prioritizing patients to receive the appropriate level of care or transportation

(B) An injury caused by an object that pierces the skin or other body structure

(C) The process of determining scene safety, the nature of the problem, total number of patients, and need for additional resources

(D) A serious injury to the body or a severe emotional shock

(E) The type of condition or complaint a medical patient has

(F) The first step in initial assessment to quickly identify what is wrong and how serious it is; a time to use instinct and draw upon past experience

(G) Procedures done in an effort to improve the patient's condition

(H) Conducted after scene size-up in order to find and manage any life-threatening conditions

(I) The forces involved or factors influencing an injury

_______ **10.** Scene Size-Up

_______ **11.** Trauma

_______ **12.** Triage

(J) Tissue compression and cavity formation caused by the pressure of a projectile entering the body

(K) Injury caused by non-penetrating forces

(L) Memory aid used to help categorize a patient's level of unresponsiveness: A= Alert, V = responds to Verbal stimuli, P= Responds to Pain, U= Unresponsive

LABELING DIAGRAM

Fill in the correct patient assessment step in the blank portions of the flow chart below.

CRITICAL STEPS IN SCENE SIZE-UP

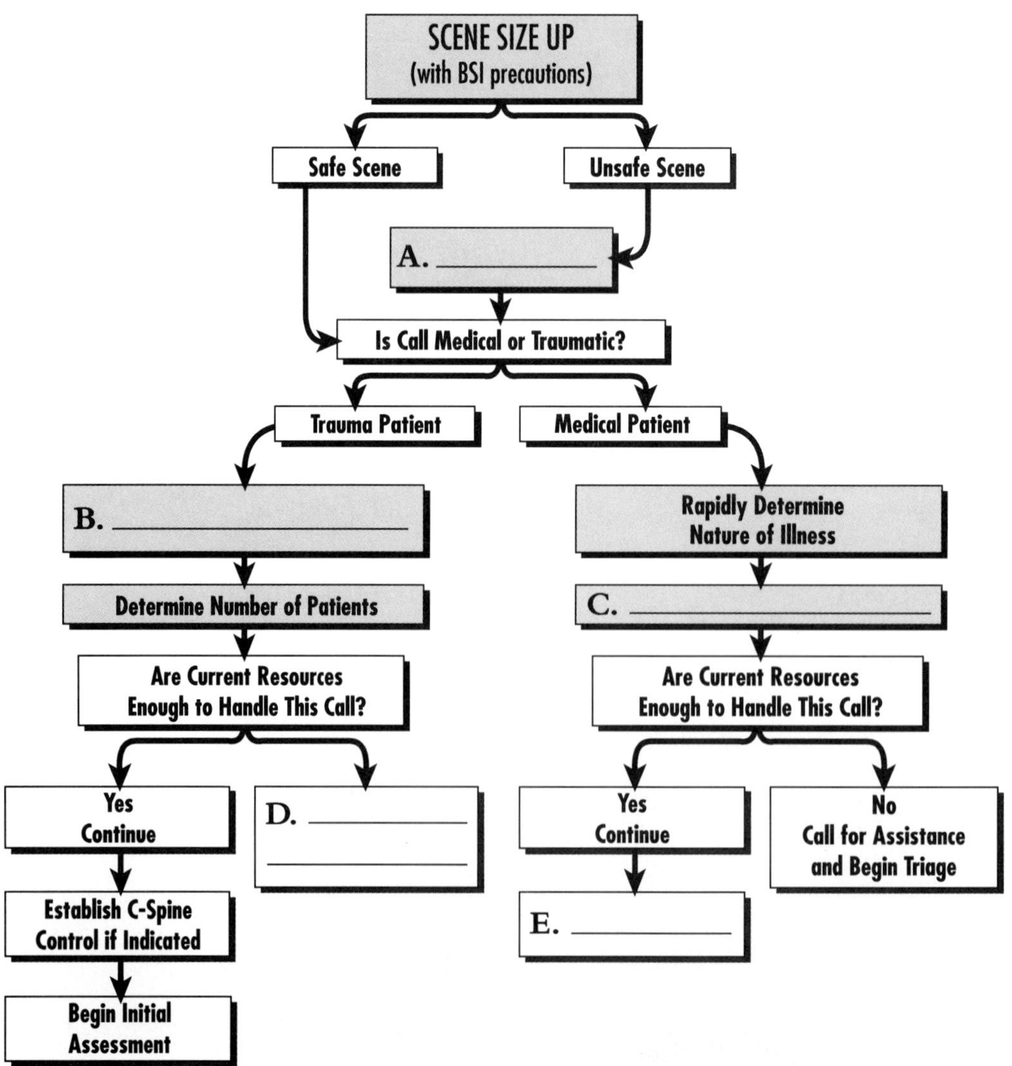

SKILLS CHECKLISTS

Check your knowledge of important EMT-B skills by marking off each step in the following skills sheet.

THE INITIAL ASSESSMENT

- [ ] Take BSI precautions.
- [ ] Form a general impression based on assessment of environment and patient's chief complaint and appearance.
- [ ] Assess mental status. Determine level of responsiveness using AVPU (alert, verbal, painful, unresponsive).
- [ ] Assess airway and breathing (assess, initiate appropriate oxygen therapy, assure adequate ventilation).
- [ ] Assess circulation (assess for and control major bleeding; assess pulse; assess skin color, temperature, and condition).
- [ ] Determine patient's treatment priority (high/low, C.V.P.S.), and make transport decision.

NOTE: Apply manual stabilization on first contact with any patient who you suspect may have an injury to the spine.

(reprinted from *Pocket Reference for The EMT-B and First Responder* by Bob Elling, Prentice Hall, 1999)

D.O.T. OBJECTIVES CHECKLIST

Use the following list of knowledge objectives to check what you've learned. Check off only those objectives that you feel you completely understand and have mastered. For any objectives not checked, go back and review that section of the text chapter. Textbook page references have been provided to help you review the text material.

- [ ] Recognize hazards/potential hazards. *(p. 256)*
- [ ] Describe common hazards found at the scene of a trauma and a medical patient. *(p. 256)*
- [ ] Determine if the scene is safe to enter. *(p. 256)*
- [ ] Discuss common mechanisms of injury/nature of illness. *(p. 263)*
- [ ] Discuss the reason for identifying the total number of patients at the scene. *(p. 270)*
- [ ] Explain the reason for identifying the need for additional help or assistance. *(p. 270)*

- [ ] Summarize the reasons for forming a general impression of the patient. *(p. 273)*
- [ ] Discuss methods of assessing altered mental status. *(p. 273)*
- [ ] Differentiate between assessing the altered mental status in the adult, child, and infant patient. *(p. 273)*
- [ ] Discuss methods of assessing the airway in the adult, child, and infant patient. *(p. 275)*
- [ ] State reasons for management of the cervical spine once the patient has been determined to be a trauma patient. *(p. 275)*
- [ ] Describe methods used for assessing if a patient is breathing. *(p. 276)*
- [ ] State what care should be provided to the adult, child, and infant patient with adequate breathing. *(p. 276)*
- [ ] State what care should be provided to the adult, child, and infant patient without adequate breathing. *(p. 276)*
- [ ] Differentiate between a patient with adequate and inadequate breathing. *(p. 276)*
- [ ] Distinguish between methods of assessing breathing in the adult, child, and infant patient. *(p. 276)*
- [ ] Compare the methods of providing airway care to the adult, child, and infant patient. *(p. 276)*
- [ ] Describe the methods used to obtain a pulse. *(p. 276)*
- [ ] Differentiate between obtaining a pulse in an adult, child and infant patient. *(p. 276)*
- [ ] Discuss the need for assessing the patient for external bleeding. *(p. 278)*
- [ ] Describe normal and abnormal findings when assessing skin color. *(p. 278)*
- [ ] Describe normal and abnormal findings when assessing skin temperature. *(p. 278)*
- [ ] Describe normal and abnormal findings when assessing skin condition. *(p. 278)*
- [ ] Describe normal and abnormal findings when assessing skin capillary refill in the infant and child patient. *(p. 278)*
- [ ] Explain the reason for prioritizing a patient for care and transport. *(p. 279)*

CHAPTER 9

Patient Assessment

CHAPTER 9 SUMMARY

If the patient has suffered a traumatic injury, perform the focused history and physical exam (FHPE) for a trauma patient. If the mechanism of injury (MOI) is significant, complete a rapid examination of the patient from head to toe (the rapid trauma assessment). If the MOI is minor, examine only the affected area with a focused examination. The transportation decision may be made early in the initial assessment or at the end of the FHPE, depending on the patient's severity.

For responsive medical patients, perform a medical focused history and physical exam. If the patient is unconscious, perform a quick head-to-toe assessment (the rapid medical assessment). Carefully evaluate unconscious patients to be sure that traumatic injury is not involved.

The detailed physical exam is usually performed while en route to the hospital. The detailed exam is a careful, more thorough assessment of the patient from head to toe. Based on the patient's chief complaint, there may be specific signs or symptoms you will look for or listen to.

While en route to the receiving facility, it is very important to perform an ongoing assessment. For unstable patients, you should perform these every 5 minutes. For stable patients, reevaluate every 15 minutes. The ongoing assessment involves repeating the initial assessment, retaking the vital signs, and checking any interventions you may have performed.

REVIEW QUESTIONS

Please circle the best answer for each question.

1. Which of the following statements about the mechanism of injury is NOT true?
   A) It will help evaluate the patient's chief complaint.
   B) It determines the exact event that caused the injury.
   C) It leads to a high index of suspicion for hidden injuries.
   D) It may involve discovery of critical injuries that are not immediately obvious.
   [Reference text pages 263, 269 , 294]

2. When assessing a patient's condition, the measurement and recording of vital signs should be performed before other procedures.
   A) True **B)** False
   [Reference text page 304]

3. Which of the following should be performed when assessing the chest?
   A) Cut away clothing and check for DCAP-BTLS.
   B) Auscultate each lung base at the midaxillary line.
   C) Assess for adequacy of breathing.
   D) All of the above.
   [Reference text page 297, 299]

4. How should open chest wounds, flail chest for example, be covered?
   A) With a light bandage and returned to after assessment is complete.
   B) Immediately with a gloved hand.
   C) With an occlusive dressing, bandaged tightly on four sides.
   D) Dealt with during the detailed physical exam.
   [Reference text page 300]

5. If a trauma patient complains of pelvic pain, it is important to perform a thorough exam of this area, including palpation.
   A) True **B)** False
   [Reference text page 302]

6. Check for pulses, motor, and sensory function in all four extremities.
   A) True **B)** False
   [Reference text page 302]

7. After performing the Rapid Trauma Assessment and taking the patient's vital signs, obtain a ________ history.
   A) brief **B)** detailed **C)** SAMPLE **D)** focused
   [Reference text page 304]

8. Vital signs in a stable patient should be monitored every ________ minutes.
A) 5 **B)** 10 **C)** 15 **D)** 20
[Reference text page 304]

9. All trauma patients require a rapid trauma assessment, regardless of the mechanism of injury.
A) True **B)** False
[Reference text page 296]

CD-ROM LINK: *Review the* Mechanism of Injury *videos in Chapter 9 of the MedEMT CD-ROM.*

10. You should not obtain a SAMPLE history on an unresponsive patient.
A) True **B)** False
[Reference text page 304]

11. Which of the following terms is used to describe a patient with symptoms caused by underlying illness such as diabetes or heart attack?
A) Medical **B)** Trauma
C) Critical **D)** None of the above
[Reference text page 304]

12. In medical patients, assess the mental status to determine if the patient is responsive or unresponsive.
A) True **B)** False
[Reference text pages 274, 304]

13. Assess the chief complaint using the acronym:
A) SAMPLE **B)** AVPU **C)** OPQRST **D)** CUPS
[Reference text page 305]

14. The Rapid Medical Assessment is a quick and systematic head-to-toe exam performed on the unresponsive medical patient.
A) True **B)** False
[Reference text page 306]

15. The focused history includes both the OPQRST questions and the SAMPLE history.
A) True **B)** False
[Reference text page 305]

16. During transport, do all of the following EXCEPT:
A) reassess vital signs every 15 minutes.
B) monitor effectiveness of all interventions.
C) try not to disturb the patient.
D) redo the focused physical exam at least once.
[Reference text page 312]

17. In the assessment of a responsive medical patient, perform the physical exam before the focused history.
A) True **B)** False
[Reference text page 305]

18. The "E" in SAMPLE history stands for ________ leading to the injury or illness.
A) elevation **B)** evaluation **C)** everything **D)** events
[Reference text pages 166, 306]

19. Transport a critically ill or injured patient as soon as possible.
A) True **B)** False
[Reference text page 307]

20. An unresponsive patient should always be transported in the recovery position to improve drainage of secretions and to help keep the airway open.
A) True **B)** False
[Reference text page 307]

21. A sign of possible respiratory distress is the use of ________ muscles.
A) rib **B)** axial **C)** accessory **D)** very few
[Reference text page 311]

22. When assessing the neck, look for:
A) jugular venous distention. **B)** a tracheostomy tube.
C) a medical identification tag. **D)** all of the above.
[Reference text pages 299, 243, 311]

23. Abnormal accumulation of fluid in the tissues causing swelling of extremities is :
A) distention. **B)** ascites. **C)** infection. **D)** edema.
[Reference text page 303]

24. In the unresponsive medical patient, baseline vital signs are obtained:
A) before the rapid medical assessment. **B)** after rapid medical assessment.
C) as often as possible. **D)** every 15 minutes.
[Reference text page 304]

25. The recovery position is used:
A) when spinal injury is suspected.
B) to improve drainage of secretions from the patient's mouth.
C) by placing the patient in the posterior recumbent position.
D) to expedite the patient's recovery.
[Reference text page 307]

26. All unconscious patients should receive airway maintenance, suctioning or assisted ventilation if necessary.
A) True **B)** False
[Reference text page 307]

27. The detailed physical exam must be completed prior to transport.
A) True **B)** False
[Reference text page 308]

28. Begin palpating the abdomen in the quadrant where the patient has indicated pain.
A) True **B)** False
[Reference text page 302]

29. Which of the following is true about the detailed physical exam?
A) It is performed completely and thoroughly on all patients.
B) It may not be completed in a patient with critical injuries.
C) It is not necessary in unresponsive patients.
D) None of the above.
[Reference text page 308]

CD-ROM LINK: *Review the* Detailed Physical Exam *video in Chapter 9 of the MedEMT CD-ROM.*

30. The occipital region is :
A) the eye socket. **B)** the back of the head.
C) examined first in a head assessment. **D)** the least injured region.
[Reference text page 310]

31. Deviation of the ________ suggests severe chest or lung injury.
A) trachea **B)** cervical spine **C)** larynx **D)** nasal bridge
[Reference text page 299]

CD-ROM LINK: *Review the* Assessment in the Ambulance *video in Chapter 9 of the MedEMT CD-ROM.*

32. Palpate the chest wall for:
A) paradoxical motion.
B) equal expansion of lungs.
C) crepitation.
D) all of the above.
[Reference text pages 300, 311]

33. Which of the following is true about a patient with a pulsatile mass in the abdomen?
A) May have an aortic aneurysm (a medical emergency)
B) Should be transported when stable
C) May have swallowed an animal
D) All of the above
[Reference text page 302]

34. An unstable pelvis requires rapid transport.
A) True **B)** False
[Reference text page 302]

35. The purpose of the ongoing assessment is to:
A) identify any injuries missed during initial assessment.
B) detect any changes in the patient's condition.
C) determine effectiveness of interventions and adjust as needed.
D) complete all of the above.
[Reference text page 309]

36. The ongoing assessment includes reassessing the mental status of the patient.
A) True **B)** False
[Reference text pages 309, 312]

37. A focused history and physical exam should be performed immediately following the:
A) scene size-up **B)** rapid assessment **C)** initial assessment **D)** ongoing exam
[Reference text page 292]

38. The ________ assessment is performed on a patient suffering a significant MOI
A) rapid medical
B) focused trauma
C) rapid trauma
D) focused medical
[Reference text page 292]

39. The extent of injury from penetrating trauma depends on all of the following EXCEPT
A) the velocity of the missile.
B) the density of the tissue.
C) the affected area of the body.
D) All of the above will affect the extent of injury.
[Reference text page 267]

40. A child pedestrian who is struck by an automobile is more likely to have a chest injury than an adult pedestrian is.
A) True **B)** False
[Reference text page 288]

41. Wearing a helmet has little effect on reducing the mortality rate from head injuries in motorcyclists.
A) True **B)** False
[Reference text page 266]

42. Usually the motorcyclist who is involved in an accident will be lying next to the motorcycle.
A) True **B)** False
[Reference text page 266]

43. Tissue compression that occurs as a result of the pressure wave of the missile is referred to as:
A) a blast injury.
B) the second wave
C) compression delay.
D) cavitation.
[Reference text page 267]

44. Gunshot wounds frequently produce severe internal bleeding, severe external bleeding, shock, and respiratory compromise.
A) True **B)** False
[Reference text page 267]

45. The region of the body penetrated, the proximity of organs and vessels, and the velocity of the missile all affect the extent of injury involved with penetrating injuries.
A) True **B)** False
[Reference text page 267]

46. What is the term for injuries received from a force that acts on the body, but does not physically penetrate the skin?
A) Blunt force trauma
B) Localized trauma
C) Piston trauma
D) Degloving injury
[Reference text page 264]

47. Which of the following is NOT one of the collisions that occur in every motor vehicle collision?
A) Vehicle impact
B) Occupant impact
C) Internal organ impact
D) Rebound impact
[Reference text pages 264, 286]

48. What is the most frequent injury suffered by a cyclist?

A) Fractured pelvis
B) Closed head injury
C) Aortic tear
D) Long bone fracture
[Reference text page 266]

49. According to the text, which of the following is NOT one of the factors that affect the outcome of a fall?
A) The distance fallen
B) The type of surface impacted
C) The part of the body that hits first
D) The gender of the patient who fell
[Reference text page 266]

50. What kind of trauma results from the penetration of the skin by an object?
A) Blunt trauma
B) Penetrating trauma
C) Localized trauma
D) Stabbing trauma
[Reference text page 267]

51. Consider ________ for a critically injured patient or a patient who begins to deteriorate.
A) Advanced Life Support
B) Air transport
C) Specialized resources
D) All of the above.
[Reference text page 292]

52. Other than direct pressure, what can reduce the amount of bleeding from an injured extremity?
A) Vasopressors
B) Elevation
C) Supination
D) Nitrates
[Reference text pages 552-53]

53. If direct pressure and elevation fail to control bleeding, use ________ by compressing the artery against a bone.
A) pressure points
B) indirect elevation
C) systemic vasopressors
D) long-bone elevations
[Reference text pages 552-53]

54. A "transection" of the aorta means that the aorta:
A) has a leak in one of its sections.
B) has sections that were repaired in surgery.
C) was transplanted from a donor aorta.
D) was torn during rapid deceleration.
[Reference text page 286]

55. When is elevation of an injured, bleeding limb not recommended?
A) When direct pressure has already been applied to the injury.
B) When the patient's breathing is rapid and shallow.
C) When the patient has an allergy to bandaging materials.
D) When the extremity is swollen, deformed, or very painful.
[Reference text page 552]

CASE STUDIES

Use a separate piece of paper to answer the case study questions. Number your answers with the case study number and question letter (1A, 1B, etc.).

1. The alarm rings for a violent assault call at an apartment complex. A sheriff's officer who is standing in a doorway hurriedly waves you up. You can see blood all over the walkway. At the door, two patients are lying on the floor covered in blood. It looks like the male shot himself beneath the chin with a large caliber gun. The female patient is slow to respond and has very labored breathing at a rate of 12 per minute. You can see obvious skull deformity just above her right eye.
   A) List ten mechanisms of injury that are considered significant in adult patients.
   B) List the steps for completing a history and physical exam of a patient with a significant mechanism of injury.
   C) Describe the steps for completing a history and physical exam when you have determined that the mechanism of injury was not significant.
2. The weather has turned ugly, and many of the rural roads will be flooded in just a few minutes. A highway patrol officer requests emergency services for a three-car crash about eight miles south of town. As you arrive on scene, two volunteers have just completed triage. They direct you to a patient who was ejected from a small pickup truck that appears to have rolled several times. The single occupant is a 16-year-old male with obvious head injuries and bilateral deformity of the lower extremities. Volunteer First Responders are maintaining spinal precautions and ventilating the patient with a pocket mask.
   A) Would this patient receive a rapid trauma assessment or focused history and physical exam? Why?
   B) How does the rapid trauma assessment differ from the focused history and physical exam?
   C) What do the letters "DCAP-BTLS" stand for? Why are they important?
   D) The EMT-Basic volunteer who is working with you is providing the patient with artificial ventilations. He has only worked with the rescue squad for two months, and is still unsure of his skills. As he begins another round of ventilations, he stops and reports that his ventilations are not causing the chest to rise. The patient is cyanotic around the lips and earlobes. What should you do in this situation?
   E) As you begin your rapid assessment of the patient's neck, what specific things will you look for?
3. The local mall is full of holiday shoppers. It takes you minutes just to make your way through the crowds to the security office. A 23-year-old female was caught shoplifting and brought to the office for processing. While being questioned, the patient began complaining of feeling sick. She had what they describe as a 20-

(A) A physical exam designed to quickly determine the nature and severity of an illness and identify necessary interventions

(B) A physical exam designed to quickly identify critical injuries and emergency interventions

(C) A shifting of the trachea to either side of the midline caused by the pressure of air trapped in the chest cavity

second seizure of her arms and lower legs. The seizure began and ended while the suspect was sitting in a chair, and she never lost consciousness. The guards moved her into a recovery position on the office floor prior to your arrival. The patient is slow to respond to questions. She denies any history of seizure activity.

A) In the initial steps of the focused history and physical exam of a medical patient, in what two categories can you place the patient?

B) Into which category does the above patient fit? How does the assessment differ between these categories?

C) What are some of the other conditions that may cause a patient to have altered mental status?

D) What questions are appropriate for obtaining the history of the chief complaint from a responsive patient?

E) What are the average vital sign ranges for this adult patient?

(D) Chest movement during breathing in which one section of the chest moves in the opposite direction from the rest; indicates multiple rib fractures (flail chest)

(E) Frequent reevaluation of a patient after initial assessment and primary interventions; to identify changes in patient condition and ensure appropriate care

(F) A crackling sensation felt and heard beneath the skin; caused by broken bone ends grating against each other or by subcutaneous air

(G) Assessment procedure used to identify conditions requiring emergency care; performed after initial assessment and lifesaving interventions

(H) Abnormal accumulation of fluid in the tissues causing swelling

(I) A careful, comprehensive examination of the body performed on critical patients, usually while en route to the receiving facility

(J) Abnormal bulging of the jugular veins indicating injury to the heart or chest

4. Fred has had a very rough life, and consequently has multiple medical problems. He does not hesitate to call 911 when he feels sick or is slightly injured, so the local EMS agency knows him very well. Fred recently finished chemotherapy, so he has been especially weak and in need of assistance. This morning, Fred's neighbor came over to visit and found him lying unresponsive on the kitchen floor. Fred appears to have fallen off a stepladder while trying to change a lightbulb. He does not respond normally to your verbal commands and has a bloody nose and some obvious bruising around his left cheek.

A) When should a detailed assessment be performed on this patient?

B) Why would you consider spinal precautions in this scenario?

C) What personal protective equipment should you wear in this case?

5. Transport times from your new response area are commonly in excess of 30 minutes. You are comfortable with ten or fifteen-minute transports found on your previous assignment, but are still learning how to handle calls that last longer. The patient in your unit has been complaining of general weakness and dizziness. She is 73 years old and denies any significant medical history. She has been vomiting for several hours and has been unable to eat since yesterday morning. Your initial assessment and physical exam have revealed no significant problems or findings. Her base-line vital signs are normal with a slight decrease from normal blood pressure.

A) What are the reasons for the ongoing assessment?
B) If the patient's condition were unstable, how often would you take vital signs? Why?
C) One step in the ongoing assessment is to check interventions. What does that step include?

KEY TERMS MATCHING

Assess your knowledge of the chapter key terms by matching the terms on the left to the definitions on the right.

______ **1.** Crepitation (krep-eh-TAY-shun)

______ **2.** Detailed Physical Exam

______ **3.** Edema (eh-DEE-muh)

______ **4.** Focused History and Physical Exam

______ **5.** Jugular Venous Distention (JVD) (JUG-yuh-ler VEE-nus di-STEN-shun)

______ **6.** Ongoing Assessment

______ **7.** Paradoxical Motion

______ **8.** Rapid Medical Assessment

______ **9.** Rapid Trauma Assessment

______ **10.** Tracheal Deviation (TRAY-kee-ul dee-vee-AY-shun)

LABELING DIAGRAMS

Fill in the corresponding term for the acronym below:

DCAP-BTLS

D = ________

C = ________

A = ________

P = ________

B = ________

T = ________

L = ________

S = ________

Fill in the correct step in the blanks in the assessment diagram on the following page.

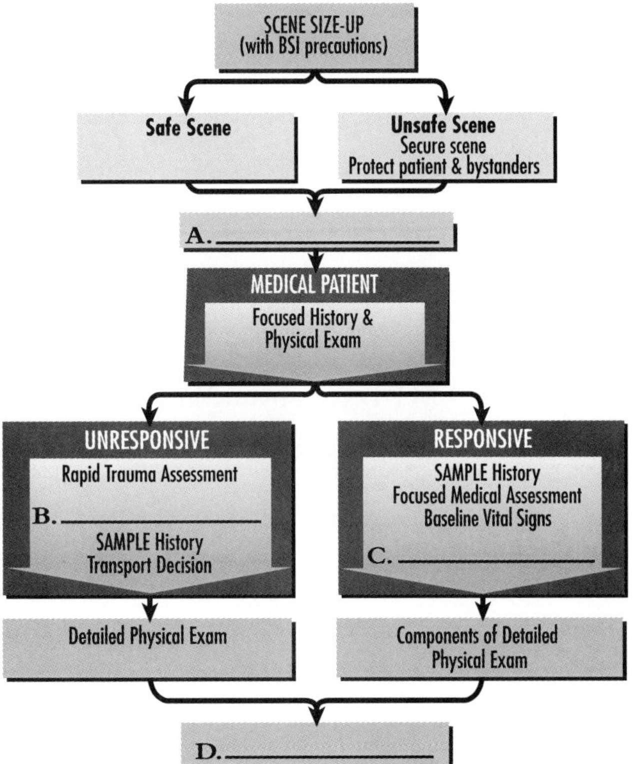

STEPS IN THE ASSESSMENT OF A MEDICAL PATIENT

SKILLS CHECKLISTS

Check your knowledge of important EMT-B skills by marking off each step in the following skills sheets.

FOCUSED HISTORY AND PHYSICAL EXAM—RESPONSIVE MEDICAL PATIENT

- [ ] Take BSI precautions.
- [ ] Gather history of present illness from patient by asking OPQRST questions.
- [ ] Gather a SAMPLE history from patient.
- [ ] Conduct a focused physical exam (focusing on the area patient complains of).
- [ ] Obtain baseline vital signs.
- [ ] Perform interventions and contact on-line medical direction as needed.
- [ ] Transport (re-evaluate transport decision).

FOCUSED HISTORY AND PHYSICAL EXAM—UNRESPONSIVE MEDICAL PATIENT

- [ ] Take BSI precautions.
- [ ] Conduct a rapid physical exam, by assessing:
  - [ ] Head.
  - [ ] Neck.
  - [ ] Chest.
  - [ ] Abdomen.
  - [ ] Pelvis.
  - [ ] Extremities.
  - [ ] Posterior.
- [ ] Obtain baseline vital signs.
- [ ] Gather history of the present illness from bystanders or family by asking OPQRST questions.
- [ ] Gather a SAMPLE history from bystanders or family.
- [ ] Perform interventions (obtain medical direction as required locally). Reassess vital signs.
- [ ] Transport (re-evaluate transport decision).

FOCUSED HISTORY AND PHYSICAL EXAM—TRAUMA PATIENT, NO SIGNIFICANT MOI

- [ ] Take BSI precautions.
- [ ] Reconsider MOI.
- [ ] Determine patient's chief complaint.
- [ ] Conduct a focused physical exam (focusing on the area patient complains of plus areas of potential injury suggested by the MOI).
- [ ] Obtain baseline vital signs.
- [ ] Take a SAMPLE history.
- [ ] Perform interventions as needed.
- [ ] Transport.

FOCUSED HISTORY AND PHYSICAL EXAM—TRAUMA PATIENT, SIGNIFICANT MOI

- [ ] Take BSI precautions.
- [ ] Reconsider MOI.
- [ ] Continue manual stabilization of head and neck.
- [ ] Consider requesting ALS personnel.
- [ ] Reconsider your transport decision.
- [ ] Reassess mental status.
- [ ] Perform a rapid trauma assessment. After assessing head and neck, apply a cervical collar and continue to maintain manual stabilization.
- [ ] Obtain baseline vital signs.
- [ ] Take a SAMPLE history.
- [ ] Perform a detailed physical exam either on scene, if there is time, or en route to the hospital.
- [ ] Perform ongoing assessment, including vital signs.
- [ ] Transport.

RAPID TRAUMA ASSESSMENT

- [ ] Take BSI precautions.
- [ ] Assess head: DCAP-BTLS + crepitation.
- [ ] Assess neck: DCAP-BTLS + jugular vein distention (JVD) and crepitation.
- [ ] Assess chest: DCAP-BTLS + paradoxical motion, crepitation, breath sounds.
- [ ] Assess abdomen: DCAP-BTLS + firmness, softness, distention.
- [ ] Assess pelvis: DCAP-BTLS + pain, tenderness, motion.
- [ ] Assess extremities: DCAP-BTLS + distal pulse, motor function, and sensation.
- [ ] Assess posterior: DCAP-BTLS.

DETAILED PHYSICAL EXAM

- [ ] Take BSI precautions.
- [ ] Examine head: DCAP-BTLS + crepitation.
- [ ] Examine scalp and cranium: DCAP-BTLS + crepitation.

CHAPTER 10

Communications and Documentation

CHAPTER 10 SUMMARY

Communication is an integral part of patient care. You must be able to gather and relay patient information as well as produce an accurate written prehospital care report (PCR) at the conclusion of each call.

Verbal communication is also an integral part of your patient care. You will communicate frequently with medical direction and dispatch, in addition to your patients and crew members.

When communicating with a receiving facility or medical direction, you must present an accurate and concise picture of your patient. Repeat word-for-word any orders or denials you are given. Question any unclear or inappropriate order.

Always communicate changes in your unit's status to dispatch (en route to call, arriving on scene, etc.).

At the conclusion of the call, you will produce a written report of the patient's condition and the medical care provided. This documentation assists in the continued care of the patient and is legal evidence of the prehospital care received. These forms are often used for quality improvement, to influence patient care decisions, and for billing purposes.

Certain situations, such as patient refusals, require careful documentation to protect you from claims of abandonment or negligence. Other situations, such as assaults, child abuse, elder abuse, domestic violence, and sexual crimes, may require you to file a report with an outside agency such as social services or law enforcement. Be familiar with local procedures.

Prehospital care reports must be honest. Carefully correct any errors. If you make an error in caring for the patient, carefully document the situation and what you did to correct the problem once it was identified.

REVIEW QUESTIONS

Please circle the best answer for each question.

1. Good communication skills are essential for:
   A) radio communications.
   B) verbal communication with hospital personnel.
   C) interpersonal communications.
   D) all of the above.
   [Reference text page 322]

2. After being given an order or a denial for any medication or procedure, you must immediately repeat the order back to medical control word-for-word.
   A) True **B)** False
   [Reference text page 327]

3. A prehospital care report must be filled out if time and the patient's condition allow.
   A) True **B)** False
   [Reference text page 331]

4. Remember this EMS saying when filling out reports: If it wasn't done, don't:
   A) do it. **B)** say it.
   C) write it down. **D)** pretend it was.
   [Reference text page 331]

5. The prehospital care report is an informal document meant to ensure continuity of care at the receiving facility.
   A) True **B)** False
   [Reference text page 331]

6. Complete documentation includes:
   A) interventions and response to interventions.
   B) trends in patient's condition.
   C) information from the scene.
   D) all of the above.
   [Reference text page 331]

7. An EMT-Basic should document patient care from initial contact through arrival at the receiving facility.
   A) True **B)** False
   [Reference text page 331]

8. The prehospital care report is considered a legal document.
A) True **B)** False
[Reference text page 337]

9. If you discover an error while completing the prehospital care report, carefully erase it and correct the document.
A) True **B)** False
[Reference text page 338]

CD-ROM LINK: *Review the* Paramedic in the Ambulance *video in Chapter 10 of the MedEMT CD-ROM.*

10. During a typical emergency response, radio transmissions are used for all of the following EXCEPT:
A) notifying dispatch of your arrival at the hospital.
B) notifying the hospital of the patient's condition.
C) calling for emergency police backup.
D) acknowledging receipt of the call from the dispatcher.
[Reference text page 323]

11. Radio communications are regulated and monitored by:
A) D.O.T.. **B)** the FCC. **C)** the EPA. **D)** OSHA.
[Reference text page 323]

12. A radio that is located at a stationary site is called a:
A) portable. **B)** repeater. **C)** mobile. **D)** base station.
[Reference text page 324]

13. A radio communications system that is widely available, has guaranteed channel access, and is most commonly used by EMS agencies is the:
A) cellular telephone band. **B)** digital transmission band.
C) VHF band. **D)** UHF band.
[Reference text page 325]

14. A radio communications system that is not widely available and dependent on a third party for channel access is the:
A) cellular telephone band. **B)** digital transmission band.
C) VHF band. **D)** UHF band.
[Reference text page 325]

15. The range of a UHF band mobile radio is generally ________ miles.
A) 1 to 2 **B)** 3 to 5 **C)** 15 to 20 **D)** 20 or more
[Reference text page 325]

16. When transmitting on a radio, you should:
A) listen to the channel before starting to talk.
B) hold the microphone 2 to 3 inches from your lips as you speak.
C) depress the microphone and wait a second before talking.
D) do all of the above.
[Reference text page 325]

17. Courtesy is assumed in radio transmission, so do not say "please" or "thank you."
A) True **B)** False
[Reference text page 326]

18. It is not necessary to repeat medical orders over the radio as this leads to lengthy conversations.
A) True **B)** False
[Reference text page 327]

19. Of the following, which is NOT an example of good communication at the scene of a call?
A) Quickly enter the residence and proceed immediately to treat the patient.
B) Be aware of how your body language may communicate to the patient.
C) Use the patient's name throughout the contact.
D) Speak clearly, slowly, and distinctly, using language the patient understands.
[Reference text page 330]

20. When communicating with children, you may need to stretch the truth to gain their trust.
A) True **B)** False
[Reference text page 331]

21. The standardized medical abbreviation for *history* is:
A) Ht. **B)** Hx. **C)** Hy. **D)** none of the above.
[Reference text page 341]

22. The standardized medical abbreviation for *rule out* is:
A) r/o. **B)** rl/ot. **C)** ru/t. **D)** none of the above.
[Reference text page 341]

23. The standardized medical abbreviation for *loss of consciousness* is:
A) lc. **B)** ALC. **C)** Los. **D)** LOC.
[Reference text page 341]

24. The abbreviation STAT means:
A) asap. **B)** prn. **C)** immediately. **D)** when available.
[Reference text page 341]

25. The abbreviation *NKDA* means:
A) not a known diabetic. **B)** needs drugs to stay alert.
C) no known drug allergies. **D)** never knows day of the week.
[Reference text page 341]

CASE STUDIES

Use a separate piece of paper to answer the case study questions. Number your answers with the case study number and question letter (1A, 1B, etc.).

DOCUMENTATION

1. The courtroom is quiet and your palms are sweaty. The attorney has just finished with your partner. The case is about a response you completed four years ago. The two occupants of the small sedan were killed instantly, but you were able to provide care for the drunk driver who hit them. The attorney is only interested in your care of the patient. Based on your written reports, the plaintiff claims that your field care was substandard. As far as you remember, the patient was only slightly injured and was able to communicate and provide information regarding his medical history.
A) What is the primary purpose of documentation?
B) What information is included as part of patient data?
C) What administrative information is included in the PCR?
D) What are common errors made when completing patient care documentation?
E) How do documentation practices change during a mass casualty incident?
F) List the cases that require you to report your findings to specific local authorities.

COMMON MEDICAL ABBREVIATIONS

2. For the two years prior to your EMT-Basic class, you worked as a First Responder volunteer with the local search and rescue team. That experience is definitely paying off. You have been identified as one of the "smart ones" in class, and several people have approached you asking for help. One area that seems particularly difficult for many students is remembering common medical abbreviations used in writing PCRs. The students have asked you to make a list of the abbreviations you have used while writing PCRs.
A) List the abbreviations for the following items:

______________ **a)** alcohol

______________ **b)** blood pressure

______________ **c)** chief complaint

_______________ **d)** estimated time of arrival

_______________ **e)** history

_______________ **f)** loss of consciousness

_______________ **g)** oxygen

_______________ **h)** past medical history

_______________ **i)** signs and symptoms

_______________ **j)** shortness of breath

_______________ **k)** vital signs

_______________ **l)** year old

3. You are dispatched for a patient having chest pains in a rural neighborhood. On arrival, you find a 46-year-old man having chest pain. The man states that the pain started about an hour ago when he was mowing the yard and has since increased in intensity. The patient has a previous history of heart disease and hypertension. He takes one aspirin every day, but requires no other medication. However, he does have nitroglycerin for use in case of chest pain. Your initial vital sign readings are: pulse 108, respirations 22, blood pressure 150/104. The patient has no allergies but is diaphoretic and pale. You immediately place the patient on oxygen. Given the patient's history, you ask for and receive permission to assist in the administration of one nitro-glycerin tablet. The patient begins to complain of a headache immediately after administration. Vital signs after administration are pulse 104, respirations 22, blood pressure 138/88. The patient states that the pain is unchanged. He says it feels like a herd of elephants is sitting on his chest and rates the pain 8 on a 1 to 10 scale. The patient responds well and you begin transport to the receiving facility. En route, the patient's pain remains unchanged. Vital signs are stable. You call the receiving hospital and give the report to the physician.

A) Using abbreviations and your knowledge of documentation, write a brief narrative of the events described above.

4. You are at the scene of a call where you believe that, due to the mechanism of injury, the patient needs to go to the hospital. His condition is not life threatening but it definitely needs to be attended to or he could get worse. The patient refuses to go, stating he does not have insurance to pay for either the ambulance bill or the hospital emergency department bill.

A) What are some of the strategies you can use to deal with this situation?
B) What should you document on the PCR if you end up not transporting?
C) Why can't you just overpower the patient and take him into the hospital?

KEY TERMS MATCHING

Assess your knowledge of the chapter key terms by matching the terms on the left to the definitions on the right.

_______ 1. Base Station

_______ 2. Minimum Data Set

_______ 3. Mobile Radio

_______ 4. Prehospital Care Report (PCR)

_______ 5. Repeaters

(A) Communications devices that receive a low-power transmission and rebroadcast the signal at higher power

(B) Documentation of the assessment and treatment of a patient in the field

(C) Patient and administrative information required to be included in a prehospital care report

(D) Two-way radios that are usually built into emergency vehicles

(E) Radio used for central dispatch operations and coordination of emergency services in an EMS communication system

FILL-IN-THE-BLANKS

Following is a list of items a standard medical report should include. Fill in the missing information.

1. The identity of your _____________ and the levels of _____________ who are present
2. Your estimated time of _____________
3. The patient's _____________ and sex
4. The chief _____________
5. A brief, pertinent history of the present _____________
6. Information on major _____________ illnesses
7. The patient's _____________ status
8. The _____________ vital signs
9. Pertinent findings from your _____________ exam
10. A summary of emergency _____________ _____________ that has been provided
11. The patient's _____________ to the emergency medical care

SKILLS CHECKLIST

Check your knowledge of important EMT-B skills by marking off each step in the following skills sheet.

PATIENT REFUSAL PROCEDURE

- [ ] Spend time effectively communicating with patient (includes reasoning, persistence, and strategies to convince patient to go to hospital).
- [ ] Clearly inform patient of consequences of not going to hospital.
- [ ] Consult with medical direction.
- [ ] Contact family to help convince patient.
- [ ] Call law enforcement who may be able to order or "arrest" serious patient in order to force patient to go to hospital.
- [ ] Try to determine why patient is refusing care.
- [ ] Complete thorough documentation of refusal, have patient sign refusal release, and have witness sign the release (e.g., bystander, police, family).

NOTE: Procedure may differ by state and jurisdiction. Always follow your medical director's advice.

(reprinted from *Pocket Reference for The EMT-B and First Responder* by Bob Elling, Prentice Hall, 1999)

D.O.T. OBJECTIVES CHECKLIST

Use the following list of knowledge objectives to check what you've learned. Check off only those objectives that you feel you completely understand and have mastered. For any objectives not checked, go back and review that section of the text chapter. Textbook page references have been provided to help you review the text material.

- [ ] List the proper methods of initiating and terminating a radio call. *(p. 324)*
- [ ] State the proper sequence for delivery of patient information. *(p. 328)*
- [ ] Explain the importance of effective communication of patient information in the verbal report. *(p. 328)*
- [ ] Identify the essential components of the verbal report. *(p. 328)*

- [ ] Describe the attributes for increasing effectiveness and efficiency of verbal communications. *(p. 324)*

- [ ] State legal aspects to consider in verbal communication. *(p. 328)*

- [ ] Discuss the communication skills that should be used to interact with the patient. *(p. 329)*

- [ ] Discuss the communication skills that should be used to interact with the family, bystanders, and individuals from other agencies while providing patient care and the difference between skills used to interact with the patient and those used to interact with others. *(p. 329)*

- [ ] List the correct radio procedures in the following phases of a typical call:

  - [ ] To the scene
  - [ ] At the scene
  - [ ] To the facility
  - [ ] At the facility
  - [ ] To the station
  - [ ] At the station *(p. 326)*

- [ ] Explain the components of the written report and list the information that should be included in the written report. *(p. 331)*

- [ ] Identify the various sections of the written report. *(p. 334)*

- [ ] Describe what information is required in each section of the prehospital care report and how it should be entered. *(p. 334)*

- [ ] Define the special considerations concerning patient refusal. *(p. 339)*

- [ ] Describe the legal implications associated with the written report. *(p. 337)*

- [ ] Discuss all state and/or local record and reporting requirements. *(p. 331)*

CHAPTER 11

General Pharmacology

CHAPTER 11 SUMMARY

An EMT-Basic can administer certain medications and assist patients to self-administer others. Most EMT-Basic services carry oxygen, instant glucose, and activated charcoal. You may also be directed to assist a patient in taking his or her own nitroglycerin, epinephrine, or prescribed inhaler. Always consult medical direction before giving these drugs.

Some medications are known by several different names. Always read label information carefully to avoid medication errors. If you are not sure, ask medical control to help you understand exactly what form of what medication you are looking at.

Before administering any drug, you must be familiar with the indications, contraindications, form, dose, administration, action, and side effects.

After administering a medication, monitor the patient's response. Document any improvements, deteriorations, or side effects on the PCR and reassess the patient's vital signs.

REVIEW QUESTIONS

Please circle the best answer for each question.

1. Only EMT-Intermediates and EMT-Paramedics may administer prescription medications.
   A) True **B)** False
   [Reference text page 350]

2. The EMT-Basic may administer oral glucose at his or her own discretion.
   A) True **B)** False
   [Reference text page 351]

3. The term "sublingual" refers to the ________ of a medication.
   A) dosage **B)** indications **C)** prescription **D)** administration
   [Reference text page 354]

4. An EMT-Basic may assist a patient with which injectable liquid?
   A) Epinephrine **B)** Glucose
   C) Albuterol **D)** Metaproterenol
   [Reference text page 351]

5. What type of emergencies may require the EMT-Basic to administer activated charcoal?
   A) Overdose **B)** Respiratory arrest
   C) Shock **D)** Allergic reaction
   [Reference text page 351]

6. Oral glucose is most commonly administered in what form?
   A) fine powder **B)** tablet **C)** gel **D)** liquid
   [Reference text page 351]

7. An example of a gas that can be administered by an EMT-Basic is:
   A) oxygen. **B)** nitroglycerin.
   C) hydrogen peroxide. **D)** albuterol.
   [Reference text page 351]

8. Which term indicates that administration of a medication may be harmful?
   A) Contraindication **B)** Complication
   C) Contradiction **D)** Therapeutic
   [Reference text pages 353-54]

9. Which of the following medications is typically administered sublingually?
   A) Oxygen **B)** Epinephrine
   C) Nitroglycerin **D)** Activated charcoal
   [Reference text pages 353-54]

10. The indications for a specific drug's use refer to:
A) A. the specific illness, signs or symptoms the drug is designed to treat
B) when not to administer the drug.
C) the most effective route of administration for the drug.
D) the allergic reactions a drug may produce.
[Reference text page 353]

11. Therapeutic effect is best achieved when a medication is administered:
A) by injection in the proper dosage.
B) by the most qualified professional.
C) in the proper dosage.
D) to an adult patient.
[Reference text page 354]

12. The side effect produced by a medication is called a/n:
A) contraindication.
B) complication.
C) indication.
D) condition.
[Reference text page 354]

13. The dosage of a medication refers to:
A) how much of the drug to give.
B) how the patient should receive the drug.
C) when to use the drug.
D) how the drug affects the body.
[Reference text page 354]

14. The actions of a medication refer to:
A) how the drug affects the body.
B) how the patient should receive the drug.
C) when to use the drug.
D) how much of the drug to give.
[Reference text pages 353-54]

15. When an EMT-Basic assists a patient with the administration of a patient's medication, the EMT-Basic's best source of information about the drug can be obtained from the:
A) patient's Do Not Resuscitate form.
B) EMS agency's standing orders.
C) what the patient or family tells the EMT-Basic.
D) staff at the supervising hospital.
[Reference text page 355]

16. After administering any medication to a patient, the EMT-Basic should:
A) ask the patient if it belongs to him or her.
B) check the label to make sure the medication has not expired.
C) check with the supervising hospital to verify any standing orders.
D) reassess the patient to see how he or she responded.
[Reference text page 355]

17. Which of the following medications are generally outside the scope of the EMT-Basic?
A) Atropine **B)** Oxygen
C) Oral glucose **D)** Activated charcoal
[Reference text page 351]

18. Written orders from the Medical Director authorizing medical treatment are known as:
A) directives. **B)** standing orders. **C)** prescriptions. **D)** policies.
[Reference text pages 26, 351]

19. Medications may have several names. Which is listed in the publication *U. S. Pharmacopoeia* (USP)?
A) Brand name **B)** Trade name **C)** Generic name **D)** Popular name
[Reference text page 352]

20. Which medication is carried on all basic ambulances?
A) Morphine **B)** Oxygen **C)** Epinephrine **D)** Nitroglycerin
[Reference text page 351]

21. The trade name of a medication refers to the:
A) name listed in the *U.S. Pharmacopoeia.*
B) name used during drug development.
C) compound's chemical makeup.
D) brand name assigned by the manufacturer.
[Reference text page 352]

22. A device that vaporizes liquids in a fixed dose is a/an:
A) nebulizer. **B)** inhaler. **C)** suspender. **D)** dispenser.
[Reference text page 353]

23. A drug's indication refers to the:
A) situations in which the medication would be harmful if administered.
B) amount of drug that is administered to achieve a therapeutic effect.
C) therapeutic effect of the medication on a patient's body or systems.
D) use of the medication for specific illnesses, signs, or symptoms.
[Reference text page 353]

24. Which of the following is not one of the "rights of medication administration"?
A) Right patient **B)** Right route
C) Right indication **D)** Right time
[Reference text page 354]

25. When a patient gets a headache after taking nitroglycerin, this is called a normal side effect of the medication.
A) True **B)** False
[Reference text page 353]

CASE STUDIES

Use a separate piece of paper to answer the case study questions. Number your answers with the case study number and question letter (1A, 1B, etc.).

GENERAL PHARMACOLOGY

1. You are on the scene with an elderly man who was complaining of chest pain. You have completed your assessment and determined that you should assist the patient in taking nitroglycerin tablets. Medical control has given its approval.
A) What questions should the EMT-Basic ask the patient immediately before administering any medication?
B) What "rights" should you check before administering any medication?

2. You are on the scene with a teenaged female who has taken an overdose. You have completed your assessment and determined that you should contact medical control for permission to administer activated charcoal to the patient. Since the patient's mental status is verbal and there is a good gag reflex, medical control has given its approval.
A) In what form does this medication come?
B) What is the route of administration for this medication?
C) What is the term used for situations in which this drug should not be used?

KEY TERMS MATCHING

Assess your knowledge of the chapter key terms by matching the terms on the left to the definitions on the right.

_____ 1. Action
_____ 2. Contraindication (KON-trah-in-duh-KAY-shun)
_____ 3. Dosage
_____ 4. Generic Name
_____ 5. Indication
_____ 6. Metered Dose Inhaler (MDI)
_____ 7. Nebulizer
_____ 8. Route of Administration
_____ 9. Side Effect
_____ 10. Trade Name

(A) Hand-held inhalation device for delivering liquid or powdered medication in premeasured doses
(B) Unwanted effect of a medication
(C) Pathway by which a medication is administered: sublingual, oral ingestion, injection, inhalation, etc.
(D) Device for administering vaporized liquid medication
(E) Manufacturer's brand name for a medication
(F) A sign, symptom, or condition for which a specific medication or treatment is given
(G) The desired effect of a medication or treatment
(H) Appropriate amount of a medication to administer; also dose
(I) Condition under which a specific medication or treatment should not be given
(J) Official common name of a medication

D.O.T. OBJECTIVES CHECKLIST

Use the following list of knowledge objectives to check what you've learned. Check off only those objectives that you feel you completely understand and have mastered. For any objectives not checked, go back and review that section of the text chapter. Textbook page references have been provided to help you review the text material.

☐ Identify which medications will be carried on the unit. *(p. 350)*

☐ State the medications carried on the unit by the generic name. *(p. 350)*

☐ Identify the medications with which the EMT-Basic may assist the patient with administering. *(p. 351)*

☐ State the medications the EMT-Basic can assist the patient with by the generic name. *(p. 351)*

☐ Discuss the forms in which the medications may be found. *(p. 353)*

CHAPTER 12

Respiratory Emergencies

CHAPTER 12 SUMMARY

Difficulty breathing is the chief complaint in many calls. Assessing the patient's breathing is very important. Look for signs of inadequate respiration. If breathing is inadequate, begin assisting ventilations immediately. If breathing is adequate, provide high-flow oxygen by non-rebreather mask.

Use the OPQRST questions to elaborate on the patient's chief complaint. Consider assisted administration of an inhaler if the patient has one and if no contraindications exist. Always consult with medical direction before assisting with an inhaler.

The use of handheld inhalers is a common treatment in children. Emergency care is the same as for adults. Be aware of anatomical differences in the respiratory system between children and adults. Cyanosis is a late sign of a respiratory emergency in a child. Don't wait for it to occur before considering treatment in the field.

REVIEW QUESTIONS

Please circle the best answer for each question.

1. Movement of air from outside the body into and out of the lungs is referred to as:
   A) exhalation. **B)** ventilation. **C)** inhalation. **D)** rescue breathing.
   [Reference text page 364]

2. The larynx is constructed mainly of ________ and muscles.
   A) bones **B)** skin **C)** tendons **D)** cartilage
   [Reference text page 112]

3. During swallowing, the epiglottis is pushed over the top of the larynx, preventing food from entering the respiratory tract.
   A) True **B)** False
   [Reference text page 363]

4. The bronchioles are held open by cartilage rings.
   A) True **B)** False
   [Reference text page 114]

5. The ________ are the functional units of the lungs, where gas exchange takes place.
   A) bronchi **B)** epiglottis **C)** alveoli **D)** bronchioles
   [Reference text pages 115, 363]

6. Each alveolus is covered by a network of ________ for gas exchange between blood and air.
   A) veins **B)** arteries **C)** red blood cells **D)** capillaries
   [Reference text pages 115, 118]

7. To begin inspiration, the air pressure within the lungs is ________ the atmospheric pressure.
   A) greater than **B)** less than
   C) equal to **D)** none of the above
   [Reference text page 117]

8. When the diaphragm expands and contracts, the thoracic cavity:
   A) becomes larger. **B)** becomes smaller.
   C) collapses. **D)** stays the same.
   [Reference text page 363]

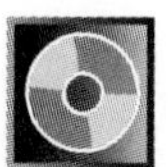

CD-ROM LINK: *Review the* Assessment of Breathing *video for the signs and symptoms of breathing difficulty in Chaper 12 of the MedEMT CD-ROM.*

9. A person in severe respiratory distress may show:
A) minimal chest wall movement. **B)** nasal flaring.
C) use of accessory muscles. **D)** all of the above.
[Reference text page 366]

10. Breathing by using the accessory muscles would generally be considered to be:
A) adequate. **B)** inadequate. **C)** unnecessary. **D)** none of the above.
[Reference text page 366]

11. Which of the following indicate a partial upper airway obstruction?
A) Stridor **B)** Crowing **C)** Snoring **D)** All of the above
[Reference text pages 366, 368, 795]

12. Which of the following are signs that a patient is in severe respiratory distress?
A) Use of accessory muscles **B)** The tripod position
C) Cyanosis **D)** All of the above
[Reference text pages 366-67]

13. In a patient who is having difficulty breathing, there is little in common between the patient's position and the degree of respiratory distress.
A) True **B)** False
[Reference text page 367]

14. A spacer device allows for more effective delivery of medication from an inhaler to the bronchioles.
A) True **B)** False
[Reference text page 374]

15. Asthma is a respiratory disease seen in children as well as in adults.
A) True **B)** False
[Reference text page 382]

16. Wheezing is often heard when auscultating the lungs of a patient who is experiencing an asthma attack.
A) True **B)** False
[Reference text page 382]

17. Cigarette smoking is a common cause of COPD.
A) True **B)** False
[Reference text page 383]

18. Because the mouth and nose of a child are ________ than in adults, they are more easily obstructed.
A) longer **B)** smaller **C)** larger **D)** flatter
[Reference text page 375]

19. Since the cartilage in the chest wall is softer, a child or an infant depends more on the ________ for breathing.
A) larynx **B)** bronchioles **C)** diaphragm **D)** alveoli
[Reference text page 376]

20. A child's tongue takes up ________ space in the pharynx compared to an adult's.
A) more **B)** less **C)** the same **D)** no
[Reference text page 375]

21. Signs of pediatric respiratory distress include:
A) retractions. **B)** grunting and head bobbing.
C) seesaw respirations. **D)** all of the above.
[Reference text page 376]

22. A toddler with breathing difficulty will be less agitated or anxious if he or she can sit on a parent's lap while being evaluated and treated.
A) True **B)** False
[Reference text page 377]

23. In children, frequent coughing, rather than wheezing, can be a sign of bronchospasm.
A) True **B)** False
[Reference text page 376]

24. An acute illness is a condition that lasts a long time, perhaps for life.
A) True **B)** False
[Reference text page 362]

25. Exchange of oxygen and carbon dioxide between the lungs and blood, which occurs in the alveoli, is called:
A) diffusion. **B)** ventilation.
C) cellular exchange. **D)** none of the above.
[Reference text page 364]

26. A generic term for emphysema is:
A) asthma. **B)** COPD.
C) bronchitis. **D)** none of the above.
[Reference text pages 364, 382]

27. A patient in the ________ position is trying to maximize respiratory effort by sitting, leaning forward with hands on the knees.
A) supine **B)** tripod **C)** Fowler's **D)** Trendelenburg
[Reference text page 367]

28. If your patient is having breathing difficulty, you should make an immediate transportation decision if he or she has:
A) an elevated pulse. **B)** pale color.
C) difficulty speaking. **D)** a slow pulse.
[Reference text page 369]

29. Albuterol, isoetharine, and terbutaline are examples of medications designed to cause:
A) bronchodilation. **B)** a faster pulse.
C) a lower BP. **D)** nausea.
[Reference text pages 372-73]

30. A device that delivers a controlled dose of finely powdered, aerosolized medication is called:
A) a non-rebreather mask. **B)** a Venturi mask.
C) an MDI. **D)** none of the above.
[Reference text page 372]

31. Albuterol is administered if the patient has:
A) signs and symptoms of respiratory distress.
B) a physician prescribed handheld inhaler.
C) medical control permission for the EMT-Basic to administer.
D) all of the above.
[Reference text page 372]

32. A complete lack of respiratory drive or pulmonary function is called:
A) respiratory failure. **B)** respiratory arrest.
C) respiratory distress. **D)** none of the above.
[Reference text page 375]

33. A time when the respiratory system cannot deliver an adequate supply of oxygen to meet the body's current demand is called:
A) respiratory failure. **B)** respiratory arrest.
C) respiratory distress. **D)** none of the above.
[Reference text page 375]

34. Difficult breathing involving an increased effort to breathe due to impaired respiratory function is called:
A) respiratory failure. **B)** respiratory arrest.
C) respiratory distress. **D)** none of the above.
[Reference text page 375]

35. A patient with a chronic cough and dyspnea who has gotten considerably worse in the last few days probably has:
A) an airway obstruction.
B) an infection.
C) a pulmonary embolism.
D) all of the above.
[Reference text page 383]

CASE STUDIES

Use a separate piece of paper to answer the case study questions. Number your answers with the case study number and question letter (1A, 1B, etc.).

1. Alarms wake you from a deep sleep. Your first day back has been especially busy. Dispatch advises you of a patient at a local bar who is having difficulty breathing. As you enter the bar, you notice a few patrons gathered in the far back. The owner tells you that the patient is one of his regular customers. He further states that the woman had been drinking all evening when she suddenly started complaining of chest pain and shortness of breath. The elderly female is anxious, pale, and unable to speak in full sentences. She has a cigarette in her hand and every few seconds takes a long drag. You also notice an inhaler sitting right next to her cigarette case.
A) What elements of the patient history become important when deciding whether to assist a patient in administering a medication?
B) During the assessment of the patient, you find that the patient has already used her inhaler four times over the past five minutes. What side effects might you note during the assessment?
C) Would you, as an EMT-Basic, consider assisting the patient with the administration of additional inhaler doses? What other treatments are indicated? Justify your answer.
D) What are the signs of inadequate breathing?
E) What are the signs of adequate breathing?

2. Several family members are gathered on the front lawn of the address dispatch posted. Many of the adults are holding each other and crying. You and your partner are guided to a 74-year-old female in slight respiratory distress. The family says this level of distress and cyanosis is normal. The family called 911 to have her transported to a hospice center. Her condition has been deteriorating over the last several months. The female patient is sitting upright in her bed, and she is slightly cyanotic about the fingertips. The patient can speak in five-to-six-word sentences. The family members advise you that the patient has a long history of chronic obstructive airway disease and lung cancer. You also are handed a "partial no-code" document signed by the patient.
A) What types of interventions would you expect to find in the patient's home?
B) Your initial assessment reveals no life-threatening conditions. Your focused history and physical exam is limited because the patient has no specific complaints. Vital signs are within tolerable limits, with slightly elevated pulse and respiratory rates. Are any interventions necessary during transport?
C) How would you address the psychological needs of this patient and family?

3. You have been dispatched to the local day care center. As you and your partner respond, the dispatcher relays that a young child was found unresponsive in his crib. Day care workers are beginning airway maneuvers and checking for a pulse. As you arrive on scene, the 6-month-old boy is attempting to cough and gag. He is unable to make sound and is in significant distress. The staff tells you they found crayons in his crib that look like they have been chewed.
   A) Why are children and infants especially prone to airway obstructions?
   B) What procedures would you follow for this child?
   C) When would you begin transport?

4. You respond to a call for a 23-year-old female who is anxious and in obvious respiratory distress. She states that she has had asthma since childhood and is not clear what set her off today. She states that her chest feels very tight.
   A) What sounds would you expect to hear when listening to her lungs?
   B) What types of medications would you expect to see in the patient's home?
   C) Prior to calling for medical control permission to assist the patient with an MDI, what should you ask her?

KEY TERMS MATCHING

Assess your knowledge of the chapter key terms by matching the terms on the left to the definitions on the right.

	Term	Definition
______	**1.** Acute Illness	**(A)** Position that helps keep the airway open and maximizes respiratory effort: sitting, leaning forward with hands on the knees
______	**2.** Asthma (AZ-muh)	**(B)** Long-term illness
______	**3.** Bronchoconstriction	**(C)** Difficulty breathing; increased effort necessary to breathe due to impaired respiratory function
______	**4.** Bronchodilator	**(D)** A complete lack of respiratory drive or pulmonary function
______	**5.** Chronic Illness	**(E)** Generic term for emphysema, chronic bronchitis, and other obstructive airway diseases
______	**6.** Chronic Obstructive Pulmonary Disease (COPD)	**(F)** When the respiratory system cannot deliver an adequate supply of oxygen to meet the body's current demand
______	**7.** Respiratory Arrest	**(G)** Reactive airway disease caused by spasmodic contraction of the bronchi; characterized by recurrent attacks of dyspnea, coughing, and wheezing
______	**8.** Respiratory Distress	**(H)** Narrowing of the air passageways due to constriction of the smooth muscle of the bronchi and bronchioles
______	**9.** Respiratory Failure	**(I)** Drug that relaxes the smooth muscle of the bronchi and bronchioles, reversing bronchoconstriction
______	**10.** Tripod Position	**(J)** Illness with a severe, rapid onset

LABELING DIAGRAM

Fill in other causes of shortness of breath in the diagram below.
[Reference text page 362]

CAUSES OF SHORTNESS OF BREATH

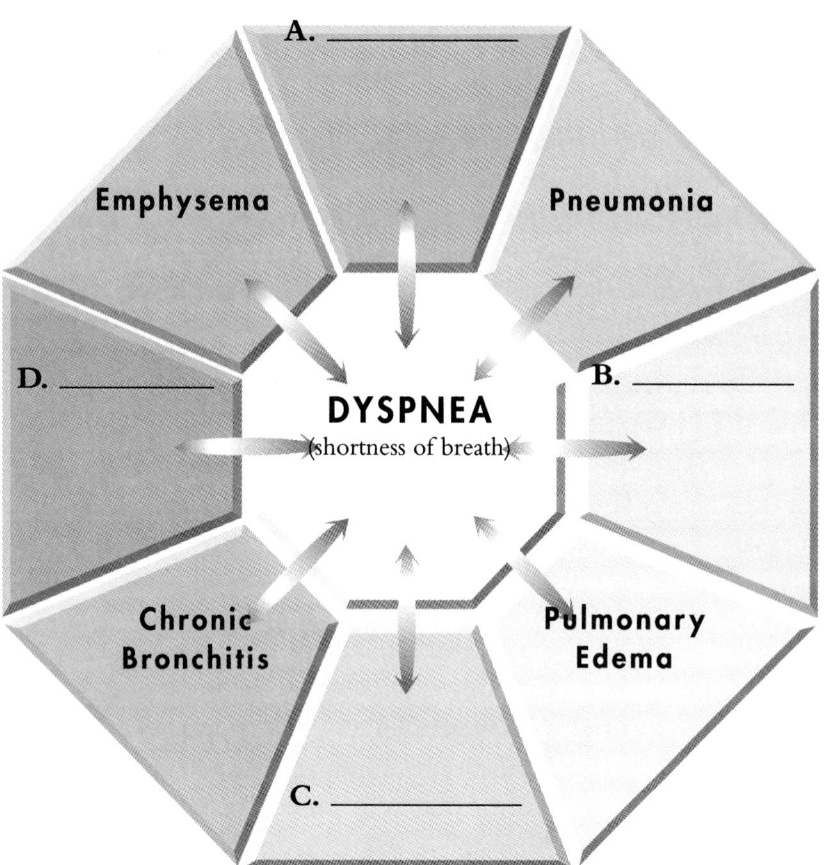

SKILLS CHECKLISTS

Check your knowledge of important EMT-B skills by marking off each step in the following skills sheets.

USING THE PULSE OXIMETER

- [ ] Review the instruction manual for the specific unit you are using.
- [ ] Properly assemble finger-clip sensor and extension to pulse oximeter.
- [ ] Properly affix finger-clip sensor to index finger. (It may be necessary to quickly remove patient's fingernail polish.)

- [ ] Turn on pulse oximeter, and record heart and oxygen readings. Spot-check mode and extended mode (30 minutes).
- [ ] When done using oximeter, shut off the unit. After each use, disassemble and store wiring and accessories in pouch provided.
- [ ] Review operation of all display indicators, pulse amplitude, low battery, pulse search, oxygen saturation, and pulse rate.
- [ ] Review all controls (i.e., measure button, battery check button, printer on/off, printer paper advance).
- [ ] Change battery and paper printout if needed.

ADMINISTRATION OF A HANDHELD METERED DOSE INHALER

- [ ] Obtain order from medical direction, either on-line or off-line.
- [ ] Assure right patient, right medication, right dose, right route, and patient alert enough to use inhaler.
- [ ] Check expiration date of inhaler.
- [ ] Check if patient has already taken any doses.
- [ ] Assure inhaler is at room temperature or warmer.
- [ ] Shake inhaler vigorously several times.
- [ ] Have patient exhale deeply.
- [ ] Have patient put lips around opening of inhaler.
- [ ] Have patient depress the handheld inhaler as he or she begins to inhale deeply.
- [ ] Instruct patient to hold breath for as long as comfortable so medication can be absorbed.
- [ ] Put oxygen back on patient.
- [ ] Allow patient to breathe a few times, and repeat second dose if so ordered by medical direction.
- [ ] If patient has a spacer device for inhaler, it should be used.

(reprinted from *Pocket Reference for The EMT-B and First Responder* by Bob Elling, Prentice Hall, 1999)

D.O.T. OBJECTIVES CHECKLIST

Use the following list of knowledge objectives to check what you've learned. Check off only those objectives that you feel you completely understand and have mastered. For any objectives not checked, go back and review that section of the text chapter. Textbook page references have been provided to help you review the text material.

☐ List the structure and function of the respiratory system. *(p. 363)*

☐ State the signs and symptoms of a patient with breathing difficulty. *(p. 366)*

☐ Describe the emergency medical care of the patient with breathing difficulty. *(p. 364)*

☐ Recognize the need for medical direction to assist in the emergency medical care of the patient with breathing difficulty. *(p. 369)*

☐ Describe the emergency medical care of the patient with breathing distress. *(p. 364)*

☐ Establish the relationship between airway management and the patient with breathing difficulty. *(p. 364)*

☐ List signs of adequate air exchange. *(p. 363)*

☐ State the generic name, medication forms, dose, administration, action, indications, and contraindications for the prescribed inhaler. *(p. 372)*

☐ Distinguish between the emergency medical care of the infant, child, and adult patient with breathing difficulty. *(p. 374)*

☐ Differentiate between upper airway obstruction and lower airway disease in the infant and child patient. *(p. 688)*

CHAPTER 13

Cardiovascular Emergencies

CHAPTER 13 SUMMARY

You will respond to many calls for "a possible heart attack" or "a patient with chest pain." Some will be episodes of sudden cardiac arrest, while others may be simple indigestion. You should not focus on the underlying cause of the pain or difficulty. Simply treat every patient with the signs and symptoms of cardiac compromise as if the condition is actually life threatening. Most chest pain patients do not become cardiac arrest patients.

Always supply oxygen to patients with signs and symptoms of cardiac compromise. If the patient's breathing is adequate, use high-flow oxygen by non-rebreather mask. If breathing is inadequate, assist ventilations and provide supplemental oxygen.

Ask OPQRST questions to elaborate on the conscious patient's chief complaint of "chest pain." If time allows, obtain information from bystanders or family members for an unresponsive patient.

Consider assisting administration of nitroglycerin if a conscious patient has physician-prescribed nitroglycerin spray or tablets. Make sure no contraindications exist and the medication is actually the patient's. Consult with medical control before assisting the patient in taking this drug. Nitroglycerin dilates the coronary arteries, allowing more oxygenated blood to reach the heart muscle. This can cause a headache and a drop in the patient's blood pressure. Never administer nitroglycerin to a patient with a systolic blood pressure below 100 mmHg or to a child. Follow local protocols where they exist.

The AED is indicated in pulseless, apneic patients who are over the age of 12 and weigh more than 90 pounds. For cardiac arrest patients less than 12 years old or 90 pounds, do CPR and transport. Never apply an AED to a patient with a pulse.

In cardiac arrest patients, apply the AED as quickly as possible and defibrillate if indicated by the AED. Begin transport of the cardiac arrest patient after 6 shocks have been administered, 3 "No Shock Advised" messages have been received, or the patient regains a pulse. Again, follow local protocols if they exist.

REVIEW QUESTIONS

Please circle the best answer for each question.

1. The arteries that feed the highest percentage of oxygen to the heart are called:
   A) cardiac veins. **B)** major vessels.
   C) coronary arteries. **D)** cardiac arteries.
   [Reference text pages 124, 388]

2. Red blood cells carry:
   A) oxygen and carbon dioxide. **B)** antibodies.
   C) the clotting factor. **D)** nutrients.
   [Reference text pages 124, 387]

3. Nitroglycerin is taken for the treatment of:
   A) angina (also called chest pain). **B)** anxiety.
   C) emotional stress. **D)** unresponsiveness.
   [Reference text pages 389, 391]

4. Which of the following is NOT a side effect of nitroglycerin?
   A) Hypotension **B)** Headache
   C) Pulse rate changes **D)** Euphoria
   [Reference text page 393]

5. Why is it necessary to use BSI precautions when assisting a patient with nitroglycerin?
   A) The possibility of absorption into the assisting EMT-Basic's body
   B) The possibility of giving too much of the medication
   C) The possibility of losing the medication
   D) The possibility of altering the strength of the medication through absorption or loss
   [Reference text page 392]

6. What is the lowest systolic blood pressure recommended for the administration of nitroglycerin?
   A) 90 mmHg **B)** 100 mmHg **C)** 110 mmHg **D)** 120 mmHg
   [Reference text page 393]

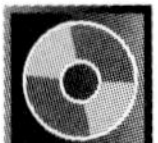

CD-ROM LINK: *Review the* Heart Attack *video in Chapter 13 of the MedEMT CD-ROM.*

7. AED stands for:
   A) Association of Emergency Departments.
   B) Automated External Defibrillator.
   C) Automatic Emergency Dispatch.
   D) Association of Emergency Dispatchers.
   [Reference text page 396]

8. There are two types of automated external defibrillators.
A) True **B)** False
[Reference text page 397]

9. The AED should never be used on a patient who is:
A) unresponsive. **B)** pulseless. **C)** conscious. **D)** apneic.
[Reference text pages 400-401]

10. While one EMT-Basic sets up the AED, his or her partner should:
A) clear the scene. **B)** call for backup.
C) perform adequate CPR. **D)** dress any wounds necessary.
[Reference text page 402]

11. After use of the AED, which of the following is NOT an indication to begin transport?
A) Six shocks have been delivered.
B) The patient's pulse returns.
C) Three consecutive *no shock advised* messages have been received.
D) The patient's pulse becomes irregular.
[Reference text page 402]

12. In emergency medicine, CAD stands for:
A) Coronary Artery Disease. **B)** Computer Aided Defibrillation.
C) Cardiac Angina Discomfort. **D)** Cerebral Artery Disease.
[Reference text page 389]

CD-ROM LINK: *Review the* Automated External Defibrillator *video in Chapter 13 of the MedEMT CD-ROM.*

13. After successful conversion of the patient using the AED, the EMT-Basic's first priority is to:
A) begin rapid transport.
B) give nitroglycerin.
C) place the patient in the rescue position.
D) maintain the patient's airway.
[Reference text page 404]

14. Cell fragments necessary for blood clotting are called:
A) plasma. **B)** platelets.
C) white blood cells. **D)** red blood cells.
[Reference text page 387]

15. The only artery that carries oxygen-poor blood in an adult is the ________ artery.
A) femoral **B)** coronary **C)** pulmonary **D)** aorta
[Reference text page 124]

16. What is the basic composition of blood?
A) Plasma and cells
B) Red and white cells
C) Lymph cells and plasma
D) None of the above
[Reference text page 387]

17. Approximately ________ people died in 1997 because of cardiovascular diseases.
A) 150,000
B) 300,000
C) 400,000
D) 700,000
[Reference text page 386]

18. The blood cells involved in fighting infection are the:
A) lymph cells.
B) white cells.
C) red cells.
D) platelets.
[Reference text page 387]

19. Of the following signs and symptoms, which is NOT characteristic of shock?
A) Delayed capillary refill in children
B) Pale, cyanotic, clammy skin
C) Fast, strong pulse
D) Restlessness
[Reference text page 388]

20. Signs and symptoms of cardiac compromise include:
A) pale, clammy skin.
B) nausea and/or vomiting.
C) abnormal or irregular pulse.
D) all of the above.
[Reference text page 389]

21. A random disorganized electrical activity of the heart is called ventricular fibrillation.
A) True
B) False
[Reference text page 389]

22. Which of the following is NOT a symptom or sign of cardiac compromise?
A) Dyspnea
B) Lower back pain
C) Sudden onset of profuse sweating
D) Nausea or vomiting
[Reference text page 389]

23. Severe pain and constriction about the heart is called:
A) a dysrhythmia.
B) acute myocardial infarction.
C) angina pectoris.
D) coronary artery disease.
[Reference text page 389]

24. Causes of chest pain include:
A) lung disease.
B) musculoskeletal disorders.
C) anxiety.
D) all of the above.
[Reference text page 390]

25. Side effects of nitroglycerin include all of the following EXCEPT:
A) hypotension. **B)** hypothermia. **C)** headache. **D)** pulse rate changes.
[Reference text page 393]

26. The links in the chain of survival include each of the following EXCEPT early:
A) access to the EMS system. **B)** CPR.
C) defibrillation. **D)** fluid therapy.
[Reference text page 395]

27. It is imperative that the EMT-Basic always carry spare batteries with an AED.
A) True **B)** False
[Reference text page 399]

28. When the AED is used on a call, the post-call QI should address:
A) timeliness of the care. **B)** actions of the EMT-Basics.
C) performance of the machine. **D)** all of the above.
[Reference text page 406]

29. If the patient is soaking wet because he or she was just pulled out of a pool, the EMT-Basic should dry off the patient prior to using the AED.
A) True **B)** False
[Reference text page 400]

30. Within ________ minutes of nitroglycerin administration, the EMT-Basic should recheck the patient's BP.
A) 2 **B)** 5 **C)** 10 **D)** 15
[Reference text page 393]

CASE STUDIES

Use a separate piece of paper to answer the case study questions. Number your answers with the case study number and question letter (1A, 1B, etc.).

1. It is a Friday evening, and you are called to a high school football stadium where a 51-year-old, 190-pound man has collapsed while coaching his team in a divisional championship. You arrive to find two football players performing CPR. Your assessment reveals the patient to be unconscious, apneic, and pulseless. You can feel a pulse with a rescuer performing chest compressions.
A) What should your immediate action be?
B) The AED has given you the message *shock advised.* What are your next steps?
C) You have just delivered the third consecutive shock. Describe an appropriate course of action.
D) When is it appropriate to transport a cardiac arrest patient?

2. You are dispatched to a local gym where a 60-year-old, 150-pound man collapsed while working out. You arrive to find a bystander attempting mouth-to-mouth resuscitation. Your assessment reveals the patient to be unconscious, apneic, and pulseless. Your partner begins delivering chest compressions. You attach the AED electrodes, stop CPR, and initiate analysis of the patient's heart rhythm. It advises that a shock should be delivered. You deliver the first and second shocks without difficulty. The AED analyzes the patient's heart rhythm and advises *no shock*.
   A) What should the EMT-Basic do immediately upon receiving a *no shock* message?
   B) The patient has a palpable carotid pulse but is still not breathing. What should you do?

3. You have just transported a patient to the hospital. You are in the back of the ambulance putting away equipment and replacement supplies when you are dispatched to another call. You arrive on scene to find a 77-year-old female who is short of breath. She is reported to have a history of heart problems for which she takes water pills. Assessment reveals she is awake, has labored breathing at a rate of 24 bpm, a bounding pulse with a rate of 126, a blood pressure of 168/102, and cool, sweaty skin. You note the presence of cyanosis about her lips and accessory muscle usage. She has trouble getting the words out but tells you that her breathing difficulty started earlier in the week and does not seem to be relieved by her medicine.
   A) Is assisted administration of nitroglycerin indicated for this patient?
   B) What interventions should you utilize in the care of this patient?
   C) While you are performing your assessment, the patient's husband repeatedly tells you to give her one of his "heart pills" (which you recognize as nitroglycerin). How do you respond to his demand?

4. It is 6:00 A.M. and you just came on duty. Although your partner wants to go for coffee, you insist on first quickly checking the oxygen, the gasoline in the ambulance, and the AED. This was a lesson you had learned the hard way a few months ago. Every day when you check out the AED, you use a checklist that has a few very important items on it to review prior to using the device each day.
   A) If there was to be a failure of the AED on a call, what would be the most probable cause of the failure?
   B) How can you prevent AED failures in the field?

5. There are four links in the AHA chain of survival. Breaking any one of the links can lead to a failed resuscitation in the field. In your community, the EMS agency has decided to help strengthen the chain.
   A) What are the four links in the chain?
   B) How can the first link be strengthened?
   C) How can the second link be strengthened?
   D) How can the third link be strengthened?

KEY TERMS MATCHING

Assess your knowledge of the chapter key terms by matching the terms on the left to the definitions on the right.

_____ 1. Acute Myocardial (my-oh-KAR-de-ul) Infarction (AMI)

_____ 2. Angina Pectoris (an-JI-nah pek-TOR-is)

_____ 3. Automated External Defibrillator (AED)

_____ 4. Cardiac Compromise

_____ 5. Chain of Survival

_____ 6. Coronary Artery Disease (CAD)

_____ 7. Defibrillation

_____ 8. Dysrhythmia (dis-RITH-me-uh)

_____ 9. Nitroglycerin (NTG)

_____ 10. Ventricular Fibrillation (VF) (ven-TRIK-yu-ler fi-bri-LAY-shun)

(A) Rapid, uncoordinated movements of the ventricle walls that replace the normal contraction; treated with defibrillation methods

(B) Medication that dilates blood vessels and decreases the workload of the heart; taken sublingually by tablet or by spray for relief of chest pain

(C) Term used for the four interventions that provide the best chance for successful resuscitation of a patient in cardiac arrest: early access, early CPR, early defibrillation, early ACLS

(D) Condition of plaque accumulation causing narrowing within coronary artery walls; leads to decreased oxygen delivery to heart muscle

(E) Defibrillation equipment designed to analyze, shock, and reanalyze cardiac dysfunction after applying electrodes to patient

(F) Any action or factor that reduces the functionality of the cardiac system

(G) A disturbance in heart rate and/or rhythm; formerly called arrhythmia

(H) Severe pain and constriction about the heart; also called angina or myocardial ischemia; often treated with nitroglycerin

(I) Electrical shock or current delivered to the heart through the patient's chest wall to help the heart restore a normal rhythm

(J) Sudden cardiac muscle death or injury due to lack of oxygen; a heart attack

LABELING DIAGRAMS

For the two diagrams that follow, fill in the correct answers in the blanks provided.

STRUCTURES OF THE CARDIOVASCULAR SYSTEM

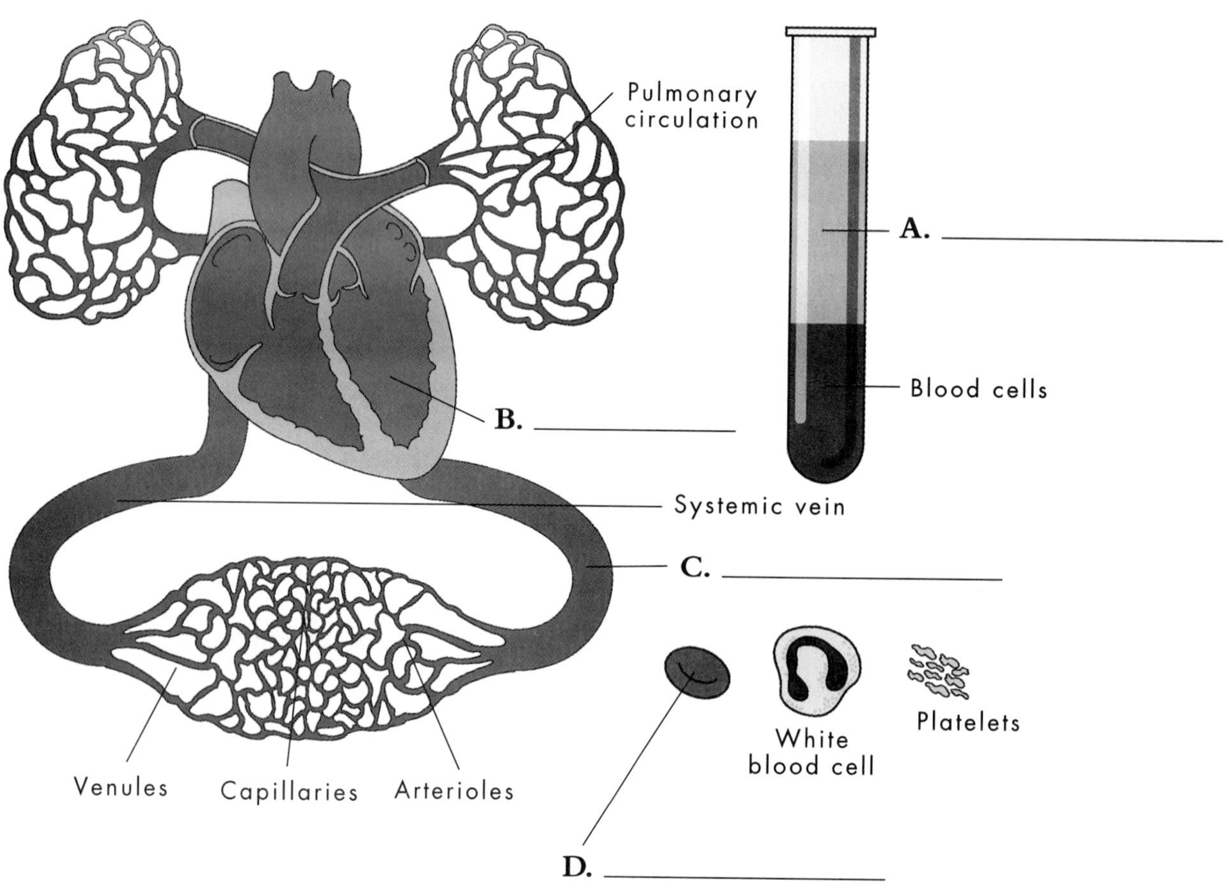

STEPS IN USING THE AED, TWO OR MORE RESCUERS, PULSELESS PATIENT

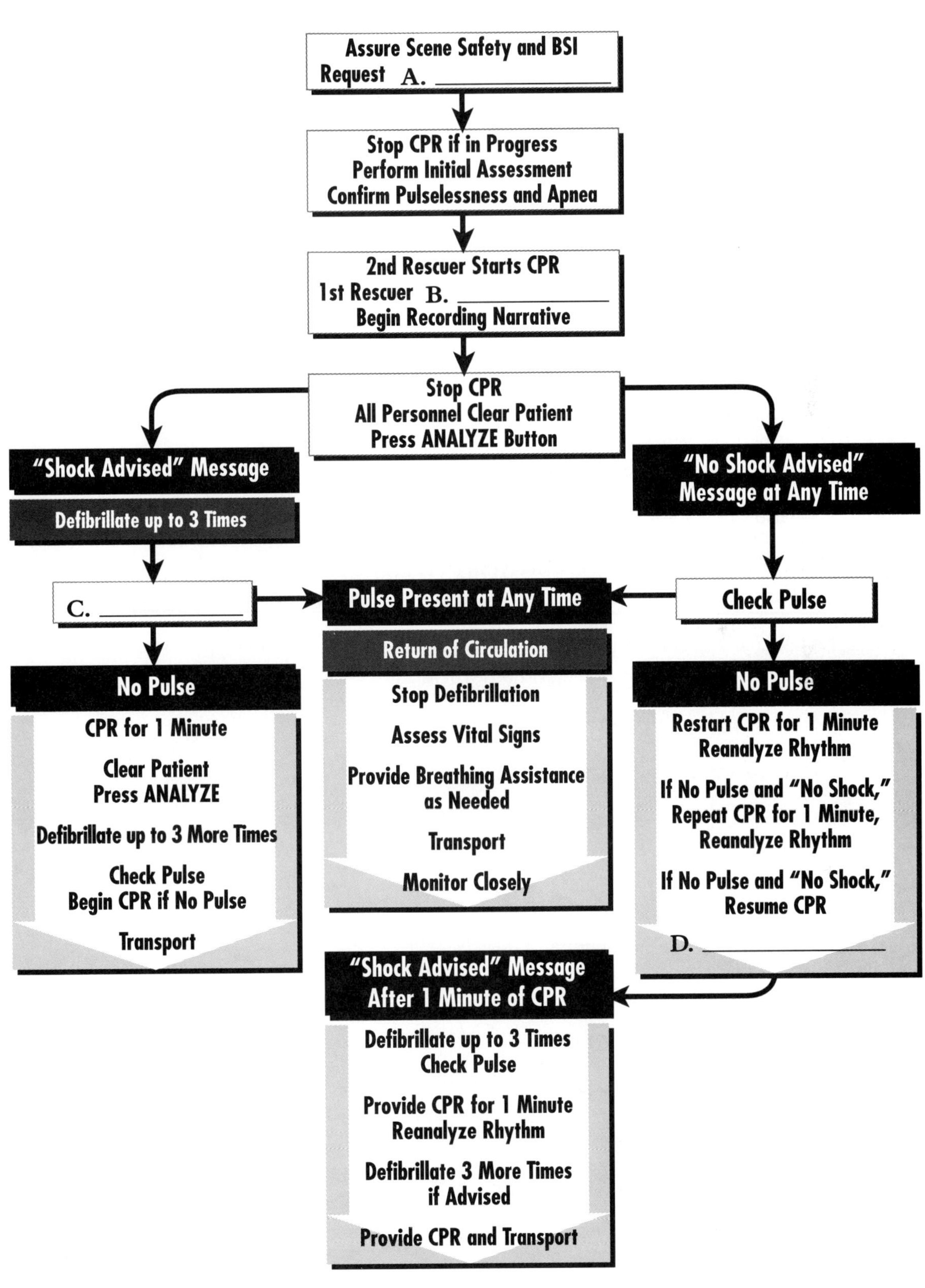

SKILLS CHECKLISTS

Check your knowledge of important EMT-B skills by marking off each step in the following skills sheets.

ADMINISTRATION OF NITROGLYCERIN

- [ ] Perform focused assessment for cardiac patient.
- [ ] Take blood pressure. (Systolic pressure must be above 100.)
- [ ] Contact medical direction if no standing orders.
- [ ] Assure right medication, right patient, right dose, right route.
- [ ] Check expiration date.
- [ ] Assure patient is alert.
- [ ] Question patient on last dose taken and effects.
- [ ] Assure understanding of route of administration.
- [ ] Ask patient to lift tongue. Place tablet or spray dose under it (while wearing gloves), or have patient place tablet or spray under it.
- [ ] Have patient keep mouth closed with tablet under tongue (without swallowing) until dissolved and absorbed.
- [ ] Recheck blood pressure within two minutes.
- [ ] Record administration, route, and time.
- [ ] Perform reassessment.

CHECKING THE AED

Check the AED for the following:

- [ ] Unit, cables, connectors for cleanliness.
- [ ] Supplies carried with AED.
- [ ] Power supply and its operation.
- [ ] Indicators on ECG display.
- [ ] ECG recorder operation.
- [ ] Charge display cycle with a simulator.

- [ ] Pacemaker feature if applicable.
- [ ] File a written report on status of AED.

NOTE: This list is derived from FDA Automated Defibrillator: Operator's Shift Checklist.

CARDIAC ARREST MANAGEMENT AND THE AED

- [ ] Take BSI precautions.
- [ ] Assess patient for breathing and pulses as stated for CPR.
- [ ] If no pulse is present, direct CPR while attaching AED to patient.
- [ ] Direct rescuer to stop CPR.
- [ ] Verify absence of spontaneous pulse.
- [ ] Turn on defibrillator power.
- [ ] Ensure all individuals are standing clear of patient.
- [ ] Initiate analysis of rhythm.
- [ ] Deliver shock (up to three successive shocks).
- [ ] Verify presence or absence of pulse.
- [ ] If pulse is absent, direct resumption of CPR for one minute. During that one minute:
    - [ ] Gather additional information on arrest events.
    - [ ] Confirm effectiveness of CPR (ventilation and compressions).
    - [ ] Direct insertion of an airway adjunct (oro- or nasopharyngeal).
    - [ ] Direct ventilation of patient with high concentration of oxygen.
    - [ ] Assure CPR continues without unnecessary/prolonged interruption.
- [ ] After one minute of CPR, re-evaluate patient.
- [ ] Repeat defibrillator sequence.
- [ ] Check carotid pulse.
- [ ] If there is a spontaneous pulse, check patient's breathing.
- [ ] If breathing is adequate, provide high-concentration oxygen by nonrebreather mask. If breathing is inadequate, ventilate patient with high-concentration oxygen.
- [ ] Transport patient without delay.

(reprinted from *Pocket Reference for The EMT-B and First Responder* by Bob Elling, Prentice Hall, 1999)

D.O.T. OBJECTIVES CHECKLIST

Use the following list of knowledge objectives to check what you've learned. Check off only those objectives that you feel you completely understand and have mastered. For any objectives not checked, go back and review that section of the text chapter. Textbook page references have been provided to help you review the text material.

- [ ] Describe the structure and function of the cardiovascular system. *(p. 386)*
- [ ] Describe the emergency medical care of the patient experiencing chest pain/discomfort. *(p. 390)*
- [ ] List the indications for automated external defibrillation (AED). *(p. 396)*
- [ ] List the contraindications for automated external defibrillation. *(p. 399)*
- [ ] Define the role of the EMT-Basic in the emergency cardiac care system. *(p. 395)*
- [ ] Explain the impact of age and weight on defibrillation. *(p. 399)*
- [ ] Discuss the position of comfort for patients with various cardiac emergencies. *(p. 390)*
- [ ] Establish the relationship between airway management and the patient with cardiovascular compromise. *(p. 390)*
- [ ] Predict the relationship between the patient experiencing cardiovascular compromise and basic life support. *(p. 390)*
- [ ] Discuss the fundamentals of early defibrillation. *(p. 396)*
- [ ] Explain the rationale for early defibrillation. *(p. 396)*
- [ ] Explain that not all chest pain patients result in cardiac arrest and do not need to be attached to an automated external defibrillator. *(p. 389)*
- [ ] Explain the importance of prehospital ACLS intervention if it is available. *(p. 395)*
- [ ] Explain the importance of urgent transport to a facility with Advanced Cardiac Life Support if it is not available in the prehospital setting. *(p. 395)*

- [ ] Discuss the various types of automated external defibrillators. *(p. 397)*
- [ ] Differentiate between the fully automated and the semiautomated defibrillator. *(p. 397)*
- [ ] Discuss the procedures that must be taken into consideration for standard operations of the various types of automated external defibrillators. *(p. 397)*
- [ ] State the reasons for assuring that the patient is pulseless and apneic when using the automated external defibrillator. *(p. 399)*
- [ ] Discuss the circumstances that may result in inappropriate shocks. *(p. 399)*
- [ ] Explain the considerations for interruption of CPR when using the automated external defibrillator. *(p. 399)*
- [ ] Discuss the advantages and disadvantages of automated external defibrillators. *(p. 397)*
- [ ] Summarize the speed of operation of automated external defibrillation. *(p. 397)*
- [ ] Discuss the use of remote defibrillation through adhesive pads. *(p. 397)*
- [ ] Discuss the special considerations for rhythm monitoring. *(p. 399)*
- [ ] List the steps in the operation of the automated external defibrillator. *(p. 401)*
- [ ] Discuss the standard of care that should be used to provide care to a patient with persistent ventricular fibrillation and no available ACLS. *(p. 404)*
- [ ] Discuss the standard of care that should be used to provide care to a patient with recurrent ventricular fibrillation and no available ACLS. *(p. 404)*
- [ ] Differentiate between the single rescuer and multi-rescuer care with an automated external defibrillator. *(p. 404)*
- [ ] Explain the reason for pulses not being checked between shocks with an automated external defibrillator. *(p. 399)*

- [ ] Discuss the importance of coordinating ACLS trained providers with personnel using automated external defibrillators. *(p. 406)*

- [ ] Discuss the importance of post-resuscitation care. *(p. 404)*

- [ ] List the components of post-resuscitation care. *(p. 404)*

- [ ] Explain the importance of frequent practice with the automated external defibrillator. *(p. 405)*

- [ ] Discuss the need to complete the Automated Defibrillator: Operator's Shift Checklist. *(p. 399)*

- [ ] Discuss the role of the American Heart Association (AHA) in the use of automated external defibrillation. *(p. 395)*

- [ ] Explain the role medical direction plays in the use of automated external defibrillation. *(p. 405)*

- [ ] State the reasons why a case review should be completed following the use of the automated external defibrillator. *(p. 405)*

- [ ] Discuss the components that should be included in a case review. *(p. 405)*

- [ ] Discuss the goal of quality improvement in automated external defibrillation. *(p. 405)*

- [ ] Recognize the need for medical direction of protocols to assist in the emergency medical care of the patient with chest pain. *(p. 406)*

- [ ] List the indications for the use of nitroglycerin. *(p. 392)*

- [ ] State the contraindications and side effects for the use of nitroglycerin. *(p. 392)*

- [ ] Define the function of all controls on an automated external defibrillator, and describe event documentation and battery defibrillator maintenance. *(p. 401)*

CHAPTER 14

Neurological, Diabetic, and Behavioral Emergencies

CHAPTER 14 SUMMARY

Altered mental states have many potential causes. The most common reasons for an altered mental state include: failure of the patient to take medications prescribed for specific conditions (e.g.: diabetes, seizures, or mental illness), alcohol abuse, drug abuse, poisoning, trauma (especially patients with head injuries), and hypoxia.

If the patient is a known diabetic, you may not know if the problem is related to high or low blood sugar. Since low blood sugar, or hypoglycemia, can rapidly affect the patient's brain, the EMT-Basic usually presumes the problem is low blood sugar.

Consider the administration of oral glucose for patients with an altered mental state and a history of medication- or diet-controlled diabetes. Before administering this product, assess the patient's ability to swallow and maintain the airway. Contact medical direction for permission to administer the medication.

When treating patients with an altered mental status and no history of diabetes, focus on maintaining the airway. Provide supplemental oxygen and transport immediately. Be prepared to assist ventilations.

The EMT-Basic should treat all seizure activity as potentially life threatening. If a patient is actively seizing, protect him or her from injury.

Behavioral emergencies, like altered mental status, can have many causes. Pay close attention to scene safety in behavioral emergencies. Never allow the patient to block your exit. Many behavioral emergencies involve suicide attempts or an attempt to hurt others. Your demeanor is important when approaching and assessing the patient. Be calm and keep the patient well informed. Provide reassurance that you are there to help. Listen empathetically and acknowledge the patient's feelings.

Know the legal procedure in your area for treating patients against their will. Restrain a patient only as a last resort. Use the least amount of physical force possible. Never restrain a patient unless there are adequate resources to conduct the task without endangering yourself, your crew, or the patient.

REVIEW QUESTIONS

Please circle the best answer for each question.

1. Altered mental status is often a symptom of an underlying illness or injury.
   A) True **B)** False
   [Reference text page 417]

2. A mildly confused patient is not considered to be exhibiting altered mental status.
   A) True **B)** False
   [Reference text page 417]

3. When there is a lack of ________, the patient's blood sugar may climb very high.
   A) insulin **B)** potassium **C)** sodium **D)** glucose
   [Reference text page 419]

4. When the body begins to break down fat rather than glucose as its energy source, this condition is known as:
   A) hypoglycemia. **B)** insulin shock. **C)** a stroke. **D)** DKA.
   [Reference text page 421]

5. A lack of insulin production or use is known as diabetes mellitus.
   A) True **B)** False
   [Reference text page 418]

6. All of the following are causes of hypoglycemia EXCEPT:
   A) excessive blood sugar. **B)** excessive exercise.
   C) too much insulin taken. **D)** insufficient food intake.
   [Reference text page 420]

7. A diabetic patient who presents with a fruity smelling breath and labored respirations most likely has hypoglycemia.
   A) True **B)** False
   [Reference text page 421]

8. Diabetics in distress are sometimes mistakenly identified as:
   A) suffering from myocardial infarction. **B)** intoxicated with alcohol or drugs.
   C) suffering from epilepsy. **D)** suffering from preeclampsia.
   [Reference text page 420]

9. Oral glucose paste should be given to the diabetic patient with an altered mental status because:
   A) it will reverse diabetic coma.
   B) it is rapidly absorbed by large vessels in the mouth.
   C) it will slow down his or her pulse.
   D) all of the above will occur.
   [Reference text page 422]

10. Oral glucose should not be given to an unresponsive patient or a patient who is unable to swallow.
   A) True **B)** False
   [Reference text pages 422-23]

11. During the postictal phase of a seizure, convulsive activity stops and the patient's level of consciousness is depressed.
   A) True **B)** False
   [Reference text page 425]

12. Seizure activity usually last less than ________ minutes.
   A) 5 **B)** 10 **C)** 15 **D)** 20
   [Reference text page 424]

13. A state of prolonged seizures or multiple seizures between which the patient does not regain consciousness is called:
   A) status athmaticus. **B)** grand mal.
   C) petit mal. **D)** status epilepticus.
   [Reference text page 425]

14. Another name for a stroke is a:
   A) heart attack.
   B) syncopal episode.
   C) brain attack.
   D) transient ischemic attack.
   [Reference text page 429]

15. Common causes of a seizure include:
   A) fever. **B)** hypoxia. **C)** poisoning. **D)** all of the above.
   [Reference text page 425]

16. Stroke is usually caused by a blockage of an artery supplying blood to one area of the brain.
   A) True **B)** False
   [Reference text page 429]

17. A transient ischemic attack is a:
A) sudden loss of neuro function that clears up in 24 hours.
B) formation of a blood clot in an artery supplying the brain.
C) rupture of an artery in the brain.
D) seizure activity.
[Reference text page 430]

18. Care of a stroke patient includes all of the following EXCEPT:
A) administering oxygen.
B) ensuring a patent airway.
C) providing a calm and compassionate attitude towards the patient.
D) giving the patient fluid by mouth.
[Reference text pages 430-31]

19. The first treatment priority of an EMT-Basic when confronted with an unconscious patient who may have had a stroke is to:
A) obtain vital signs.
B) administer glucose paste.
C) place the patient on his or her side.
D) secure a patent airway.
[Reference text page 430]

20. Which is most typically characterized by a feeling of helplessness and hopelessness?
A) Anxiety
B) Paranoia
C) Depression
D) Manic-depressive disorder
[Reference text page 432]

21. A patient who has attempted suicide should be restrained.
A) True
B) False
[Reference text page 436]

22. A depressed individual with alcohol and a gun should be considered a suicide risk.
A) True
B) False
[Reference text page 436]

23. You may NOT transport a patient who refuses care.
A) True
B) False
[Reference text page 437]

24. If a legal guardian or legally responsible adult is unavailable to provide consent, you may be allowed to begin lifesaving treatment based on the principle of:
A) implied consent.
B) emancipation.
C) informed consent.
D) required consent.
[Reference text pages 68, 437]

25. A patient having a stroke may also be referred to as having a brain attack.
A) True **B)** False
[Reference text page 429]

26. Signs and symptoms of hyperglycemia include:
A) weak, thready pulse. **B)** low blood sugar.
C) weakness and headache. **D)** all of the above.
[Reference text page 421]

27. A patient presents with excess salivations, twitching of one area of the body, and repetitive speech. This patient probably has:
A) a TIA. **B)** a seizure. **C)** a CVA. **D)** hypoglycemia.
[Reference text page 424]

28. Causes of a seizure include:
A) epilepsy. **B)** hypoxia. **C)** tumor. **D)** all of the above.
[Reference text page 425]

29. If the airway is filled with secretions or vomit that cannot be cleared by suctioning, turn the backboard and the patient together to clear the airway.
A) True **B)** False
[Reference text page 427]

30. A syncopal episode may be preceded by:
A) general weakness. **B)** visual field closing in.
C) lightheadedness. **D)** all of the above.
[Reference text page 428]

31. Which of the following is not a serious cause of syncopy?
A) Fainting spell **B)** Abnormal heart rate
C) Hypovolemia from dehydration **D)** Cardiac pumping failure
[Reference text page 428]

32. A completely irrational fear of people, things, or events is called:
A) phobia. **B)** depression. **C)** bipolar disorder. **D)** schizophrenia.
[Reference text page 432]

33. Behavior characterized by widely exaggerated mistrust or suspiciousness is called:
A) phobia. **B)** schizophrenia. **C)** paranoia. **D)** anxiety.
[Reference text page 432]

34. To attempt to calm a behavioral emergency patient, the EMT-Basic should:
A) focus on physical contact.
B) tell the patient the truth.
C) avoid eye contact.
D) not discuss the patient being upset.
[Reference text page 433]

35. In assessing a patient's risk of violence, watch for:
A) verbal abuse or threats.
B) yelling.
C) clenched fists.
D) all of the above.
[Reference text page 435]

36. General risk factors for suicide include:
A) individuals between 18 and 40 years of age.
B) married persons.
C) recent diagnosis of serious or terminal illness.
D) no history of destructive behavior.
[Reference text pages 435-36]

37. Patients who have tools or materials to complete the plan of action, such as guns, ropes, or large amounts of medications, are high risk for suicide.
A) True
B) False
[Reference text page 436]

38. The amount of force that is reasonable should be determined by:
A) patient's size, strength, and gender.
B) type of abnormal behavior.
C) mental state of patient.
D) all of the above.
[Reference text page 438]

39. A person intent on suicide may have no reservations about taking the lives of others.
A) True
B) False
[Reference text page 435]

40. Extreme levels of agitation, fear, and restlessness may be due to:
A) depression.
B) anxiety or panic.
C) schizophrenia.
D) paranoia.
[Reference text page 432]

CASE STUDIES

Use a separate piece of paper to answer the case study questions. Number your answers with the case study number and question letter (1A, 1B, etc.).

1. As you pull the rescue unit up to the loading dock of a local office building, a supervisor requests that you follow her to a private area in the back of the facility. You find a 22-year-old female lying on a blanket. She is slurring her words and occasionally laughing uncontrollably. The supervisor is aware of Sandra's diabetic condition and had noticed Sandra acting out of character a few hours earlier. Sandra is not responding to questions, and her behavior has remained abnormal despite efforts to "bring her around." Sandra is also wearing a small medical identification necklace that identifies her as an insulin-dependent diabetic.

A) What actions might have allowed Sandra's blood glucose to drop to an unsafe level?
B) Is oral glucose appropriate for Sandra?
C) What are the common signs and symptoms of a patient suffering a diabetic emergency?
D) List the treatment steps for a patient who has a history of diabetes and is currently suffering from an altered mental status.
E) On the way out of the building, the office manager stops your crew. He demands to know what is wrong and implies that he thinks Sandra must have been drinking alcohol on the job. How do you respond to this situation?

2. You've been hired right out of your EMT-Basic program to work at a local theme park as a seasonal EMT-Basic. You and your partner are responsible for responding to all requests for first aid. As the summer warms up, you have been treating a lot of people for heat exhaustion and sunburns. A 19-year-old female has been found lying face down on her towel by the tide pools. Her friends were unable to get her to wake up. These friends admit that she was drinking large amounts of alcohol prior to entering the park.

A) What causes might be behind her altered mental status?
B) What complications could arise from alcohol intoxication?
C) Since you are not involved in the transport of the patient to the hospital, what is your primary focus in treating this patient?

3. You are dispatched to assist a police unit. You arrive on scene to find a concerned officer and a patient who is under arrest. The police officer was on scene for less than three minutes when the person he was arresting began having a full-body seizure. The officer estimates the seizure lasted less than 15 seconds. The patient then became talkative and alert immediately after the seizure. The family claims the patient has a long history of seizures, and she stopped taking her medicine about three weeks ago. Now that the ambulance has arrived, the patient is slow to respond and will not stand up.

A) What might have caused the seizure witnessed by the police officer?
B) Can the EMT-Basic determine whether or not a patient is faking an illness?
C) Describe the postical state found in most patients.

4. The senior center has just finished a weekend craft fair and all the volunteers are exhausted. No one even noticed that Sonna did not return from a trip to the stockroom. After about 20 minutes, the entire group began searching and calling for her. After several minutes of searching, Sonna is found behind an inventory shelf in the back of the stockroom. As you and your partner arrive on scene, you notice that Sonna is conscious and looking around, although she is unable to move or communicate. Your assessment reveals obvious deficits on the left side. Although it appears that she fell, you see no signs of head trauma.

A) Aside from the usual assessments and interventions, what special considerations should you have for stroke patients?
B) What are typical signs and symptoms of a stroke?
C) Describe the emergency medical care you would give Sonna.

5. You are dispatched to a private residence for an overdose. Upon arrival, the 25-year-old female patient is still verbally responsive and tells you she took a full bottle of Tylenol about 20 minutes ago. She has also been drinking all night. She states she wants to kill herself because her life has become hopeless. Apparently she has had a series of broken relationships and the latest breakup, yesterday, was too much for her to handle.
   A) What should be the first priority in treating this patient?
   B) What is the definition of depression?
   C) Once you are assured that her ABCs have been managed, what things should you say to the patient?
   D) What should you NOT do or say to her?

KEY TERMS MATCHING

Assess your knowledge of the chapter key terms by matching the terms on the left to the definitions on the right.

_____ **1.** Altered Mental Status (AMS)

_____ **2.** Behavioral Emergency

_____ **3.** Cerebrovascular (se-REE-bro-VAS-kyu-ler) Accident (CVA)

_____ **4.** Diabetes Mellitus (di-uh-BEE-teez muh-LEE-tus)

_____ **5.** Glucose

_____ **6.** Hyperglycemia (high-per-gly-SEE-me-uh)

_____ **7.** Hypoglycemia (high-po-gly-SEE-me-uh)

_____ **8.** Insulin

(A) A sudden loss of neurological functions that clears up within 24 hours; the symptoms are similar to a CVA; also called a ministroke

(B) Common term for a cerebrovascular accident

(C) Sudden onset of a temporary loss of consciousness caused by low blood pressure in the brain; fainting

(D) A state of prolonged seizures or multiple seizures between which the patient does not regain consciousness

(E) Condition in which blood sugar is too low; results from too much insulin or not enough glucose in the blood

(F) A patient's condition after a seizure, during which the patient may appear sleepy, confused, or unresponsive

(G) Hormone secreted by the pancreas that regulates blood sugar levels

(H) Chaotic electrical activity in the brain that can lead to a momentary break in the stream of thought, muscular spasms, or a complete loss of consciousness

(I) Condition in which blood sugar is too high; results from inadequate insulin in the blood for glucose metabolism

______ **9.** Postictal (post-IK-tul) State

______ **10.** Seizure

______ **11.** Status Epilepticus (STA-tus ep-uh-LEP-ti-kus)

______ **12.** Stroke

______ **13.** Syncope (sin-KO-pee)

______ **14.** Transient Ischemic (is-KEE-mik) Attack (TIA)

(J) A situation in which the patient exhibits behavior that others consider unacceptable or intolerable

(K) A disease characterized by inadequate production or use of insulin

(L) Stroke or brain attack; occurs when a blood vessel in the brain becomes blocked or ruptures

(M) A simple sugar that is the body's basic source of energy

(N) Broad term indicating a change in normal thinking or clarity of thought; behavior may range from mild confusion to complete unresponsiveness

LABELING DIAGRAM

Fill in other causes of altered mental status in the blanks in the diagram below. *[Reference text page 416]*

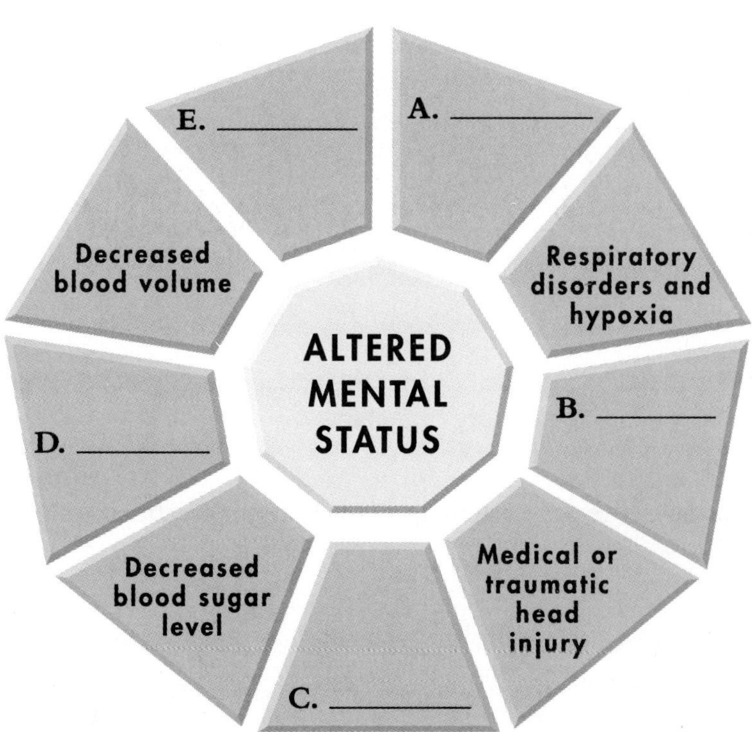

CAUSES OF ALTERED MENTAL STATUS

SKILLS CHECKLIST

Check your knowledge of important EMT-B skills by marking off each step in the following skills sheet.

ADMINISTRATION OF GLUCOSE

- [ ] Assure signs and symptoms of altered mental status with a known history of diabetes.
- [ ] Assure patient is awake with a gag reflex.
- [ ] Administer glucose:
    - [ ] Place on tongue depressor between cheek and gum.
    - [ ] Self-administered between cheek and gum.
    - [ ] Perform ongoing assessment.

(reprinted from Pocket Reference for The EMT-B and First Responder by Bob Elling, Prentice Hall, 1999)

D.O.T. OBJECTIVES CHECKLIST

Use the following list of knowledge objectives to check what you've learned. Check off only those objectives that you feel you completely understand and have mastered. For any objectives not checked, go back and review that section of the text chapter. Textbook page references have been provided to help you review the text material.

- [ ] Identify the patient taking diabetic medications with altered mental status and the implications of a diabetes history *(p. 418)*
- [ ] State the steps in the emergency medical care of the patient taking diabetic medicine with an altered mental status and a history of diabetes. *(p. 421)*
- [ ] Establish the relationship between airway management and the patient with altered mental status. *(p. 417)*
- [ ] State the generic and trade names, medication forms, dose, administration, action, and contraindications for oral glucose. *(p. 422)*

- [ ] Evaluate the need for medical direction in the emergency medical care of the diabetic patient. *(p. 421)*

- [ ] Define behavioral emergencies. *(p. 431)*

- [ ] Discuss the general factors that may cause an alteration in a patient's behavior. *(p. 431)*

- [ ] State the various reasons for psychological crises. *(p. 431)*

- [ ] Discuss the characteristics of an individual's behavior that suggest the patient is at risk for suicide. *(p. 435)*

- [ ] Discuss special medical/legal considerations for managing behavioral emergencies. *(p. 437)*

- [ ] Discuss the special considerations for assessing a patient with behavioral problems. *(p. 434)*

- [ ] Discuss the general principles of an individual's behavior that suggest he or she is at risk for violence. *(p. 435)*

- [ ] Discuss methods to calm behavioral emergency patients. *(p. 433)*

CHAPTER 15

Allergic Reactions

CHAPTER 15 SUMMARY

Allergic reactions are exaggerated responses to common substances. Insect bites/stings, food (e.g., nuts and shellfish), plants, and medicines (e.g., penicillin, codeine, and sulfa drugs) are among the most common causes.

Patients with anaphylaxis may present to the EMT-Basic with or may devevelop aireay and respiratory compromise, and/or shock.

Patients with a known history of severe reactions often carry a physician-prescribed epinephrine auto-injector (EpiPen®). Consider assisting with administration of the drug rapidly if signs and symptoms of shock or respiratory distress develop. Consult medical control before assisting the patient to administer epinephrine. Transport a symptomatic patient with a history of serious reactions immediately if he or she does not have an epinephrine auto-injector. Epinephrine has no contraindications in a life-threatening situation.

REVIEW QUESTIONS

Please circle the best answer for each question.

1. Only a person with a childhood history of allergies is likely to suffer a severe allergic reaction.
   A) True **B)** False
   [Reference text page 449]

2. Severe allergic reactions may be associated with ________ compromise.
   A) heart rate **B)** cardiac **C)** airway **D)** mental status
   [Reference text page 449]

3. A patient having an anaphylactic reaction might experience:
   A) tightness in chest or throat.
   B) decreased blood pressure.
   C) pale, clammy skin.
   D) all of the above.
   [Reference text page 453]

4. Rapid onset of allergic symptoms:
   A) indicates a reaction that will pass quickly.
   B) is often associated with a severe reaction.
   C) can be aggravated by administering oxygen.
   D) should not cause the patient much anxiety.
   [Reference text page 449]

5. The injected drug of choice for severe anaphylactic allergic reactions is:
   A) aspirin. **B)** benadryl. **C)** epinephrine. **D)** lasix.
   [Reference text page 456]

6. Which of the following are central nervous system signs and symptoms of an allergic reaction?
   A) Hallucinations and cyanosis
   B) Increasing mental status and a runny nose
   C) Disorientation and seizures
   D) Ringing in the ears and a cough
   [Reference text page 452]

7. Patients with known allergies sometimes carry a prescribed auto-injector. The medication carried in the auto-injector is:
   A) albuterol. **C)** oral glucose.
   B) oxygen. **D)** epinephrine.
   [Reference text pages 455-56]

8. Which of the following are respiratory signs and symptoms of anaphylactic shock?
A) Pale, clammy skin
B) Wheezing
C) Increased heart rate
D) Decreased mental status
[Reference text page 453]

9. Predicting the exact course of an allergic reaction is difficult.
A) True
B) False
[Reference text page 452]

10. Which of the following is NOT a symptom of anaphylaxis?
A) Itching
B) Difficulty breathing
C) Weak or absent pulse
D) Tightness in the throat or chest
[Reference text page 453]

11. Epinephrine is also called:
A) amorphine.
B) adrenaline.
C) acetocholine.
D) actifed.
[Reference text page 456]

12. When managing the patient having an anaphylactic shock, the EMT-Basic should be prepared to use the AED and CPR.
A) True
B) False
[Reference text page 455]

13. Epinephrine is contraindicated in a child having a severe allergic reaction.
A) True
B) False
[Reference text page 456]

14. The route that epinephrine is most often administered to the patient having a severe allergic reaction is:
A) as a gel in the mouth.
B) sublingual.
C) as an injection into the thigh.
D) as a capsule taken twice a day.
[Reference text page 457]

15. Epinephrine is indicated for:
A) a patient who shows signs and symptoms of a severe allergic reaction.
B) patients who have their own prescribed medication.
C) situations where medical direction has authorized the use for this patient.
D) all of the above.
[Reference text page 456]

16. A single dose of an adult EpiPen® delivers:
A) 0.15 mg.
B) 0.3 mg.
C) 1.5 mg.
D) 3 mg.
[Reference text page 456]

17. The pediatric dose of epinephrine is twice that of the adult's since children are more prone to anaphylaxis.
A) True **B)** False
[Reference text page 456]

18. After administering epinephrine in the field, the EMT-Basic should reevaluate the patient and watch for:
A) decreasing mental status.
B) increasing breathing difficulty.
C) decreasing BP.
D) all of the above.
[Reference text page 457]

19. The drug response of epinephrine lasts for:
A) about 2 hours.
B) about 1 hour.
C) about 20 minutes.
D) the rest of the day.
[Reference text page 456]

20. Some health care providers have developed a sensitivity and allergic reaction to:
A) stainless steel.
B) the air in the back of an ambulance.
C) latex products.
D) epinephrine.
[Reference text page 451]

CASE STUDIES

Use a separate piece of paper to answer the case study questions. Number your answers with the case study number and question letter (1A, 1B, etc.).

ALLERGIC REACTIONS

1. You have been called to a campsite where a 41-year-old female was stung by a bee. According to her husband, she was gathering firewood when she suddenly grasped her leg and screamed. Assessment reveals that she is awake but disoriented, has labored breathing at a rate of 20 breaths per minute, a weak pulse at rate of 130 beats per minute, a blood pressure of 100/74, and flushed skin. You notice that there is facial swelling particularly around the eyes and cyanosis about the lips. You can hear wheezing as the patient breathes. You determine that the patient is allergic to bee stings and has a prescription from her physician for EpiPen®. Examination of the patient's back and posterior arms reveals several large red welts. You note the presence of alcohol on the patient's breath.
A) Explain what medical condition your patient is experiencing.
B) Your emergency treatment for this patient includes:
1. Inserting a nasopharyngeal airway
2. Placing her into a supine position and elevating her legs
3. Contacting medical command to get permission to administer epinephrine via prescribed auto-injector
4. Administering oxygen at 10 to 15 liters via non-rebreather mask

Select the correct answer.

A) 2, 3 and 4
B) 3 and 4
C) 4 only
D) 1,2 and 4

2. You respond to a restaurant for a call involving a patient who passed out. Upon your arrival, you find a 19-year-old female who is very pale and wheezing. Apparently she just ate some sauce that had shrimp in it, which she tells you she is not supposed to eat.
   A) Where in the body are allergy symptoms most prominent?
   B) Besides shellfish, what are other foods that commonly can cause an allergic reaction?
   C) What signs would indicate that this is a serious systemic reaction as opposed to a minor local reaction?
   D) How should this patient be managed?

KEY TERMS MATCHING

Assess your knowledge of the chapter key terms by matching the terms on the left to the definitions on the right.

______ **1.** Adrenaline

______ **2.** Allergen

______ **3.** Allergic Reaction

______ **4.** Anaphylactic (an-eh-feh-LAK-tik) Shock

______ **5.** Anaphylaxis

______ **6.** Antibody

______ **7.** Antigen

______ **8.** Epinephrine

______ **9.** Hives

______ **10.** Immune Response

(A) A series of reactions that are the body's defense mechanism against invading viruses, bacteria, and toxins

(B) Another name for anaphylactic shock

(C) Hormone secreted in response to stress; causes tachycardia and vasoconstriction; used as an injected medication to relieve severe allergic reactions

(D) An antigen, such as dust, mold, or pollen, that causes an allergic reaction

(E) A protein produced by the immune system that combines with a specific antigen and helps to destroy it

(F) Severe allergic reaction in which blood vessels dilate rapidly, causing a drop in blood pressure and respiratory distress

(G) Raised, red blotches associated with allergic reactions

(H) An exaggerated immune response to a substance that is normally harmless

(I) A foreign substance that enters the body and causes an immune response.

(J) Another name for epinephrine

SKILLS CHECKLIST

Check your knowledge of important EMT-B skills by marking off each step in the following skills sheet.

ADMINISTRATION OF EPINEPHRINE

- [ ] Obtain patient's prescribed auto-injector. Ensure prescription is written for the patient who is experiencing the severe allergic reaction. Ensure medication is not discolored (if visible).
- [ ] Obtain order from medical direction, either on-line or off-line.
- [ ] Remove cap from auto-injector. Place tip of auto-injector against patient's thigh (lateral portion, midway between waist and knee).
- [ ] Push the injector firmly against the thigh until the injector activates.
- [ ] Hold the injector in place until the medication is injected (at least 10 seconds).
- [ ] Record activity and time.
- [ ] Dispose of injector in biohazard container.

(reprinted from *Pocket Reference for The EMT-B and First Responder* by Bob Elling, Prentice Hall, 1999)

D.O.T. OBJECTIVES CHECKLIST

Use the following list of knowledge objectives to check what you've learned. Check off only those objectives that you feel you completely understand and have mastered. For any objectives not checked, go back and review that section of the text chapter. Textbook page references have been provided to help you review the text material.

- [ ] Recognize the patient experiencing an allergic reaction. (p. 451)
- [ ] Describe the emergency medical care of the patient with an allergic reaction. *(p. 453)*
- [ ] Establish the relationship between the patient with an allergic reaction and airway management. *(p. 451)*
- [ ] Describe the mechanisms of allergic response and the implications for airway management. *(p. 451)*
- [ ] State the generic and trade names, medication forms, dose, administration, action, and contraindications for the epinephrine auto-injector. *(p. 456)*
- [ ] Evaluate the need for medical direction in the emergency medical care of the patient with an allergic reaction. *(p. 453)*
- [ ] Differentiate between the general category of those patients having an allergic reaction and those patients having an allergic reaction and requiring immediate medical care, including immediate use of an epinephrine auto-injector. *(p. 453)*

CHAPTER 16

Poisoning and Overdose

CHAPTER 16 SUMMARY

Poisons may enter the body by one of four ways: ingestion, inhalation, absorption, or injection. Poisoning is common in young children, and many times it is caused by poisons being stored in containers that look similar to household products. Poisons should always be stored out of the reach of children.

Your safety is always a top priority. Never expose yourself to toxic or poisonous substances in an attempt to rescue the patient. Before transporting any potentially hazardous substance, verify that doing so is safe.

Always record the name of the suspected poison if known. Record the route of exposure, the quantity of poison that entered the body, the time period in which the exposure occurred, and any interventions done before you arrived. Knowing the patient's weight is important to determine the amount of activated charcoal to use if indicated.

Contact medical direction or poison control early, so that poison-specific treatment can begin as early as possible.

Activated charcoal can be administered in cases of ingested poison. Activated charcoal binds to certain poisons. This prevents the body from absorbing them. Never administer activated charcoal to patients with an altered mental status, those who have ingested strong alkalis or acids, or patients who are unable to swallow.

REVIEW QUESTIONS

Please circle the best answer for each question.

1. A poison can enter the body through ingestion, __________, injection, or absorption.
   A) infection **B)** inhalation **C)** eating **D)** convection
   [Reference text page 465]

2. The effect of a poison may vary depending upon which of the following?
   A) The amount of poison **B)** The route of exposure
   C) The age and health of the patient **D)** All of the above
   [Reference text page 465]

3. If the patient vomits after administration of activated charcoal, you should:
   A) repeat the dose.
   B) shake the bottle and repeat the dose.
   C) wait four hours after poison ingestion.
   D) contact medical direction.
   [Reference text page 470]

4. If there is no discarded syringe at the scene, you can rule out injected poisoning.
   A) True **B)** False
   [Reference text page 474]

5. Routes of entry for poisons to enter the body include:
   A) circulation. **B)** abduction. **C)** ingestion. **D)** digestion.
   [Reference text page 465]

6. Centers that maintain up-to-date information on chemical compounds, their effects on the body, and ways to treat overdoses or poisonings are:
   A) poison control centers. **B)** medical direction centers.
   C) emergency ingestion centers. **D)** centers for disease control.
   [Reference text page 467]

7. Signs and symptoms of poisoning:
   A) are typically limited to nausea and vomiting.
   B) only occur from poison ingestions.
   C) vary dramatically depending on the poison.
   D) are rarely considered serious to the patient.
   [Reference text page 465]

8. Of the poisonings that occur, more than ________ percent of the reported exposures occurred in the home.
A) 10 **B)** 90 **C)** 25 **D)** 50
[Reference text page 464]

9. A food, plant, chemical, or drug that has an adverse effect on the body is a/n:
A) medication. **B)** oral agent. **C)** poison. **D)** inhalant.
[Reference text page 465]

10. A liquid or solid toxic substance that is swallowed is called a/n:
A) toxin. **B)** ingested poison.
C) inhalant. **D)** antidote.
[Reference text page 467]

11. An agent that blocks or reverses the effect of a poison is called a/n:
A) antidote. **B)** toxin. **C)** oral agent. **D)** inhalant.
[Reference text page 467]

12. The most common route of poisoning is:
A) injection. **B)** inhalation. **C)** ingestion. **D)** absorption.
[Reference text page 467]

13. Ingested poisons enter the bloodstream through the capillaries in the intestinal lining.
A) True **B)** False
[Reference text page 467]

14. Examples of commonly ingested nonprescription medications are:
A) aspirin. **B)** vitamins with iron.
C) pain relievers. **D)** all of the above.
[Reference text page 468]

15. Examples of commonly ingested prescription medications are:
A) sedatives. **B)** cold medications.
C) aspirin. **D)** rubbing alcohol.
[Reference text page 468]

16. Which of the following is NOT a sign or symptom of ingestions poisoning?
A) Nausea and/or vomiting **B)** Cherry red skin color
C) Altered heart rate **D)** Abdominal tenderness
[Reference text page 469]

17. Inhaled poisons enter the bloodstream through the capillaries in the linings of the lungs.
A) True **B)** False
[Reference text page 471]

18. A side effect of activated charcoal is:
A) hypotension. **B)** rapid pulse. **C)** black stools. **D)** headache.
[Reference text page 471]

19. Contraindications for the use of activated charcoal include:
A) the patient is unable to swallow.
B) the patient swallowed a strong acid or alkali.
C) the patient has an altered mental status.
D) all of the above.
[Reference text page 471]

20. A toxic substance that is breathed in is called:
A) a fume. **B)** a vapor. **C)** a spray. **D)** all of the above.
[Reference text page 471]

21. One of the most common poisonous gases is:
A) hydrogen sulfide. **B)** carbon monoxide.
C) sulfur dioxide. **D)** chlorine.
[Reference text page 472]

22. If you suspect toxic fumes, you should park your vehicle downhill and downwind of the residence.
A) True **B)** False
[Reference text page 472]

23. If a firefighter has singed nasal hair after fighting a fire, you should suspect:
A) carbon monoxide. **B)** nitrous oxide.
C) ammonia. **D)** freon.
[Reference text page 472]

24. Bright cherry red color is an early sign of a significant CO exposure.
A) True **B)** False
[Reference text page 473]

25. A poison that enters the bloodstream through a puncture injury is called an ________ poison.
A) inhaled **B)** absorbed **C)** injected **D)** infected
[Reference text page 474]

26. As you gather history of an injection poisoning patient, be sure to ask:
   A) if the patient is allergic to any insects.
   B) if the patient has a history of illicit drug use.
   C) if the patient has been bitten by anything.
   D) all of the above.
   [Reference text page 475]

27. The removal or cleansing of dangerous chemicals and other dangerous or infectious materials is called:
   A) decontamination.
   B) reabsorption.
   C) inhalation.
   D) none of the above.
   [Reference text page 477]

28. The signs and symptoms of absorption poisoning include:
   A) delayed capillary refill.
   B) burns and itching.
   C) blue color and tearing.
   D) edema and ringing in the ears.
   [Reference text page 477]

29. Poisons that are _______ enter the bloodstream through capillaries in the skin.
   A) inhaled
   B) injected
   C) absorbed
   D) none of the above
   [Reference text page 476]

30. If a chemical is spilled into the patient's eyes, how long should the EMT-Basic flush?
   A) 5 minutes
   B) 20 minutes
   C) 45 minutes
   D) Not at all
   [Reference text page 477]

CASE STUDIES

Use a separate piece of paper to answer the case study questions. Number your answers with the case study number and question letter (1A, 1B, etc.).

POISONING

1. You respond to a home on one of the first days of winter. There are three family members who are complaining of headaches, nausea, vomiting, and are very sleepy.
   A) What should you suspect whenever there are multiple patients with medical complaints of this nature?
   B) If a gas was involved, what is the most likely substance and how did it probably occur?
   C) What would a late indicator of this problem present as in this patient?
2. You respond to a gardening supply shop where the patient has been handling fertilizers all day. He states that his skin is irritated and itching. You can see it is blotchy red in places on his hands and arms.
   A) What do you suspect may have happened to the patient?

B) What should be done to the patient prior to transport?
C) If any of the substance may have gotten into his eyes, what should you do?

3. You are treating a 27-year-old male patient who ingested a poisonous substance. Medical control has agreed to allow you to administer activated charcoal to the patient since his vital signs are stable.
   A) What is this patient's mental status?
   B) What side effects may accompany the charcoal administration?
   C) What is the normal adult dose to be administered to this patient?
   D) What are some of the trade names of the substance you are giving the patient?

KEY TERMS MATCHING

Assess your knowledge of the chapter key terms by matching the terms on the left to the definitions on the right.

______ **1.** Absorbed Poison

______ **2.** Activated Charcoal

______ **3.** Antidote

______ **4.** Decontamination

______ **5.** Ingested Poison

______ **6.** Inhaled Poison

______ **7.** Injected Poison

______ **8.** Poison

______ **9.** Toxin

(A) A food, plant, chemical, or drug that has an adverse effect on the body

(B) A substance that is poisonous to cells or tissues

(C) A toxic substance that enters the body through a puncture in the skin; injection may be by needle, animal bite, or insect sting

(D) A liquid or solid toxic substance that is swallowed

(E) A toxic substance such as a gas, fumes, vapor, or spray that is breathed in

(F) The removal or cleansing of dangerous chemicals and other dangerous or infectious materials

(G) An agent that blocks or reverses the effect of a poison

(H) A toxic substance taken into the body across unbroken skin or mucous membranes

(I) Substance that hinders the absorption of ingested poisons and enhances their elimination from the body, preventing further damage

SKILLS CHECKLISTS

Check your knowledge of important EMT-B skills by marking off each step in the following skills sheets.

MANAGEMENT OF ABSORBED POISONS

- [ ] Size up situation and take the necessary precautions to prevent injury to yourself and your crew.
- [ ] Remove patient from source. Avoid contaminating yourself with poison.
- [ ] Conduct an initial assessment.
- [ ] Maintain an open airway.
- [ ] Administer high-concentration oxygen.
- [ ] Perform a focused history and physical exam, including SAMPLE history and vital signs.
- [ ] Brush powders from patient. Be careful not to abrade patient's skin.
- [ ] Remove contaminated clothing and other articles, such as shoes and jewelry.
- [ ] Quickly gather information about product.
- [ ] If appropriate, irrigate with large amounts of clear water for at least 20 minutes. Call medical direction.
- [ ] Perform ongoing assessment.
- [ ] Be alert for shock, and transport as soon as possible.

MANAGEMENT OF INGESTED POISONS

- [ ] Take BSI precautions.
- [ ] Conduct an initial assessment.
- [ ] Maintain an open airway.
- [ ] Perform a focused history and physical exam, including SAMPLE history and vital signs.
- [ ] Quickly gather information about substance.
- [ ] Call medical direction on scene or en route.
- [ ] If directed, administer activated charcoal.

- [ ] Position patient for vomiting and save all vomitus. Have suction ready.
- [ ] Perform ongoing assessment.
- [ ] Transport as soon as possible.

MANAGEMENT OF INHALED POISONS

- [ ] Size-up the situation and take the necessary precautions to prevent injury to yourself and your crew.*
- [ ] Remove patient from the source. Avoid contaminating yourself with poison.
- [ ] Maintain open airway. Stay alert for vomiting. Properly position the patient and have suction equipment ready.
- [ ] Conduct an initial assessment.
- [ ] Administer high-concentration oxygen by nonrebreather mask.
- [ ] Perform a focused history and physical exam, including a SAMPLE history.
- [ ] Remove contaminated clothing and other articles (e.g., shoes, jewelry).
- [ ] Assess baseline vital signs.
- [ ] Quickly gather information about product (containers, bottles, and labels).
- [ ] Call medical direction on the scene or en route.
- [ ] Transport as soon as possible.
- [ ] Perform ongoing assessment en route.

***SAFETY NOTE:** In the presence of hazardous fumes or gases, wear protective clothing and a self-contained breathing apparatus or wait for those who are properly trained and equipped to enter scene and remove patient to a safe area.

ADMINISTRATION OF ACTIVATED CHARCOAL

- [ ] Consult medical direction.
- [ ] Shake container thoroughly.
- [ ] Since medication looks like mud, patient may need to be persuaded to drink it. Providing a covered container and a straw will prevent patient from seeing the medication and so may improve patient compliance.
- [ ] If patient does not drink the medication right away, the charcoal will settle. Shake or stir it again before administering.

☐ Record the name, dose, route, and time of administration of the medication.

(reprinted from *Pocket Reference for The EMT-B and First Responder* by Bob Elling, Prentice Hall, 1999)

D.O.T. Objectives Checklist

Use the following list of knowledge objectives to check what you've learned. Check off only those objectives that you feel you completely understand and have mastered. For any objectives not checked, go back and review that section of the text chapter. Textbook page references have been provided to help you review the text material.

☐ List various ways that poisons enter the body. *(p. 465)*

☐ List signs/symptoms associated with poisoning. *(p. 468)*

☐ Discuss the emergency medical care for the patient with possible overdose. *(p. 469)*

☐ Describe the steps in the emergency medical care for the patient with suspected poisoning. *(p. 469)*

☐ Establish the relationship between the patient suffering from poisoning or overdose and airway management. *(p. 466)*

☐ State the generic and trade names, indications, contraindications, medication form, dose, administration, actions, side effects, and reassessment strategies for activated charcoal. *(p. 470)*

☐ Recognize the need for medical direction in caring for the patient with poisoning or overdose. *(p. 466)*

CHAPTER 17

Environmental Emergencies

CHAPTER 17 SUMMARY

Environmental emergencies are commonly found in conjunction with other medical or traumatic complaints. Certain factors can predispose a patient to an environmental emergency including: extremes in climate; patient age; preexisting medical conditions; the presence of drugs, medications, or poisons in the patient's system. The key element of managing environmental emergencies is removal of the patient from the environment.

Generalized hypothermia involves the whole patient. Remove any wet clothing and cover with warm blankets. Handle the patient gently, as rough handling may cause cardiac arrest. Actively rewarm the patient if he or she is alert and responding appropriately by placing warm packs on the neck, the armpits, and the groin. If the patient has an altered mental status, rewarm passively using warm blankets only.

Localized cold injuries often occur to the face, ears, and extremities. It is important that you protect the area from further injury and remove any jewelry or clothing that may cause problems when swelling begins. Do not massage the area or reexpose it to the cold. If transport is long or delayed, consider rewarming the area by immersing in a warm water bath.

Heat emergencies may present with a wide variety of signs and symptoms. Your treatment is based primarily on the patient's skin condition. Consider patients with hot skin as having a life-threatening emergency. It is appropriate to cool the patient using cool packs to the neck, armpits, and groin. Patients with signs and symptoms of a heat emergency that have normal or cool temperature skin should be moved to a cool environment; remove or loosen any restrictive clothing. If the patient is not nauseated and has a secure airway, allow him or her to drink water or other liquid authorized by medical direction.

When dealing with water-related emergencies, always consider safety a top priority. All rescuers near the edge of the water should consider using a personal flotation device. Never attempt a water rescue unless properly trained and equipped. Suspect spinal injury if diving is involved or if the cause is unknown. Always attempt resuscitation on cold-water drowning victims.

Bites and stings are common environmental emergencies involving injected poisons. Evaluate the patient carefully for signs and symptoms of an allergic reaction and treat for such if indicated. If there are no signs of an allergic reaction, remove jewelry or restrictive clothing from the injured area. Do not apply cold. Place the injection site slightly below the patient's heart. Consult with medical direction for additional treatment instructions.

REVIEW QUESTIONS

1. Altered mental status, rapid pulse, and decreased respirations may be seen in cases of hypothermia.
   A) True **B)** False
   [Reference text page 489]

2. There are four basic mechanisms for transferring heat. They are conduction, convection, radiation and:
   A) retention. **B)** inflation. **C)** evaporation. **D)** transference.
   [Reference text page 485]

3. Transfer of heat from a warmer object in contact with a colder object is called:
   A) conduction. **B)** convection. **C)** radiation. **D)** inflation.
   [Reference text page 485]

4. Heat released by an object into the surrounding air as waves of infrared radiation is called:
   A) conduction. **B)** convection. **C)** radiation. **D)** evaporation.
   [Reference text page 485]

5. A person suffering from hypothermia will always be shivering.
   A) True **B)** False
   [Reference text page 490]

6. Why is age a predisposing factor for hypothermia?
   A) Older people do not wear enough clothing.
   B) Older people have less body fat and muscle mass.
   C) Older people are usually sick.
   D) Older people are not predisposed to hypothermia.
   [Reference text page 487]

7. The EMT-Basic should suspect hypothermia if the patient has:
   A) been immersed in water for a long time.
   B) been outdoors, in the cold, for a long time without a hat.
   C) been pinned in a vehicle for a long extrication.
   D) any of the above.
   [Reference text page 487]

8. The air temperature surrounding the patient is called the:
   A) wind-chill factor. **B)** convection temperature.
   C) ambient temperature. **D)** environmental formula.
   [Reference text page 487]

9. After removing a generalized hypothermia patient from the harmful environment and determining there are no injuries, you should encourage the patient to walk around to help warm the body.
   A) True **B)** False
   [Reference text page 491]

10. In the late stages of hypothermia, the patient may have:
   A) shivering. **B)** a rapid pulse rate.
   C) pale, cyanotic, or white skin. **D)** rapid breathing.
   [Reference text page 489]

11. Which of the following factors do not exaggerate the severity of hypothermia?
   A) A history of heatstroke **B)** Ingestion of large quantities of alcohol
   C) Severe trauma **D)** Outdoor resuscitation attempts
   [Reference text page 488]

12. Why can a head injury make hypothermia worse?
   A) The patients forget to wear a coat.
   B) Head injured patients have less muscle mass.
   C) Damage may occur to the thermoregulatory center of the brain.
   D) The patients begin to hyperventilate early in a head injury.
   [Reference text page 488]

13. Signs and symptoms that indicate deterioration of body temperature regulation include:
   A) weakness and/or exhaustion. **B)** altered mental status.
   C) dizziness and/or fainting. **D)** all of the above.
   [Reference text page 495]

14. As the relative humidity rises, the body's ability to rid itself of heat by sweat evaporation diminishes.
   A) True **B)** False
   [Reference text page 494]

15. Hyperthermia can be amplified by all of the following conditions EXCEPT:
   A) underweight for age. **B)** dehydration.
   C) fatigue. **D)** fever.
   [Reference text page 494]

16. If the relative humidity exceeds ________ percent, sweating becomes ineffective.
   A) 10 **B)** 20 **C)** 55 **D)** 75
   [Reference text page 494]

17. A hyperthermia patient with an open airway and no nausea should be allowed to drink water or an electrolyte solution.
A) True **B)** False
[Reference text page 496]

18. Drownings can occur in bathtubs and:
A) spas.
B) irrigation canals.
C) recreational facilities.
D) any of the above.
[Reference text page 497]

19. A near-drowning is:
A) a patient who is able to swim out of a body of water.
B) a patient who survives for at least 24 hours following an immersion.
C) a rescue involving a patient who could not swim.
D) none of the above.
[Reference text page 497]

20. If the skin is hot to the touch, you should aggressively attempt to cool the patient.
A) True **B)** False
[Reference text page 496]

21. Based on reports from resuscitated survivors, after exhaustion they probably were unable to hold their breath no longer than ________ seconds.
A) 15 **B)** 30 **C)** 45 **D)** 60
[Reference text page 498]

22. The most common stings are from:
A) black widow spiders.
B) stingrays and jellyfish.
C) bees and wasps.
D) snakes and scorpions.
[Reference text page 499]

23. When examining a sting site, if a venom sac is found, you should:
A) remove the sac carefully with a credit card.
B) squeeze the sac prior to removing.
C) attempt to pull the sac out.
D) do all of the above.
[Reference text page 501]

24. A drowning victim has been submerged in cold water for an hour. There is no pulse or breathing. The EMT-Basic should follow local protocol and begin resuscitation techniques.
A) True **B)** False
[Reference text page 498]

25. When treating a snakebite in the field, maintain the extremity at a position lower than the heart and be sure to:
A) suck out the venom.
B) cut out the venom.
C) consult with medical direction concerning the use of a venous tourniquet.
D) do all of the above.
[Reference text page 501]

CASE STUDIES

Use a separate piece of paper to answer the case study questions. Number your answers with the case study number and question letter (1A, 1B, etc.).

COLD-RELATED EMERGENCIES

1. It's January, and you and your partner are enjoying the unseasonably warm weather. Usually in January the ground is covered with at least two feet of snow. You are tempted to get out of the rig and spend a few minutes just soaking in the sunshine. Just as you unbuckle your seatbelts, the mobile terminal beeps three times. The call is for a man down. The caller is a neighbor of a frequent user of EMS services in your community. As you enter his home, you notice a chill in the air. First Responders have found the 55-year-old male lying in the kitchen on a concrete floor. He is wearing only his underwear and from the looks of things he has been on the floor for a few days. The patient is slow to respond to your commands. His skin is extremely cold to the touch.
A) List and describe the five basic ways in which body heat can be lost.
B) In what ways has this patient lost body heat?.
C) What other factors contribute to the above patient's hypothermia?

2. The local lake and mountain trails are a favorite for tourists on rented snowmobiles. As the local rescue squad, you have been to the area for injuries caused by minor snowmobile collisions. As the tones go off, you are surprised to learn that a snowmobile has broken through the ice in one of the smaller ponds and bystanders are currently searching for the operator. As you arrive on scene, you notice several young adults gathered around a patient lying supine in the snow. Bystanders say they located the operator within one to two minutes and pulled him out from underneath the ice. The patient is unresponsive and breathing very rapidly.
A) List the typical vital signs in the early stages of hypothermia caused by a cold environment.
B) How would you treat the patient in this case?
C) Given the same scenario, what additional medical concerns would you have if the patient was elderly?

3. The senior living center does a good job keeping track of all the residents. However, on occasion an elderly resident has been known to leave the grounds despite continuous monitoring and security precautions. On this occasion, a resident has missed an evening meal and the nursing staff quickly discovers that the patient is missing. A search is initiated. As a member of the search and rescue squad, you have some serious concerns for the safety of the missing resident, given cold weather conditions and the likelihood that the missing man is not properly dressed for the outdoors. Just around 2:30 A.M. your search team finds the elderly male lying at the entrance to a summer cabin in the nearby foothills. The patient is unresponsive and cold to the touch. Initial assessment finds signs of late hypothermia.

A) Describe the vital signs you would expect to find in this patient.

4. Despite cold weather, the local amusement park has been full of visitors all day. As part of the security and emergency response team, you have responded to over 45 requests for services, ranging from skinned elbows to gang skirmishes. After your shift as you make your way to the employee parking lot, you notice something move in your peripheral vision. As you get closer, it looks as if a young woman is lying beneath some bushes growing just inside the gate. The woman is slow to respond to your questions and appears to have several bruises on her arms and face. Despite the cold weather and improper clothing, the woman is not shivering or complaining of the cold.

A) Would you treat this patient as a trauma patient or medical patient? Why?

B) What treatment would you provide for this patient?

5. The ranger academy was a great learning experience. You particularly liked the EMT-Basic portion of the training and looked forward to using your new skills to help someone in need. Your first official assignment is to monitor the winter campsites on the remote eastern side of the park. As you pull up to check on yet another closed cabin, you notice some footprints in the snow. They seem to wander around almost in circles. As you check the cabin, you find the back door has been forced open. You carefully enter the cabin and find two young men lying on the floor. Both are unresponsive and appear to be in their early teens. They are extremely cold to the touch. You immediately contact dispatch and request additional support.

A) What rewarming steps might apply to these unresponsive patients?

B) Would aeromedical transport be an option for these patients?

6. You and your best friend have been working outside for over an hour, repairing the pump motor on his well and water system. It looks as if several of the bearings are frozen. The extremely cold weather is the culprit. The freezing temperature isn't abnormal, but it seems just a little colder when you are outside and working with steel parts. Several times over the last hour, both you and your friend have had to remove your gloves to work with some of the smaller moving parts. As you finish one side of the motor, your friend complains of some severe pain in his fingers and wrists. You take a look at his fingers and see that the skin is white and waxy, feeling frozen to the touch. You tell your friend its time to quit and get him some help.

A) Describe the typical signs and symptoms associated with late or deep tissue injury caused by exposure to the cold.

B) List the steps required for emergency care for late or deep and localized cold injuries.

C) Your friend wants to run his hand under hot water. Why should you stop him?

D) As you enter his farmhouse, it dawns on you that with the current weather and road conditions it may take over an hour before the ambulance or rescue unit can arrive. Given this situation, describe the steps to the rewarming process you would consider as part of your emergency treatment.

HEAT-RELATED EMERGENCIES

7. You are just finishing restocking the unit from the last response when the tones sound and dispatch requests a response to the local high school for a man down on the track. The air-conditioning inside the ambulance is working overtime just to keep the cab cool. Estimates are that the ambient temperature exceeds 100 degrees Fahrenheit. As you arrive on scene, you can see several people gathered around a middle-aged male sitting against the fence. Bystanders advise that the man was running on the track when he suddenly stopped and began vomiting. He has remained conscious and responsive. The patient denies any problems and just thinks he overexerted himself. The patient's skin is pale, moist, and cool to the touch.

A) Describe the basic emergency treatment appropriate for this patient.

B) How can you tell if the patient can safely take replenishing fluids?

8. You have just graduated from the EMT-Basic program and received your lifeguard certification. Your new summer lifeguard position at the local resort is a dream come true. Over the last few weeks, you have had a few rescues but nothing serious that has required your EMT-Basic skills. Sitting high above the beach, you suddenly notice a group of young teenagers screaming and waving to catch your attention. You notify dispatch, signal to the neighboring guards, and grab your response kit. As you approach the group, you see a teenaged female lying on a towel. She is not responding to her friends. The patient's skin is bright red and moist to the touch. She is breathing and has a rapid, weak carotid pulse.

A) Identify the proper emergency treatment for this patient.

WATER-RELATED EMERGENCIES

9. Every summer, high school kids from around the county gather at the river. Despite repeated efforts to educate them, someone always ends up jumping from the cliffs or the small bridge into the water below and getting injured. You are responding to the latest of these incidents. As you pull out of the station, dispatch advises that bystander CPR is being initiated on a 14-year-old male near-drowning victim. You are new to EMS and your partner asks you to manage the airway while he performs advanced life support interventions. As you arrive on scene, you see several people standing around and two people performing CPR. As your partner begins her assessment, you learn that the patient jumped from the bridge and did not resurface. A few minutes later, friends found the boy floating on top of the water slightly downstream. They immediately moved him to the shore and began CPR.

A) Given the possible mechanism of injury and history of the event, what would you immediately want your partner to recognize?

B) Gastric distention is common in near-drowning victims. How can it interfere with your resuscitation efforts?

C) You recognize the signs of gastric distention as you ventilate the patient, and it becomes extremely difficult to obtain chest rise and fall. Describe the steps necessary to help reduce or relieve gastric distention in your patient.

BITES AND STINGS

10. You decided to take an EMT-Basic class after working in the lumber business as a safety officer for over ten years. In the past, you could only provide some basic first aid and wait for rescue units. You have convinced the company management staff that you need more medical training and better emergency medical supplies. They agreed. Although you have been flushing out a lot of eyes full of sawdust, you are waiting for a more serious emergency. The yard supervisor requests that you assess a man complaining of general weakness and numbness around his mouth. The man states he was moving some wood chips when he was attacked by a large group of wasps. He believes he was stung more than a dozen times. You see a few red marks on his arms, neck, and forehead. The patient also begins to complain of a sore throat.

A) Describe your emergency treatment for this patient.
B) Describe the steps necessary to properly remove a stinger.

KEY TERMS MATCHING

Assess your knowledge of the chapter key terms by matching the terms on the left to the definitions on the right.

_____ **1.** Ambient Temperature

_____ **2.** Conduction

_____ **3.** Convection

_____ **4.** Drowning

_____ **5.** Evaporation

_____ **6.** Hyperthermia

_____ **7.** Hypothermia

_____ **8.** Localized Cold Injury

_____ **9.** Near-Drowning

_____ **10.** Radiation

_____ **11.** Wind Chill

(A) An immersion situation from which the patient is resuscitated and survives for at least 24 hours

(B) Death resulting from suffocation or cardiac arrest while submerged in water

(C) Abnormally high core body temperature

(D) Transfer of heat from a warmer object in contact with a colder object

(E) The air temperature surrounding the patient

(F) Transfer of heat from a warm object to cooler air moving past its surface

(G) Heat released by an object into the surrounding air as waves of infrared radiation

(H) The combined cooling effect of wind speed and ambient temperature

(I) The process of converting a liquid to a gas in which heat is lost

(J) Abnormally low core body temperature

(K) A cold injury confined to a limited area of the body; more severe cases are called frostbite

SKILLS CHECKLISTS

Check your knowledge of important EMT-B skills by marking off each step in the following skills sheets.

ACTIVE RAPID REWARMING OF FROZEN PARTS

- [ ] Take BSI precautions.
- [ ] Conduct an initial assessment.
- [ ] Conduct focused history and physical exam, including taking baseline vital signs.
- [ ] Consider administering oxygen by non-rebreather mask.
- [ ] Heat water to a temperature between 100°F and 105°F.
- [ ] Fill container with heated water and prepare injured part by removing clothing, jewelry, bands, or straps.
- [ ] Fully immerse injured part. Do not allow injured area to touch sides or bottom of container. Do not place any pressure on affected part. Continuously stir the water. When water cools below 100°F, remove affected part and add more warm water. The patient may complain of moderate pain as the affected area rewarms or may experience periods of intense pain.
- [ ] If you complete rewarming of the part, gently dry the affected area and apply a dry sterile dressing.
- [ ] Place dry sterile dressings between fingers and toes before dressing hands/feet.
- [ ] Cover the site with blankets or whatever is available to keep affected area warm. Do not allow these coverings to come in contact with injured area or to put pressure on site.
- [ ] Keep patient at rest. Do not allow patient to walk if a lower extremity has been frostbitten or frozen.
- [ ] Keep entire patient warm.
- [ ] Continue to monitor the patient.
- [ ] Assist circulation according to local protocol. (Some systems recommend rhythmically and carefully raising and lowering affected limb.)
- [ ] Do not allow limb to refreeze.
- [ ] Transport patient as soon as possible, with affected limb slightly elevated.

WATER RESCUE: POTENTIAL SPINE INJURY

- [ ] Take BSI precautions.
- [ ] Conduct an initial assessment.
- [ ] Splint head and neck with arms.
- [ ] Roll patient over into supine position.
- [ ] Assess airway and breathing. (Note: If patient is not breathing, remove him or her from water on a backboard as soon as possible.)
- [ ] Provide manual stabilization of head/neck.
- [ ] Assess pulses, motor ability, and sensory response (PMS) in four extremities.
- [ ] Slide backboard under patient.
- [ ] Apply a properly sized rigid extrication collar.
- [ ] Tie down torso, then head/neck with straps.
- [ ] Float board to edge of the water.
- [ ] Remove patient from water with as much assistance as needed.
- [ ] Obtain baseline vital signs.
- [ ] Conduct focused history and physical exam.
- [ ] Reassess PMS in four extremities.
- [ ] Apply oxygen and prepare to transport.

(reprinted from *Pocket Reference for The EMT-B and First Responder* by Bob Elling, Prentice Hall, 1999)

D.O.T. Objectives Checklist

Use the following list of knowledge objectives to check what you've learned. Check off only those objectives that you feel you completely understand and have mastered. For any objectives not checked, go back and review that section of the text chapter. Textbook page references have been provided to help you review the text material.

- [ ] Describe the various ways that the body loses heat. *(p. 485)*
- [ ] List the signs and symptoms of exposure to cold. *(p. 489)*
- [ ] Explain the steps in providing emergency medical care to a patient exposed to cold. *(p. 490)*
- [ ] List the signs and symptoms of exposure to heat. *(p. 494)*
- [ ] Explain the steps in providing emergency care to a patient exposed to heat. *(p. 495)*
- [ ] Recognize the signs and symptoms of water-related emergencies. *(p. 496)*
- [ ] Describe the complications of near-drowning. *(p. 496)*
- [ ] Discuss the emergency medical care of bites and stings. *(p. 500)*

CHAPTER 18

Obstetrics and Gynecology

CHAPTER 18 SUMMARY

Childbirth is a natural event. It is not necessarily a medical emergency. In an emergency, remember that the best way to save the life of the infant is to save the life of the mother.

Predelivery emergencies may be caused by miscarriage, vaginal bleeding, seizures, or trauma. Manage vaginal bleeding and suspected miscarriages with external pads. Treat for shock based on the patient's signs and symptoms. Bring any fetal tissues passed to the hospital. Treat pregnant victims of trauma the same as other trauma patients.

If delivery is imminent and crowning is present, prepare for immediate delivery. However, recognizing your own limitations is important. Transport immediately if any difficulty arises, even if delivery occurs during transport.

After delivery, dry, warm, suction and stimulate the infant. Complete the APGAR scoring one minute and five minutes after delivery if possible. Some infants will require resuscitation, especially if premature. Newborn resuscitation follows an inverted pyramid.

Meconium is a dark green or brown substance that indicates fetal distress during labor. It can obstruct the airway of a newborn. If meconium is present, apply suction before stimulating the infant to breathe. Maintain the airway, and transport as soon as possible.

Abnormal deliveries can endanger the life of the fetus and the mother if not managed correctly. If any part other than the infant's head presents with crowning, begin rapid transport immediately. Place the mother in the head-down, pelvis-up position. If the umbilical cord presents, insert a sterile, gloved hand into the vagina. Gently press the fetus up to remove pressure on the cord.

In cases of alleged sexual assault, try to have an EMT-Basic who is the same gender as the patient provide necessary care. Remember that sexual assaults often cause tremendous and long-term psychological injury. Be calm, professional, and compassionate. Be aware of reporting requirements for criminal assault. Limit your exam to life-threatening concerns. Discourage the patient from bathing, voiding, or changing clothes.

REVIEW QUESTIONS

Please circle the best answer for each question.

1. Prehospital childbirth situations occur:
   A) frequently.
   B) infrequently.
   C) never; you must get the mother to the hospital first.
   D) only if the EMT-Basic delays field care.
   [Reference text page 508]

2. An EMT-Basic must be able to demonstrate how and when to cut an umbilical cord.
   A) True **B)** False
   [Reference text pages 520–521]

3. The second stage of labor begins with:
   A) uterine contractions, and ends with full dilation of the cervix.
   B) crowning, and ends with delivery of the baby.
   C) the birth of the baby, and ends with delivery of the placenta.
   D) completion of dilation, and ends with delivery.
   [Reference text page 511]

4. It is possible for a woman to be pregnant without being aware of it.
   A) True **B)** False
   [Reference text pages 512, 537]

5. Symptoms of pregnancy include all of the following EXCEPT:
   A) breast tenderness. **B)** nausea and fatigue.
   C) recent normal menstrual period. **D)** enlarged abdomen.
   [Reference text page 513]

6. The EMT-Basic must try to determine the viability of a miscarried fetus.
   A) True **B)** False
   [Reference text page 515]

7. For a pregnant woman who has been in a car accident, the EMT-Basic should perform:
   A) a medical patient assessment. **B)** a trauma patient assessment.
   C) both of the above. **D)** neither of the above.
   [Reference text page 518]

8. It is important to position any pregnant patient flat on her back for transport.
   A) True **B)** False
   [Reference text page 518]

9. A discharge of a small amount of blood-tinged mucus from the vagina at the onset of labor is called a/n:
A) uterine rupture. **B)** bloody show. **C)** amniotic sac. **D)** placenta previa.
[Reference text page 511]

10. The "bag of waters" is a layperson's term for the:
A) uterus. **B)** placenta. **C)** amniotic sac. **D)** umbilicus.
[Reference text page 508]

11. You should attempt to stop serious vaginal bleeding by packing the vagina.
A) True **B)** False
[Reference text page 515]

12. Placement of sterile drapes on the patient who is imminent for delivery is:
A) to protect the patient's modesty.
B) done as part of BSI precautions.
C) done to create a sterile field for delivery of the fetus.
D) not necessary.
[Reference text page 523]

CD-ROM LINK: *Review the* Assisting a Birth *videos in Chapter 18 of the MedEMT CD-ROM.*

13. The organ that enables the exchange of nutrients, oxygen, and metabolic wastes between the maternal and fetal circulatory systems is the:
A) placenta. **B)** amniotic sac. **C)** uterus. **D)** umbilicus.
[Reference text page 508]

14. Clear straw-colored fluid, which acts as a protective cushion for the fetus, is called ________ fluid.
A) meconium **B)** placenta **C)** uterine **D)** amniotic
[Reference text page 508]

15. You are close to the receiving facility with a patient in labor. You see the fetal head crowning, but the amniotic sac has not ruptured. You should not rupture the membrane manually.
A) True **B)** False
[Reference text page 520]

16. An abnormal delivery where the infant's buttocks or lower extremities deliver first is called a:
A) shoulder dystocia. **B)** prolapsed cord.
C) breech birth. **D)** sunny-side-up birth.
[Reference text page 530]

17. If the infant is having difficulty exiting the birth canal because the shoulder is wedged under the mother's pubic bone, the EMT-Basic should:
A) support the head.
B) put the mother in the McRobert's position.
C) have a second EMT-Basic apply some pressure above the pubic bone.
D) do all of the above.
[Reference text page 529]

18. Always suction the infant's airway in the mouth first, then in the nostrils.
A) True **B)** False
[Reference text page 524]

19. If you need to temporarily delay delivery due to a complication in the field, the EMT-Basic can try to:
A) place the mother in the Trendelenburg position.
B) pack the vagina.
C) place the mother in the knee-chest position.
D) have the mother stand.
[Reference text page 531]

20. Dark green fetal waste material found in the amniotic fluid is called:
A) cervical fluid. **B)** meconium. **C)** fetal blood. **D)** bile from the fetus.
[Reference text page 531]

21. If the amniotic fluid is greenish, you should stimulate the infant's breathing as soon as possible.
A) True **B)** False
[Reference text page 531]

22. Uterine massage can help decrease uterine:
A) cancer. **B)** infection. **C)** bleeding. **D)** swelling.
[Reference text page 527]

23. Shoulder dystocia can be assessed once crowning is complete.
A) True **B)** False
[Reference text page 529]

24. Shoulder dystocia can lead to:
A) death. **B)** brain damage. **C)** bone fracture. **D)** all of the above.
[Reference text page 529]

25. One danger in a breech delivery is deprivation of ________ to the fetus.
A) oxygen **B)** sugar **C)** blood **D)** warmth
[Reference text page 530]

26. When you recognize a breech birth, you must try to delay delivery until the fetus has been turned around.
A) True **B)** False
[Reference text page 530]

27. A common complication in a multiple birth is:
A) late delivery.
B) use of fertility medicine.
C) breech delivery of both infants.
D) breech delivery of one infant.
[Reference text page 532]

28. When a newborn's breathing is shallow, you should immediately evaluate the APGAR score to characterize the problem.
A) True **B)** False
[Reference text page 534]

29. Tactile stimulation helps to initiate a good ________ effort in a newborn.
A) feeding **B)** warming **C)** breathing **D)** sucking
[Reference text page 526]

30. A newborn has good breathing effort and a pulse of 98. The EMT-Basic should:
A) begin assisted artificial ventilations.
B) evaluate the APGAR score.
C) begin chest compressions.
D) assess the patient's color.
[Reference text page 533]

31. A healthy-looking newborn with good breathing effort and pulse exhibits a bluish trunk color. The EMT-Basic should:
A) begin assisted artificial ventilations.
B) evaluate the APGAR score.
C) begin chest compressions.
D) administer free-flow oxygen.
[Reference text page 533]

32. Artificial ventilation affects the breathing rate, not the heart rate.
A) True **B)** False
[Reference text page 537]

33. An infant born before the ________ week is considered premature.
A) 22nd **B)** 25th **C)** 34th **D)** 38th
[Reference text page 532]

34. It is important to immediately examine the genitalia of a possible sexual assault victim as part of the medical evidentiary exam.
A) True **B)** False
[Reference text pages 538–539]

35. You have a 25-year-old female patient who is six months pregnant. She has suffered penetrating trauma as a result of a knife attack. How should you transport her?
A) Normally, in c-spine. **B)** On her left side in c-spine.
C) On her right side in c-spine. **D)** Prone in c-spine.
[Reference text page 518]

36. Generally speaking, the best initial EMT-Basic response to meconium is to:
A) suction immediately.
B) stimulate the baby, then suction.
C) stimulate the baby, open the airway, restimulate as necessary, then suction.
D) call the base station for advice.
[Reference text page 531]

37. Eclampsia is a/n ________ emergency.
A) harmless **B)** ectopic **C)** life-threatening **D)** traumatic
[Reference text page 517]

38. When sizing up a scene and taking a history, it is important to determine if female patients are possibly pregnant. Why?
A) Some women may not know they are pregnant.
B) Pregnancy is generally life threatening.
C) Pregnancy often causes maternal mortality.
D) Pregnancy generally results in ectopic pregnancy.
[Reference text page 512]

39. The EMT-Basic should ________ perform an internal vaginal assessment of the mother.
A) possibly **B)** not **C)** always **D)** routinely
[Reference text page 512]

40. The "bag of waters" is also known as the:
A) uterus. **B)** placenta. **C)** umbilical sac. **D)** amniotic sac.
[Reference text page 508]

41. The second stage of labor is characterized by:
A) the fetus descending through the dilated cervix and vagina.
B) the contractions increasing in strength and frequency.
C) delivery of the placenta from the birth canal.
D) the passage of a clump of blood-tinged mucus.
[Reference text page 511]

42. How should the EMT-Basic transport a patient who presents with a prolapsed cord?
A) in a supine position **B)** in a left lateral position
C) in a right lateral position **D)** in a knee-chest position
[Reference text pages 528–529]

43. An EMT-Basic should do all of the following when assessing a women in labor EXCEPT:
A) scene size-up and initial assessment.
B) ask her questions about the pregnancy.
C) stay calm and reassure the patient.
D) perform an internal vaginal assessment.
[Reference text page 512]

44. Since newborns can lose heat quickly, an EMT-Basic should:
A) run warm water over the infant's chest and limbs.
B) dry and wrap the infant in a warm blanket.
C) dry and wrap the infant in the wet linens.
D) transport the infant without warming techniques.
[Reference text pages 526–527]

45. Hypotension in the third trimester mother when she lies down is usually due to:
A) eclampsia.
B) a compressed vena cava.
C) a normally decreased blood volume.
D) a hyperactive fetus.
[Reference text page 517]

CASE STUDIES

Use a separate piece of paper to answer the case study questions. Number your answers with the case study number and question letter (1A, 1B, etc.).

PREDELIVERY EMERGENCIES

1. You are dispatched to a small apartment complex. On arrival, you find a 26 year-old woman complaining of lower abdominal pain and moderate vaginal bleeding.
A) What questions would you ask the woman?

The patient informs you that her L.M.P. was seventeen weeks ago. She tells you that she took a home pregnancy test, which showed she was pregnant. Upon questioning, you discover that the patient has had several prior miscarriages. The patient becomes emotionally distressed during your examination.
B) What are appropriate treatment steps for this patient?

2. You arrive at a house in a rural neighborhood to find a 32-year-old woman complaining of severe abdominal pain. The patient is obviously pregnant and tells you her due date is three weeks away. She states she has a small amount of vaginal bleeding, but the pain is sharp and almost unbearable.
A) What conditions might this represent?
B) What is your appropriate course of action?

3. You are dispatched to a call in a rural part of your service area. On arrival, you find a 20-year-old pregnant female who is nearing her due date. She is experiencing almost continuous contractions. She states that she had a bloody discharge several hours before. This is her third pregnancy, and she has two living children.

A) What signs would indicate that delivery is imminent?

On visual inspection, you see the wrinkled scalp of an infant bulging through the external genitalia. The mother tells you "the baby is coming" and she is going to push, whether you want her to or not.

B) What steps should you take to prepare for delivery?

4. You are called to transport an obstetrical patient to the local hospital. On arriving at the scene, you discover that the patient is three days past her due date. Contractions are two minutes apart. The bedsheets are stained where the patient's membranes ruptured, and you notice green staining. Upon physically examining the patient, you observe crowning.

A) Is delivery imminent?

B) As you deliver the head, you notice dark green staining around the mouth and nose. The head delivers without incident. What is the green staining and what does it represent?

C) What should you do for the meconium-stained newborn during delivery?

ABNORMAL DELIVERIES

5. You are dispatched to a residence you are very familiar with. The patient is a 14-year-old girl undergoing her first pregnancy. She has called 911 after numerous episodes of false labor, and her due date is still two months away. Upon arrival, the girl states she wants to go to the bathroom and initially refuses your request to examine her. Contractions are two to three minutes apart and appear regular, according to her boyfriend. She reluctantly agrees to let you examine her. You observe significant crowning, and her membranes rupture during your observation.

A) What is your best course of action in this situation?

B) Shortly after beginning transport to the local hospital, the fetus delivers normally. The newborn is extremely small and not breathing. What is your course of action?

KEY TERMS MATCHING

Assess your knowledge of the chapter key terms by matching the terms on the left to the definitions on the right.

______	**1.** Abortion	**(A)**	Female reproductive organ in which menstruation and fetal development occur; also womb
______	**2.** Amniotic (am-nee-OT-ik) Sac	**(B)**	Female genital structure; the lower portion of the birth canal
______	**3.** APGAR Score	**(C)**	Structure that connects the fetus to the placenta; contains arteries and veins responsible for the exchange of materials between fetal and maternal circulation
______	**4.** Breech Presentation	**(D)**	Maternal hypotension caused when the mother is lying on her back and the weight of the fetus compresses her inferior vena cava
______	**5.** Crowning	**(E)**	Discharge of small amount of blood-tinged mucus from the vagina at the onset of labor; also bloody show

______ **6.** Fetus

______ **7.** Gynecology

______ **8.** Labor

______ **9.** Limb Presentation

______ **10.** Meconium (meh-KO-ne-um)

______ **11.** Miscarriage

______ **12.** Obstetrics (ob-STET-rics)

______ **13.** Perineum (pair-eh-NEE-em)

______ **14.** Placenta

______ **15.** Presenting Part

______ **16.** Prolapsed Cord

______ **17.** Show

______ **18.** Supine Hypotensive Syndrome

______ **19.** Umbilical (um-BILL-ik-ul) Cord

______ **20.** Uterus

______ **21.** Vagina

(F) Presentation of the umbilical cord before the infant's head at delivery; may cause fetal death due to constriction of blood flow through the cord.

(G) The part of a newborn that comes out of the birth canal first

(H) Organ that enables the exchange of nutrients, oxygen, and metabolic wastes between the maternal and fetal circulatory systems

(I) The area of skin between the vagina and anus in females and between the scrotum and anus in males

(J) The medical specialty concerned with the care of women during pregnancy and childbirth

(K) The medical specialty concerned with conditions of the female reproductive organs

(L) Dark green fetal waste material that passes into the amniotic fluid; if inhaled, it will cause fetal distress

(M) Abnormal delivery in which a limb of the infant is the initial part to deliver through the birth canal

(N) Physical processes of childbirth; begins with uterine contractions and leads to delivery of the fetus and the placenta

(O) Delivery of an embryo or fetus prior to viability; spontaneous abortion

(P) Developing, unborn offspring in the uterus; called an embryo for the first eight weeks after conception

(Q) The stage of delivery in which the head of the fetus is first visible as it stretches the vaginal opening

(R) Abnormal delivery in which the infant's buttocks or lower extremities are the presenting part; places infant at high risk for prolapsed cord and oxygen deprivation

(S) Method for assessing newborns based on five ratings: Appearance, Pulse, Grimace, Activity, and Respiration

(T) Sac that holds the fetus suspended in amniotic fluid; also called "bag of waters"

(U) Delivery of the products of conception early in a pregnancy; may be spontaneous or medically induced

LABELING DIAGRAMS

NEWBORN RESUSCITATION MEASURES: FREQUENCIES AND PRIORITIES

Label the pyramid by filling in the sections that have been left blank.

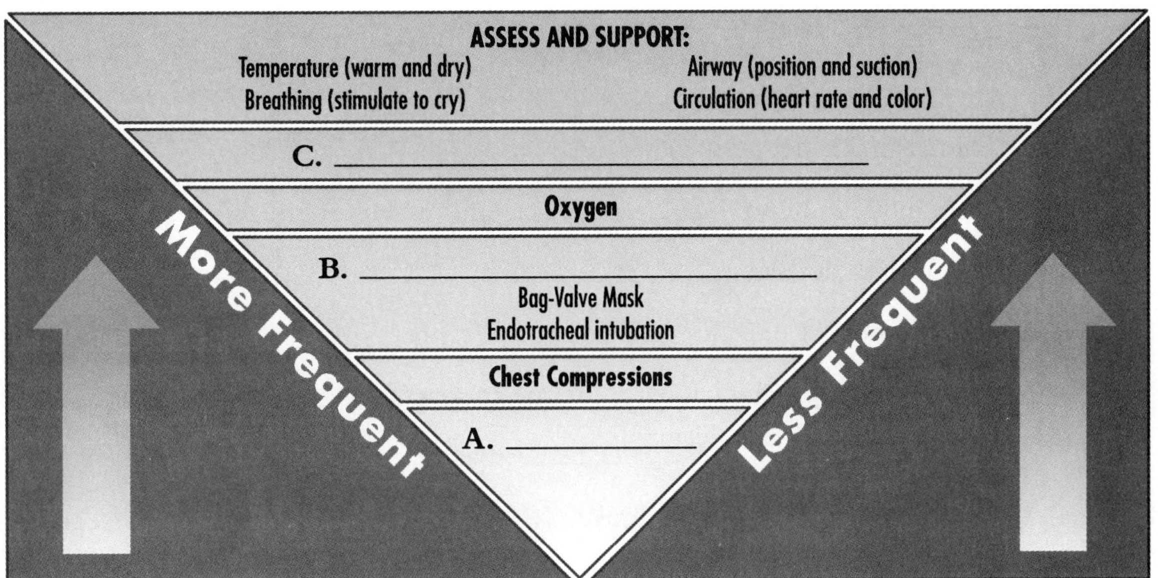

STAGES OF LABOR

Fill in the correct terms in the sequence below.

A. **First stage:** beginning of ______ to full cervical ______

B. **Second stage:** baby enters birth ______ and is born

C. **Third stage:** delivery of the ______

SKILLS CHECKLISTS

Check your knowledge of important EMT-B skills by marking off each step in the following skills sheet.

ASSESSMENT OF THE MOTHER FOR IMMINENT DELIVERY

- ☐ Take BSI precautions.
- ☐ Conduct an initial assessment.
- ☐ Obtain mother's history to determine active labor. History includes:
  - ☐ Length of term.
  - ☐ Number of previous pregnancies and births.
  - ☐ Frequency and duration of uterine contractions.
  - ☐ Recent vaginal discharge or hemorrhage.
  - ☐ Whether or not "water broke" yet.
  - ☐ Presence of strain or urge to move bowels.
- ☐ With mother's permission, examine for crowning.
- ☐ Feel for uterine contractions when she says she is having one.
- ☐ Take a set of vitals and make decision: prepare for delivery or begin transport.

(reprinted from *Pocket Reference for The EMT-B and First Responder* by Bob Elling, Prentice Hall, 1999)

D.O.T. OBJECTIVES CHECKLIST

Use the following list of knowledge objectives to check what you've learned. Check off only those objectives that you feel you completely understand and have mastered. For any objectives not checked, go back and review that section of the text chapter. Textbook page references have been provided to help you review the text material.

- ☐ Identify the following structures: uterus, vagina, fetus, placenta, umbilical cord, amniotic sac, perineum. *(p. 508)*
- ☐ Identify and explain the use of the contents of an obstetrics kit. *(p. 522)*
- ☐ Identify predelivery emergencies. *(p. 514)*

- [ ] State indications of an imminent delivery. *(p. 510)*
- [ ] Differentiate the emergency medical care provided to a patient with predelivery emergencies from a normal delivery. *(p. 514)*
- [ ] State the steps in the predelivery preparation of the mother. *(p. 523)*
- [ ] Establish the relationship between body substance isolation and childbirth. *(p. 523)*
- [ ] State the steps to assist in the delivery. *(p. 523)*
- [ ] Describe care of the baby as the head appears. *(p. 523)*
- [ ] Describe how and when to cut the umbilical cord. *(p. 526)*
- [ ] Discuss the steps in the delivery of the placenta. *(p. 526)*
- [ ] List the steps in the emergency medical care of the mother post-delivery. *(p. 526)*
- [ ] Summarize neonatal resuscitation procedures. *(p. 535)*
- [ ] Describe the procedures for the following abnormal deliveries: breech birth, prolapsed cord, limb presentation. *(p. 528)*
- [ ] Differentiate the special considerations for multiple births. *(p. 531)*
- [ ] Describe special considerations of meconium. *(p. 531)*
- [ ] Describe special considerations of a premature baby. *(p. 532)*
- [ ] Discuss the emergency medical care of a patient with a gynecological emergency. *(p. 537)*

CHAPTER 19

Bleeding and Shock

CHAPTER 19 SUMMARY

Bleeding is a common sign of traumatic injury. Severe bleeding can result in shock or hypoperfusion. The body will normally control bleeding by constricting of blood vessels and clotting. Arterial bleeding, identified by distinct spurting and bright red color, is difficult to control. This type of bleeding is often a life-threatening injury. Venous bleeding is usually easier to control, but significant blood loss is possible. Bleeding is controlled by applying direct pressure, elevation, pressure points, or a tourniquet as a last resort.

The use of the pneumatic anti-shock garment is discussed and demonstrated in this chapter. Its use is controversial and should follow local EMS system protocols.

Most serious bleeding is internal, making the assessment of shock a very important skill of the EMT-Basic. Always consider internal bleeding to be potentially life threatening. Suspect internal bleeding based on the signs and symptoms, and mechanism of injury.

Trauma patients develop shock or hypoperfusion from external and/or internal blood loss. This type of shock is referred to as hypovolemic, or hemorrhagic, shock.

REVIEW QUESTIONS

Please circle the best answer for each question.

1. The average adult male has ________ liters of circulating blood.
   A) 2 **B)** 4 **C)** 6 **D)** 8
   [Reference text page 549]

2. The sudden loss of 1000 mL of blood in an adult is considered serious.
   A) True **B)** False
   [Reference text page 549]

3. A 1-year-old has approximately ________ mL of blood.
   A) 200 **B)** 500 **C)** 800 **D)** 1000
   [Reference text page 549]

4. Methods of bleeding control include:
   A) direct pressure. **B)** elevation. **C)** pressure points. **D)** all of the above.
   [Reference text page 551]

5. Perfusion is the adequate circulation of blood through an organ structure.
   A) True **B)** False
   [Reference text page 548]

6. A steady stream of dark blood flows continuously from a/an:
   A) capillary. **B)** vein. **C)** artery. **D)** lymph node.
   [Reference text page 550]

7. Bleeding that occurs from an abrasion to the outer layers of the skin is called:
   A) capillary. **B)** venous.
   C) arterial. **D)** none of the above.
   [Reference text page 550]

8. The left and right anterior tibial arteries supply blood to the lower forearm.
   A) True **B)** False
   [Reference text page 553]

9. Of each of the following methods of bleeding control, which should be used first?
   A) tourniquet **B)** splints **C)** pressure points **D)** elevation
   [Reference text page 551]

10. Although its use is controversial, PASG may be helpful in which condition(s)?
A) Anaphylactic shock
B) Hypotension due to suspected pelvic fracture
C) Severe traumatic hypotension
D) Any of the above
[Reference text page 554]

11. To control bleeding located in the lower extremities, compress the brachial artery against the humerus.
A) True **B)** False
[Reference text pages 552-53]

CD-ROM LINK: *Review the* Arterial Bleeding *video in Chapter 19 of the MedEMT CD-ROM.*

12. Internal bleeding can:
A) be missed if not suspected.
B) result from blunt trauma.
C) cause abdominal distention.
D) do all of the above.
[Reference text page 560]

13. The PASG is contraindicated in each of the following cases EXCEPT:
A) cardiac tamponade.
B) acute myocardial infarction.
C) anaphylactic shock.
D) pulmonary edema.
[Reference text page 554]

14. A nosebleed is usually not serious, but significant blood loss is possible.
A) True **B)** False
[Reference text page 558]

15. The medical term for a nosebleed is:
A) rhinorear. **B)** epistaxis. **C)** epidural. **D)** rhinostasis.
[Reference text page 557]

16. Sinusitis or an upper respiratory tract infection can cause epistaxis.
A) True **B)** False
[Reference text page 557]

17. External bleeding is typically the most obvious and life-threatening injury the EMT-Basic will see.
A) True **B)** False
[Reference text page 548]

18. Application of a tourniquet:
   A) involves using a piece of wire.
   B) is an initial step in bleeding control.
   C) is a last resort method.
   D) can be done by applying an air splint to the arm.
   [Reference text page 556]

19. Signs of blunt trauma include all of the following EXCEPT:
   A) abrasions. **B)** edema. **C)** contusions. **D)** deep, sharp cuts.
   [Reference text page 559]

20. When managing wounds spurting blood, wearing disposable gloves and protective eyewear adequately protects the EMT-Basic.
   A) True **B)** False
   [Reference text page 549]

CD-ROM LINK: *Review the* Bleeding Control *video in Chapter 19 of the MedEMT CD-ROM.*

21. When using elevation to control bleeding, the extremity should be kept level with the heart.
   A) True **B)** False
   [Reference text page 552]

22. The ________ artery pulse can be used to control bleeding in the upper extremities.
   A) radial **B)** femural **C)** brachial **D)** pedal
   [Reference text page 553]

23. When using a pressure point, you should compress the artery against the bone with your fingertips.
   A) True **B)** False
   [Reference text pages 552-53]

24. All three compartments of the PASG should be inflated for suspected pelvic or abdominal hemorrhage.
   A) True **B)** False
   [Reference text pages 553-55]

25. The PASG should only be removed under the direction of and in the presence of a:
   A) family member. **B)** physician. **C)** paramedic. **D)** witness.
   [Reference text page 555]

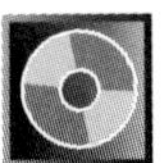

CD-ROM LINK: *Review the* Pneumatic Anti-Shock Garment *video in Chapter 19 of the MedEMT CD-ROM.*

26. Gunshot wounds frequently produce severe internal bleeding, severe external bleeding, shock, and respiratory compromise.
A) True **B)** False
[Reference text page 559]

27. Other than direct pressure, what can reduce the amount of bleeding from an injured extremity?
A) Vasopressors **B)** Elevation **C)** Supination **D)** Nitrates
[Reference text page 551]

28. If direct pressure and elevation fail to control bleeding, use ________ by compressing the artery against a bone.
A) pressure points
B) indirect elevation
C) systemic vasopressors
D) long bone elevations
[Reference text page 551]

29. Of the following signs and symptoms of shock, which is a late indicator?
A) Anxiety
B) Rapid pulse
C) Decreased systolic BP
D) Pale, cool, clammy skin
[Reference text page 563]

30. When is elevation of a bleeding, injured limb not recommended?
A) When direct pressure has already been applied to the injury
B) When the patient's breathing is rapid and shallow
C) When the patient has an allergy to bandaging materials
D) When the extremity is swollen, deformed, or very painful
[Reference text page 552]

CASE STUDIES

Use a separate piece of paper to answer the case study questions. Number your answers with the case study number and question letter (1A, 1B, etc.).

1. You respond to a frontal impact auto collision. The front seat unrestrained driver seems to have followed an up-and-over-pathway, as you notice there is visible damage to the steering wheel and windshield. The patient is initially unconscious as you approach the vehicle.
A) List the suspected injuries that you may find in a patient involved in this type of collision.
B) The driver starts to wake up and speak to you. He is verbally responsive but not quite alert just yet. A state police officer, who has EMT-Basic training, is assisting you by maintaining cervical immobilization from the back seat. You perform an initial

assessment while your partner obtains baseline vital signs. What treatment do you plan to take with this patient based on what you know so far?

C) Your partner states the patient's pulse is rapid (at 130) and thready, respiratory rate is 28 and shallow, and blood pressure is 90/70. Upon rapid exam, you note blunt chest contusion as well as discoloration over the left upper quadrant. What are your concerns at this time?

D) How would you treat this patient?

2. You are dispatched to a private residence for a patient who has a nosebleed. Apparently the patient has been seen twice this past week in the emergency department for the same problem. She tells you that the doctor said to come right back if her nose started to bleed profusely. The patient has been bleeding for about two hours and is getting weak and nauseous. She also looks pale and is clammy.

A) What are some of the causes of epistasis?

B) What is the proper way to manage this patient?

3. You are treating a patient who has a deep laceration of the femoral artery from an accident with a chain saw.

A) What signs and symptoms would be early indicators of hypoperfusion or hypovolemic shock?

B) What signs and symptoms would be late indicators of hypovolemia or hypoperfusion?

KEY TERMS MATCHING

Assess your knowledge of the chapter key terms by matching the terms on the left to the definitions on the right.

_____ **1.** Epistaxis (ep-eh-STAK-ses)

_____ **2.** Hemorrhagic (hem-or-AJ-ik) Shock

_____ **3.** Hypovolemic Shock

_____ **4.** Pressure Point

_____ **5.** Tourniquet

(A) Shock caused by inadequate circulatory volume; may be due to loss of blood or depletion of other body fluids

(B) A device that is wrapped around an extremity to prevent blood flow to or from the distal area

(C) A place where an artery passes near the surface of the body and over a bone; pressure here can stop or reduce bleeding

(D) Hemorrhage from the nose; a nosebleed

(E) Hypoperfusion syndrome caused by excessive blood loss; a type of hypovolemic shock; the most common cause of shock in a trauma patient

LABELING DIAGRAM

Fill in the blanks in the diagram that follows with the correct artery names.

PRESSURE POINTS

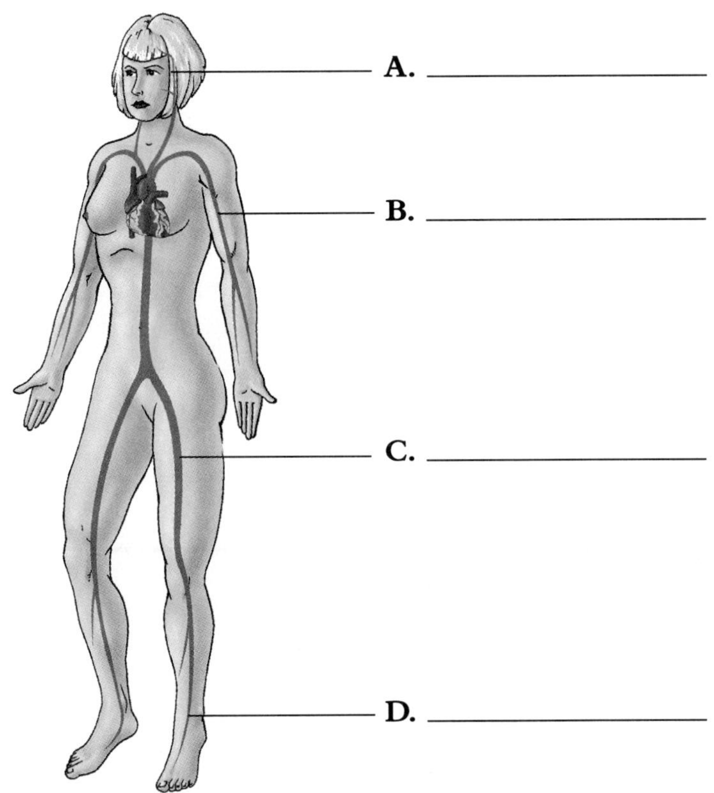

SKILLS CHECKLISTS

Check your knowledge of important EMT-B skills by marking off each step in the following skills sheets.

BLEEDING CONTROL/SHOCK MANAGEMENT

- [ ] Take BSI precautions.
- [ ] Apply direct pressure to wound.
- [ ] Elevate the extremity.
- [ ] Apply a dressing to wound.
- [ ] If wound continues to bleed, apply an additional dressing to wound.

- [ ] If wound continues to bleed, locate and apply pressure to appropriate arterial pressure point.
- [ ] Apply high-concentration oxygen.
- [ ] Properly position patient.
- [ ] Initiate steps to prevent heat loss from patient.
- [ ] Indicate need for immediate transport.

APPLICATION OF PASG

- [ ] Take BSI precautions.
- [ ] Assure patient meets local protocol for PASG.
- [ ] Check for contraindications (e.g., pulmonary edema or penetrating chest injury).
- [ ] Remove clothing and check for sharp objects.
- [ ] Quickly assess areas that will be under PASG.
- [ ] Position PASG with top of abdominal section at or below last set of ribs.
- [ ] Secure PASG around patient.
- [ ] Attach hoses.
- [ ] Check patient's blood pressure.
- [ ] Begin inflation sequence.
- [ ] Stop inflation sequence at 106 mm Hg or pop-off valve.
- [ ] Operate PASG to maintain air pressure in device.
- [ ] Reassess patient's vital signs.

WARNING: Do not actually inflate a PASG on a mock victim in class.

NOTE: MAST (military antishock trousers) is another name for the PASG.

(reprinted from *Pocket Reference for The EMT-B and First Responder* by Bob Elling, Prentice Hall, 1999)

D.O.T. OBJECTIVES CHECKLIST

Use the following list of knowledge objectives to check what you've learned. Check off only those objectives that you feel you completely understand and have mastered. For any objectives not checked, go back and review that section of the text chapter. Textbook page references have been provided to help you review the text material.

- [ ] List the structures and functions of the circulatory system. *(p. 548)*
- [ ] Differentiate between arterial, venous, and capillary bleeding. *(p. 550)*
- [ ] State methods of emergency medical care of external bleeding. *(p. 551)*
- [ ] Establish the relationship between body substance isolation and bleeding. *(p. 549)*
- [ ] Establish the relationship between airway management and the trauma patient. *(p. 551)*
- [ ] Establish the relationship between mechanism of injury and internal bleeding. *(p. 558)*
- [ ] List the signs of internal bleeding. *(p. 558)*
- [ ] List the steps in the emergency medical care of the patient with signs and symptoms of internal bleeding. *(p. 560)*
- [ ] List signs and symptoms of shock (hypoperfusion). *(p. 562)*
- [ ] State the steps in the emergency medical care of the patient with signs and symptoms of shock (hypoperfusion). *(p. 562)*

CHAPTER 20

Soft Tissue Injuries

CHAPTER 20 SUMMARY

Soft tissue injuries include both closed (blunt) and open injuries (penetrating). A hematoma and a contusion are examples of closed injuries. Lacerations, abrasions, avulsions, amputations, and punctures are open injuries. Crush injuries may be open or closed.

Special types of soft tissue injuries include: chest wounds, eviscerations, impaled objects, amputations, and open neck injuries. Chest wounds should be covered with an occlusive dressing to eliminate additional air from entering the chest cavity. Eviscerations should be covered with sterile, moist dressing and secured in place. Do not attempt to "stuff the contents back" into the abdominal cavity. Impaled objects need to be left in place and the object secured with a bulky dressing. The only time an impaled object is removed in the field is if it interferes with the airway, chest compressions, or prevents transport.

Amputations are another type of special soft tissue injury. The EMT-Basic should wrap the amputated part in a sterile dressing, place in plastic, and keep it cool. Avoid freezing the amputated part as this will destroy the tissue. Transport the amputated part with the patient so they do not get separated, wasting precious time. Open neck injuries need to be covered immediately with an occlusive dressing to prevent air from entering the large vein, creating an embolism.

This chapter also covers burns. Burns can be superficial, partial thickness, or full thickness. Consider a burn to be critical if it falls into one of the following types of injuries: burns to the hands, feet, face or genitalia; burns associated with a respiratory injury; full-thickness burns over more than 10% of the body; partial-thickness burns over more than 30% of the body; burn complicated by a painful, swollen, or deformed extremity; moderate burns in children under 5 years or adults over 55 years; and burns encompassing an entire body part.

When caring for a burned patient, always stop the burning first. Remove jewelry or clothing if possible. Cover burns with dry, sterile dressings to prevent infection. Because burned skin loses its ability to regulate temperature, treat infants and children for generalized hypothermia as well.

When dealing with chemical burns, take all necessary safety precautions. Brush off any dry powder. Flush continuously with large amounts of water. When caring for patients with electrical burns, be alert to the possibility of cardiac arrest. Recognize that electrical burns may cause very little external injury. However, severe internal injuries may be present.

REVIEW QUESTIONS

Please circle the best answer for each question.

1. The dermis is generally thinner than the epidermis.
   A) True **B)** False
   [Reference text page 572]

2. The functions of the integumentary system are: protection, sensation, excretion, vitamin D synthesis, and ________ regulation.
   A) vessel **B)** excretion **C)** temperature **D)** motor
   [Reference text page 572]

3. The layer of the skin that consists of mostly fatty cells and connective tissue is called the:
   A) epidermis. **B)** dermis.
   C) subcutaneous layer. **D)** cutaneous layer.
   [Reference text page 572]

4. A patient who has sustained a bruise can expect the wound to be ________ in 5 to 7 days.
   A) red **B)** purple **C)** green **D)** yellow
   [Reference text page 573]

5. A patient who has sustained a bruise can expect the wound to be ________ in 1 to 2 days.
   A) red **B)** purple **C)** green **D)** brown
   [Reference text page 573]

6. Swelling or mass of blood caused by breaking of a blood vessel is called a hematoma.
   A) True **B)** False
   [Reference text page 574]

7. A linear, or stellate, cut in the skin is called a/n:
   A) abrasion. **B)** avulsion. **C)** crush injury. **D)** laceration.
   [Reference text page 575]

8. A cold pack should be placed directly on the wound to reduce swelling.
   A) True **B)** False
   [Reference text page 575]

9. Aside from the oozing of blood from capillaries, abrasions have a potential for:
   A) massive hemorrhage. **B)** underlying blunt trauma.
   C) serious infection. **D)** none of the above.
   [Reference text page 576]

10. A laceration is best described as a puncture wound through the skin and underlying tissue resulting from piercing with a sharp object.
A) True **B)** False
[Reference text page 577]

11. An injury where the skin is pulled off an extremity is called a/n:
A) degloving. **B)** laceration. **C)** abrasion. **D)** puncture.
[Reference text page 577]

12. There is a potential for internal bleeding or life-threatening injuries to internal organs from a/n:
A) laceration. **B)** puncture. **C)** abrasion. **D)** avulsion.
[Reference text page 577]

13. A bullet's exit wound is usually smaller than the entrance wound.
A) True **B)** False
[Reference text page 578]

14. Extreme pressure from blunt trauma usually causes a ________ injury.
A) blunt **B)** puncture **C)** crush **D)** degloving
[Reference text page 580]

15. Air in the chest cavity between the lung and chest wall is called a/an:
A) hemothorax. **B)** pneumothorax. **C)** evisceration. **D)** air embolism.
[Reference text page 582]

16. Signs and symptoms of an open pneumothorax include:
A) sucking sound on inspiration. **B)** respiratory distress.
C) subcutaneous emphysema. **D)** all of the above.
[Reference text page 582]

17. A sign or symptom found in a tension pneumothorax, yet not present with a pneumothorax is:
A) respiratory distress. **B)** decreased breath sounds on one side.
C) jugular venous distention. **D)** none of the above.
[Reference text page 583]

18. The treatment of an open pneumothorax includes an occlusive bandage.
A) True **B)** False
[Reference text page 583]

19. Signs and symptoms of a hemothorax include:
A) respiratory distress.
B) associated rib fractures.
C) absent breath sounds on the injured side.
D) all of the above.
[Reference text page 584]

20. Bleeding within the pericardium from an injury to the heart is called:
A) a hemothorax. **B)** a tension pneumothorax.
C) a cardiac tamponade. **D)** none of the above.
[Reference text page 584]

21. When abdominal organs protrude through a laceration, this is called a/an:
A) puncture. **B)** tamponade. **C)** evisceration. **D)** crush injury.
[Reference text page 585]

22. When treating protruding abdominal organs, have the patient flex his or her knees and hips to relieve tension on the abdominal wall.
A) True **B)** False
[Reference text page 585]

23. In many cases, a patient will have already pulled out an impaled object prior to the arrival of EMS personnel.
A) True **B)** False
[Reference text page 586]

24. Because both eyes move together, bandage both eyes if the patient has an impaled object or injury to one eye.
A) True **B)** False
[Reference text page 588]

25. With large open neck injuries, the EMT-Basic should suspect:
A) massive hemorrhage. **B)** a potential air embolism.
C) a potential spine injury. **D)** all of the above.
[Reference text page 589]

26. Burn severity depends on each of the following factors EXCEPT:
A) percentage of body surface burned.
B) depth and degree of the burn.
C) the type of object that was burning.
D) the patient's age and preexisting medical condition.
[Reference text page 591]

27. A third-degree burn is also called a ________ burn.
A) full-thickness
B) complete-destruction
C) partial-thickness
D) superficial
[Reference text page 591]

28. A patient has sustained second-degree burns on the front of his torso and the front of his right leg. What percentage of his body surface area is burned?
A) 18
B) 27
C) 36
D) 45
[Reference text page 593]

29. A patient has sustained a third-degree burn on the back of her torso and the back of her left arm. What percentage of her body surface area is burned?
A) 9
B) 18
C) 22.5
D) 36
[Reference text page 593]

30. Most commonly, open soft tissue injuries are caused by an injury from the inside outward.
A) True
B) False
[Reference text page 572]

31. What is the term for injuries received from a force that acts on the body, but does not physically penetrate the skin?
A) Blunt force trauma
B) Localized trauma
C) Piston trauma
D) Degloving injury
[Reference text pages 573-74xxs]

CASE STUDIES

Use a separate piece of paper to answer the case study questions. Number your answers with the case study number and question letter (1A, 1B, etc.).

LACERATIONS

1. You respond to an assault in an alleyway downtown late on a Friday night. Your patient is a well-dressed middle-aged businessman who apparently was assaulted as he was making a night drop in the bank for his liquor store. The patient states the attacker grabbed him from behind and when he resisted handing over the money bag, the attacker slashed his neck. The patient was seen by a passing motorist struggling into the alleyway.
A) Aside from bleeding control, what is an immediate concern with this type of injury?
B) What other treatment should this patient receive?

BURNS

2. You respond to a private residence for a patient who attempted to start his gas grill with a cup of gasoline. There was a quick flash and his face, chest and both arms were burned to the second degree. Upon your arrival, his family members have removed his T-shirt and are hosing him down.
   A) Approximately what percentage of his body is burned if the front of his head, both entire arms, and his chest are all burned?
   B) Should this patient be taken to a burn center?
   C) Once the patient is cooled off with the hose, what type of bandage should be applied?

AMPUTATIONS

3. You respond to the subway for a "man-under" call. There were many people in the station and a 37-year-old male was pushed off the platform just prior to the arrival of the train. Apparently he was not able to hide completely under the platform, since his right leg was run over by the train.
   A) Would you expect severe bleeding from the amputation?
   B) After the scene has been made safe and the power turned off, you climb down onto the tracks to evaluate the patient. Although the wound is grotesque, what is your initial concern for the patient?
   C) What additional treatment should be done?

KEY TERMS MATCHING

Assess your knowledge of the chapter key terms by matching the terms on the left to the definitions on the right.

_____ **1.** Abrasion

_____ **2.** Amputation

_____ **3.** Avulsion

_____ **4.** Bandage

_____ **5.** Closed Soft Tissue Injury

_____ **6.** Contusion

_____ **7.** Crush Injury

(A) Damage to muscle, vessels or skin; outer skin remains intact

(B) Burn involving only the top layer of the skin (epidermis); first-degree burn

(C) Free of microorganisms (bacteria, viruses, spores) that can cause infection

(D) Air in the chest cavity between the lung and chest wall

(E) Burn involving both the epidermis and the dermis, but not involving underlying tissue; second-degree burn

(F) Open wound in which muscle, vessels, and/or skin is damaged

______ **8.** Dressing

______ **9.** Evisceration (eh-VIS-er-ay-shun)

______ **10.** Full-Thickness Burn

______ **11.** Hematoma (hee-muh-TO-muh)

______ **12.** Impaled Object

______ **13.** Laceration

______ **14.** Occlusive Dressing

______ **15.** Open Soft Tissue Injury

______ **16.** Partial-Thickness Burn

______ **17.** Pneumothorax (NU-mo-THOR-aks)

______ **18.** Sterile

______ **19.** Superficial Burn

(G) A dressing that forms an airtight seal; often applied to open neck, chest or abdominal wounds; items commonly used include defibrillation pads or thick plastic wrap

(H) Wound or irregular tear of the skin

(I) An object that pierces the skin

(J) Swelling or mass of blood caused by breaking a blood vessel

(K) Protective covering applied directly to a soft tissue wound

(L) Abdominal organs (viscera) protruding through an open wound

(M) Burn extending through all dermal layers; may involve the subcutaneous tissues, muscle, bone, or organs; third-degree burn

(N) Open or closed soft tissue injury resulting from bilateral blunt trauma forces

(O) Bruise; a wound in which the epidermis remains intact, but the cells and blood vessels in the dermis become damaged

(P) A superficial scrape injury to the top layer of skin

(Q) Holds a dressing in place (self-adherent, gauze rolls, triangular, air splint)

(R) A tearing off or tearing away of a skin flap or body part

(S) Removal of an extremity through trauma or surgery

LABELING DIAGRAM

Label the diagram with the percentage of body surface area to which each line is pointing.

RULE OF NINES

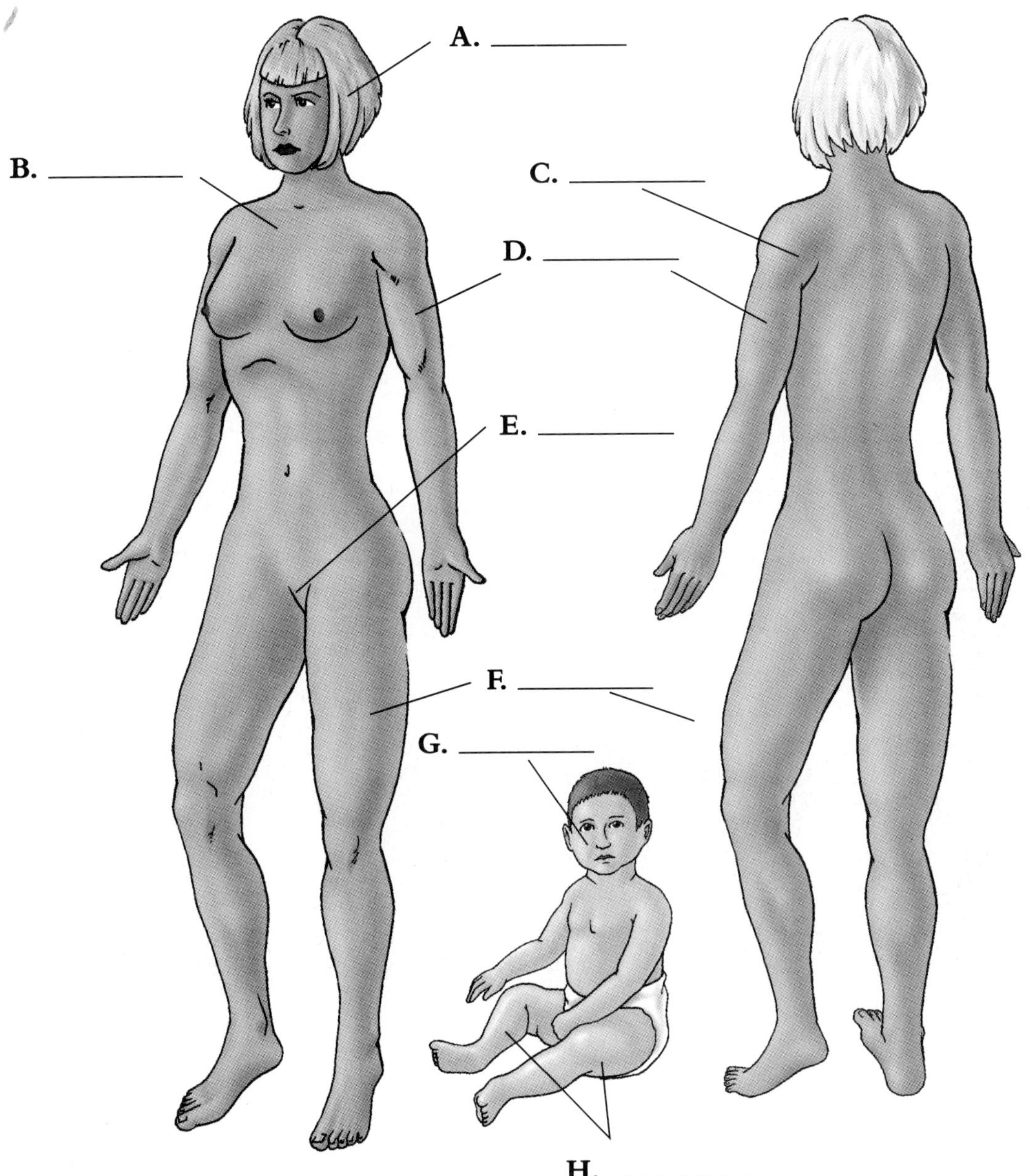

SKILLS CHECKLIST

Check your knowledge of important EMT-B skills by marking off each step in the following skills sheet.

BLEEDING CONTROL

- ☐ Take BSI precautions.
- ☐ Apply direct pressure to wound.
- ☐ Elevate the extremity.
- ☐ Apply a dressing to wound.
- ☐ If wound continues to bleed, apply an additional dressing to wound.
- ☐ If wound continues to bleed, locate and apply pressure to appropriate arterial pressure point.
- ☐ Apply high-concentration oxygen.
- ☐ Properly position patient.
- ☐ Initiate steps to prevent heat loss from patient.
- ☐ Indicate need for immediate transport.

(reprinted from *Pocket Reference for The EMT-B and First Responder* by Bob Elling, Prentice Hall, 1999)

D.O.T. OBJECTIVES CHECKLIST

Use the following list of knowledge objectives to check what you've learned. Check off only those objectives that you feel you completely understand and have mastered. For any objectives not checked, go back and review that section of the text chapter. Textbook page references have been provided to help you review the text material.

- ☐ State the major functions of the skin. *(p. 572)*
- ☐ List the layers of the skin. *(p. 572)*
- ☐ Establish the relationship between body substance isolation (BSI) and soft tissue injuries. *(p. 572)*
- ☐ List the types of closed soft tissue injuries. *(p. 573)*

- [ ] Describe the emergency medical care of the patient with a closed soft tissue injury. *(p. 574)*
- [ ] State the types of open soft tissue injuries. *(p. 575)*
- [ ] Describe the emergency medical care of the patient with an open soft tissue injury. *(p. 580)*
- [ ] Discuss the emergency medical care considerations for a patient with a penetrating chest injury. *(p. 582)*
- [ ] State the emergency medical care considerations for a patient with an open wound to the abdomen. *(p. 585)*
- [ ] Differentiate the care of an open wound to the chest from an open wound to the abdomen. *(p. 585)*
- [ ] List the classifications of burns. *(p. 591)*
- [ ] Define superficial burn. *(p. 591)*
- [ ] List the characteristics of a superficial burn. *(p. 591)*
- [ ] Define partial-thickness burn. *(p. 591)*
- [ ] List the characteristics of a partial-thickness burn. *(p. 591)*
- [ ] Define full-thickness burn. *(p. 591)*
- [ ] List the characteristics of a full-thickness burn. *(p. 591)*
- [ ] Describe the emergency medical care of the patient with a superficial burn. *(p. 595)*
- [ ] Describe the emergency medical care of the patient with a partial-thickness burn. *(p. 595)*
- [ ] Describe the emergency medical care of the patient with a full-thickness burn. *(p. 595)*

- [ ] List the functions of dressing and bandaging. *(p. 599)*
- [ ] Describe the purpose of a bandage. *(p. 600)*
- [ ] Describe the steps in applying a pressure dressing. *(p. 551)*
- [ ] Establish the relationship between airway management and the patient with chest injury, burns, blunt and penetrating injuries. *(p. 582)*
- [ ] Describe the effects of improperly applied dressings, splints, and tourniquets. *(p. 601)*
- [ ] Describe the emergency medical care of a patient with an impaled object. *(p. 586)*
- [ ] Describe the emergency medical care of a patient with an amputation. *(p. 589)*
- [ ] Describe the emergency care for a chemical burn. *(p. 595)*
- [ ] Describe the emergency care for an electrical burn. *(p. 598)*

CHAPTER 21

Musculoskeletal Injuries

CHAPTER 21 SUMMARY

When caring for a patient with a suspected musculoskeletal injury, determining whether the injury is a fracture, sprain, or strain is not important. Emergency treatment is based on the signs and symptoms of a painful, swollen, deformed extremity.

Splints prevent movement from bone fragments, bone ends, the adjacent joints, and angulated joints. Preventing motion reduces damage to muscles, nerves, and blood vessels. It prevents a closed injury from becoming an open one. Splints also help to control bleeding and pain.

Always immobilize the joint above and below the injury. Never secure a tie or strap directly over the injury. Use a splint on extremity injuries only if they are isolated. If you suspect a severe mechanism of injury and possible spinal injury, splint the extremity to the long backboard during spinal immobilization. Assess the injured extremity for the presence of distal pulses, motor movement, and sensation before and after splinting. If a deformity is severe or if the pulse is absent, you can attempt to straighten the extremity. Follow local protocols.

REVIEW QUESTIONS

Please circle the best answer for each question.

1. The key functions of the musculoskeletal system include:
   A) support. **B)** protection. **C)** movement. **D)** all of the above.
   [Reference text page 608]

2. The largest bone in the body is the:
   A) tibia. **B)** femur. **C)** humerus. **D)** spine.
   [Reference text page 608]

3. The management of all bone and joint injuries is very similar.
   A) True **B)** False
   [Reference text page 609]

CD-ROM LINK: *Refer to the* Broken Femur *video, which shows a team of EMT-Basics treating an elderly woman who has fallen in her home. This can be found in Chatper 21 of the MedEMT CD-ROM.*

4. A force that causes injury to a body part at the site of impact is called a/an ________ force.
   A) indirect **B)** twisting **C)** direct **D)** continuing
   [Reference text page 610]

5. A joint injury that involves stretching or tearing of a ligament is called a:
   A) dislocation. **B)** fracture. **C)** sprain. **D)** strain.
   [Reference text page 610]

6. A bone dislodged from its normal alignment in a joint is called a:
   A) dislocation. **B)** fracture. **C)** sprain. **D)** strain.
   [Reference text page 610]

7. A broken bone is a:
   A) fracture. **B)** dislocation. **C)** sprain. **D)** strain.
   [Reference text page 610]

8. A twisting force injury is common among athletes.
   A) True **B)** False
   [Reference text page 611]

9. A grating sensation or sound found in a fractured limb is called:
   A) subcutaneous emphysema. **B)** crackles.
   C) crepitation. **D)** rhonchi.
   [Reference text page 611]

10. What is an open fracture?
A) A broken bone with an open wound
B) Dislocation of bones at the joints
C) Penetrating wounds to joints
D) None of the above
[Reference text pages 609-10]

11. A transmitted force that causes injury some distance away from the point of impact is a/n:
A) twisting force. **B)** indirect force. **C)** direct force. **D)** indirect impact.
[Reference text page 610]

12. Deformity, angulation, pain, and tenderness are signs and symptoms of:
A) fractures. **B)** dislocations. **C)** sprains. **D)** any of the above.
[Reference text page 611]

13. Injuries to bones and joints usually do not require splinting before moving the patient.
A) True **B)** False
[Reference text page 613]

14. Reasons for splinting include:
A) reducing increased pain caused by movement of bone ends.
B) preventing excessive bleeding.
C) preventing compression of an artery.
D) all of the above.
[Reference text page 613]

15. Broken bone fragments can damage the surrounding tissue, including:
A) muscles. **B)** nerves. **C)** blood vessels. **D)** all of the above.
[Reference text page 613]

16. Reasons for splinting include all of the following EXCEPT:
A) prevention of excessive pain.
B) reducing the risk of paralysis.
C) it takes time to apply a splint.
D) preventing excessive bleeding.
[Reference text page 613]

CD-ROM LINK: *Refer to the* General Splinting Rules *video, which shows a demonstration of splinting the tibial fracture. This can be found in Chapter 21 of the MedEMT CD-ROM.*

17. Excessive movement during splinting may aggravate the injury.
A) True **B)** False
[Reference text page 615]

18. After applying a splint to a patient's limb, the EMT-Basic should assess the:
A) patient's vital signs.
B) patient's level of consciousness.
C) pulse, motor, & sensory function of limb.
D) none of the above.
[Reference text pages 615, 617]

19. Do not apply a traction splint if the:
A) femur is not broken.
B) lower leg or ankle is injured.
C) injury involves the hip.
D) all of the above.
[Reference text page 619]

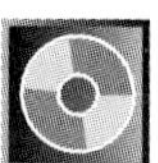

CD-ROM LINK: *Refer to the* Bipolar Traction Splint *video, which shows the steps in the application of the device. This can be found in Chapter 21 of the MedEMT CD-ROM.*

20. A unipolar traction splint can only be applied to one leg.
A) True
B) False
[Reference text page 620]

CASE STUDIES

Use a separate piece of paper to answer the case study questions. Number your answers with the case study number and question letter (1A, 1B, etc.).

1. You are called to the scene of a bad fall. When you arrive, the patient's wife is frantic. She explains that her husband fell off the ladder while cleaning the rain gutters, and she thinks he broke his leg. You and your partner put on your gloves as you approach a 35-year-old man lying on his back in his driveway. Due to the mechanism of injury, your partner maintains cervical immobilization while you perform a rapid trauma assessment. The patient, Robert, tells you that he fell 6 feet when he lost his footing at the top of the ladder. He landed on his left leg first, twisting it, and then hit the ground with his leg and buttocks. He denies head, neck, back injuries, or loss of consciousness, but complains of severe pain, swelling and deformity in his left thigh. You determine that his ABCs are stable and his injuries are localized to the left leg. The mid left thigh is painful, swollen, and deformed. His vital signs are as follows: BP 146/90, P 110, RR 24.
A) What is your next step in managing this patient?
B) Femur fractures can result in significant blood loss at the injury site. True or False?
C) What are the reasons for splinting injured extremities?
D) What type of splint would be beneficial in this patient?
E) What are indications and contraindications to a traction splint?
F) Describe the procedure for bipolar traction splinting.

2. You respond to a skating ring where you find a 12-year-old female patient who apparently twisted her ankle while skating. She is holding her ankle and crying from the pain. Your partner takes a set of baseline vitals while you continue to do the initial assessment followed by a focused trauma exam.
A) Should the skate be removed in the field?

B) She has a painful, deformed, swollen ankle. What should be done prior to applying a splint?

C) Besides immobilizing the bone ends with a splint, what else should the EMT-Basic do for this patient?

3. You are downhill skiing when suddenly a skier flies past you, appearing out of control. He goes off the trail into a tree. Fortunately he did not hit his head when he suddenly stopped after going airborne into the woods. As you approach him, you notice the bone sticking out from his right lower leg's ski pants as well as drops of blood in the snow. After sending a friend to alert the ski patrol, you begin to assess the patient. He says he previously broke the other leg but this is the first time the bone was sticking out. He is anxious and keeps moving around as you spend most of your energy trying to persuade him to keep the limb still to avoid any further injury.

A) What bones are most likely broken?

B) In what position should the long bone fracture be splinted?

C) Aside from applying a splint to the patient and skiing him down in the toboggan, what additional treatment do you feel is appropriate to do?

4. You arrive on the scene of an accident where a patient has fallen down a flight of stairs. Upon examination of the patient, it is apparent that his right midshaft femur has been fractured. Although the break is a closed fracture, the limb is starting to spasm and you are afraid of the movement causing an open fracture.

A) When would the traction splint be contraindicated for a patient with a femur fracture?

B) Can this type of injury involve significant blood loss?

C) Will the PASG be an acceptable splint for this injury?

KEY TERMS MATCHING

Assess your knowledge of the chapter key terms by matching the terms on the left to the definitions on the right.

______ **1.** Direct Force

______ **2.** Indirect Force

______ **3.** Splint

______ **4.** Twisting force

(A) Equipment used to prevent or reduce movement of body joints or injured tissue

(B) Occurs when one part of an extremity remains in place while the rest moves or twists

(C) A force that causes injury to a body part at the site of impact

(D) A transmitted force that causes injury some distance away from the point of impact

LABELING DIAGRAM

Write in the correct anatomical terms in the blanks.

DIRECT IMPACT INJURY

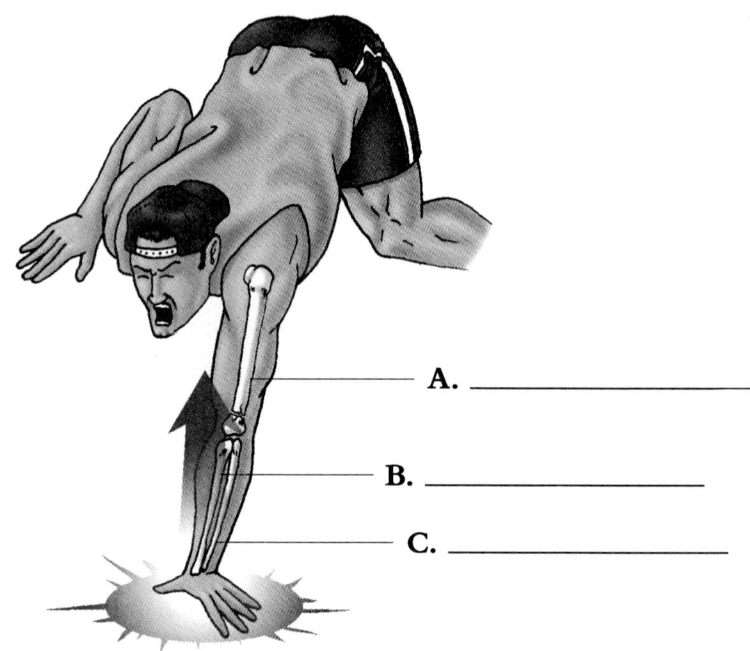

SKILLS CHECKLISTS

Check your knowledge of important EMT-B skills by marking off each step in the following skills sheets.

IMMOBILIZATION: LONG BONE

- [ ] Take BSI precautions.
- [ ] Direct application of manual stabilization.
- [ ] Assess distal pulses, motor ability, and sensory response (PMS).
- [ ] Measure splint.
- [ ] Apply splint.
- [ ] Immobilize joints above and below injury.

- [ ] Secure entire injured extremity from distal to proximal direction.
- [ ] Immobilize hand/foot in functional position.
- [ ] Reassess distal PMS.

REALIGNING AN EXTREMITY

- [ ] Take BSI precautions.
- [ ] Assess distal pulses, motor ability, and sensory response (PMS).
- [ ] Rescuer A grasps distal extremity, while Rescuer B places one hand above and below injury site.
- [ ] Rescuer B supports injury site, while Rescuer A pulls gentle manual traction in direction of long axis of body. If resistance is felt or if it appears that bone ends will come through skin, stop realignment and splint extremity in position found.
- [ ] If no resistance is felt, maintain gentle traction until extremity is properly splinted.
- [ ] Reassess distal PMS.

IMMOBILIZATION: JOINT INJURY

- [ ] Take BSI precautions.
- [ ] Direct application of manual stabilization of injury.
- [ ] Assess distal pulses, motor ability, and sensory response (PMS).
- [ ] Select proper splinting device.
- [ ] Immobilize the site of injury and the bones above and below.
- [ ] Reassess distal PMS.

IMMOBILIZATION: TRACTION SPLINT

- [ ] Take BSI precautions.
- [ ] Direct manual stabilization of injured leg.
- [ ] Assess distal pulses, motor ability, and sensory response (PMS).
- [ ] Direct application of manual traction.
- [ ] Adjust and position splint at the injured leg.

- [ ] Apply proximal securing device (e.g., ischial strap).
- [ ] Apply distal securing device (e.g., ankle hitch).
- [ ] Apply mechanical traction.
- [ ] Position and secure support straps.
- [ ] Reassess distal PMS.
- [ ] Secure patient's torso and traction splint to long backboard for transport.

APPLICATION OF PASG

- [ ] Take BSI precautions.
- [ ] Assure patient meets local protocol for PASG.
- [ ] Check for contraindications (e.g., pulmonary edema or penetrating chest injury).
- [ ] Remove clothing and check for sharp objects.
- [ ] Quickly assess areas that will be under PASG.
- [ ] Position PASG with top of abdominal section at or below last set of ribs.
- [ ] Secure PASG around patient.
- [ ] Attach hoses.
- [ ] Check patient's blood pressure.
- [ ] Begin inflation sequence.
- [ ] Stop inflation sequence at 106 mm Hg or pop-off valve.
- [ ] Operate PASG to maintain air pressure in device.
- [ ] Reassess patient's vital signs.

WARNING: Do not actually inflate a PASG on a mock victim in class.

NOTE: MAST (military antishock trousers) is another name for the PASG.

(reprinted from *Pocket Reference for The EMT-B and First Responder* by Bob Elling, Prentice Hall, 1999)

D.O.T. OBJECTIVES CHECKLIST

Use the following list of knowledge objectives to check what you've learned. Check off only those objectives that you feel you completely understand and have mastered. For any objectives not checked, go back and review that section of the text chapter. Textbook page references have been provided to help you review the text material.

- [ ] Describe the function of the muscular system. *(p. 608)*
- [ ] Describe the function of the skeletal system. *(p. 608)*
- [ ] List the major bones or bone groupings of the spinal column; the thorax; the upper extremities; the lower extremities. *(p. 608)*
- [ ] Differentiate between an open and a closed painful, swollen, deformed extremity. *(p. 609)*
- [ ] State the reasons for splinting. *(p. 613)*
- [ ] List the general rules of splinting. *(p. 615)*
- [ ] List the complications of splinting. *(p. 615)*
- [ ] List the emergency medical care for a patient with a painful, swollen, deformed extremity. *(p. 612)*

CHAPTER 22

Head and Spine Injuries

CHAPTER 22 SUMMARY

A patient may have a spinal injury even if he or she can walk, move his or her extremities, or feel normal sensation. Likewise, absence of pain in the back or spinal column does not rule out the possibility of injury. Management of airway and breathing are essential to the patient's survival and recovery from head or spine injuries.

Loss of movement or sensation in extremities is a key indication of spinal cord injury. Spinal cord injuries may cause paralysis and inadequate breathing. If the mechanism of injury suggests spinal injury, immediately control the cervical spine. Adequate immobilization is essential. This prevents worsening or aggravation of hidden spinal injuries during transport.

Apply a rigid cervical collar any time you suspect a spinal injury. To be effective, a rigid cervical collar must rest on the shoulder girdle. The rigid cervical collar alone does not adequately immobilize the spinal column. It must be used in conjunction with a long board, short board, or vest-type immobilization device.

The rigid short board and the flexible vest-style device (like the Kendrick Extrication Device, or KED) are interim devices used to stabilize the head, neck, and torso. Because the KED is a flexible piece of equipment, it can be used with contoured car seats or in other confined spaces where a short spine board will not fit. Whether a short spine board or a flexible vest is used, secure the torso first and head last.

Long board immobilization devices are full-body spinal immobilization devices.

Indicators of possible head injuries include alteration in mental status (especially combativeness), skull deformity, blood or CSF draining from the ears or nose, raccoon eyes, Battle's sign, contusions, lacerations, and hematomas.

Remove a helmet if it interferes with your ability to assess or manage the patient's airway or breathing, or if the helmet is loose. Most of the time the patient will have already removed the helmet prior to your arrival.

REVIEW QUESTIONS

Please circle the best answer for each question.

1. The brain and spinal cord are parts of the:
   A) automatic nervous system. **B)** central nervous system.
   C) peripheral nervous system. **D)** skeletal system.
   [Reference text page 632]

2. The sensory and motor nerves that extend from the brain throughout the body are part of the:
   A) automatic nervous system. **B)** central nervous system.
   C) peripheral nervous system. **D)** skeletal system.
   [Reference text page 632]

3. The skeletal system cushions and protects the central nervous system.
   A) True **B)** False
   [Reference text page 632]

4. The EMT-Basic must maintain a high index of suspicion for spine injuries in instances of:
   A) motor vehicle collisions. **B)** motorcycle accidents.
   C) diving accidents **D)** all of the above.
   [Reference text page 633]

CD-ROM LINK: *Review the* Fallen Climber *video in Chapter 22 of the MedEMT CD-ROM.*

5. Which of the following is not generally considered a high index of suspicion for spine injuries?
   A) Blunt trauma **B)** Chest trauma
   C) Hangings **D)** Unconscious trauma patients
   [Reference text page 633]

6. Extreme movement of the neck sideways can cause flexion injuries.
   A) True **B)** False
   [Reference text page 634]

7. Extreme stretching or pulling of the neck are the cause of ________ injuries.
   A) flexion **B)** lateral bending **C)** distraction **D)** compression
   [Reference text page 634]

8. A spinal injury caused when a strong force is transmitted up or down the length of the body is called a ________ injury.
   A) rotation **B)** flexion **C)** compression **D)** distraction
   [Reference text page 635]

9. The EMT-Basic should suspect cervical spine injury if the patient is injured above the clavicle.
   A) True **B)** False
   [Reference text page 635]

10. Which of the following is not a potential sign or symptom of a spine injury?
    A) Pain associated with movement
    B) Tenderness along the spine
    C) Lack of sensation on the right side of the body
    D) Numbness and tingling in the legs
    [Reference text page 635]

11. Abnormal sensation of tingling, numbness, burning, or coldness in the extremities is called:
    A) paraplegia. **B)** paraesthesia. **C)** transection. **D)** compression.
    [Reference text page 636]

12. Signs and symptoms of a spinal injury may include:
    A) incontinence. **B)** priapism.
    C) inadequate breathing. **D)** any of the above.
    [Reference text page 636]

CD-ROM LINK: *Review the* Spine Immobilization—Initial Physical Exam *video in Chapter 22 of the MedEMT CD-ROM.*

13. Whenever a potential spinal injury is suspected, regardless of the location of injury, you must secure the entire spinal column.
    A) True **B)** False
    [Reference text page 636]

14. A sensory and motor exam should be completed:
    A) before spinal immobilization.
    B) after spinal immobilization.
    C) only if you are sure the patient has an injury.
    D) on all patients with potential spine or head injuries.
    [Reference text page 637]

15. You arrive at an MVA to find the steering wheel bent, and a spider-web crack in the windshield. Immediately, you should be considering injuries to the head, neck, chest, and spine.

A) True **B)** False

[Reference text page 636]

16. When securing a patient to a long backboard, the:

A) head should be secured to the board first.
B) head should be secured last, after the torso.
C) legs should be secured first.
D) order you secure body parts is not important.

[Reference text pages 650-51]

17. The scalp is very vascular and may bleed profusely when cut.

A) True **B)** False

[Reference text page 639]

18. Fluid that fills the ventricles of the brain and spinal cord is called ________ fluid.

A) lymphatic **B)** amniotic **C)** cerebro-spinal **D)** cervical

[Reference text page 639]

19. Bruising behind the ears or mastoid process due to a basilar skull fracture is called:

A) raccoon eyes. **B)** Battle's sign. **C)** Doll's eyes. **D)** Bernicki's sign.

[Reference text page 639]

20. Bruising or discoloration around the eyes is called:

A) raccoon eyes. **B)** Battle's sign. **C)** Doll's eyes. **D)** Korsokoff's sign.

[Reference text page 639]

21. When an alert, seated patient who has been involved in a collision, complains of a salty taste in the throat, this may be due to:

A) Planter's syndrome. **B)** a subdural hematoma.
C) cerebrospinal fluid. **D)** any of the above.

[Reference text page 640]

22. The major problem with a brain injury is the potential for bleeding within the rigid skull.

A) True **B)** False

[Reference text page 641]

23. A temporary disruption of normal brain function, usually caused by blunt trauma to the head is called a:

A) contusion. **B)** concussion. **C)** hematoma. **D)** subdural.

[Reference text page 641]

24. The treatment for a brain injury includes:
A) providing high-flow oxygen.
B) controlling the airway.
C) rapid transport.
D) all of the above.
[Reference text page 643]

25. A loss of cognitive and intellectual functions caused by a variety of disorders is called dementia.
A) True
B) False
[Reference text page 642]

26. Which of the following is NOT a sign or symptom of a head injury?
A) Irregular breathing pattern
B) Unequal pupil size
C) Very low BP with a fast pulse
D) Paralysis on one side of the body
[Reference text page 642]

27. If time allows, the EMT-Basic should consider using the Glascow Coma Scale to evaluate the patient's mental status.
A) True
B) False
[Reference text page 643]

28. The best rigid cervical collars only reduce motion by 50%.
A) True
B) False
[Reference text page 645]

CD-ROM LINK: *In Chapter 22 of the MedEMT CD-ROM, review the* Spine Immobilization—Reclining Patient *video, which demonstrates sizing and applying a cervical collar.*

29. To be effective, a rigid cervical collar must:
A) be expensive.
B) be disposable.
C) rest on the shoulder girdle.
D) be soft and comfortable for the patient.
[Reference text page 646]

30. If a patient is found walking around at the scene of a collision and you see the windshield was starred from his head, you should:
A) convince him to lay down on your stretcher.
B) backboard him standing up.
C) walk him into the ambulance.
D) use the standing takedown procedure.
[Reference text page 650]

CASE STUDIES

Use a separate piece of paper to answer the case study questions. Number your answers with the case study number and question letter (1A, 1B, etc.).

1. You are dispatched to the scene of an collision involving a motorcycle and a full-sized automobile. You and your partner put on your gloves, while information is given to you by a police officer on the scene. The driver of the car did not see the motorcycle and pulled out in front of it. The motorcycle hit the car broadside at about 25 mph, and the cyclist flew over the car landing on his back 12 feet from the site of impact. The motorcyclist is wearing a helmet. He complains of severe mid-thoracic back pain with numbness and weakness in his legs. He denies loss of consciousness, head or neck pain, or any other injuries. The driver of the car is uninjured.
   A) How do you proceed from here?
   B) Under what conditions should the helmet be removed?
   C) Under what conditions should the helmet be left in place?
   D) The helmet is oversized and is making it difficult to maintaining proper in-line cervical immobilization. The patient is having difficulty breathing with the helmet in place and you are unable to maintain an open airway. Should you remove the helmet?
   E) Describe step-by-step how you would remove the helmet in this patient.
2. You arrive at the scene of a two-car collision. Apparently one vehicle was stopped at a light waiting to make a left turn when suddenly another vehicle plowed into the first vehicle's rear end. As you exit the ambulance, you notice that the windshield of the first car has two stars in it, one on each side. The driver is seated behind the wheel, complaining of head, neck, and chest pain. The front seat passenger of the first car is out and walking around. The third patient is in the back of the police car with no medical complaints. According to the police, he is going to be arrested for DWI.
   A) The scene is safe, but do you have enough resources with you and your partner?
   B) The patient in the front of the car has minor complaints except neck soreness and some tingling down his legs. His vitals are stable. How should he be removed from the car?
   C) The patient who is walking around does not look good. His skin is pale and he is clammy and appears to be avoiding any movement to his neck. He is very concerned about his friend, the driver of the vehicle, as you begin to assess him. What treatment should be done to him?
   D) Should the intoxicated patient be cleared to go with the police to jail?
3. You respond to a call for a diving accident. Apparently there was a party going on and a person who rarely drinks had three beers in a short amount of time. After consuming the alcohol, he dove into the shallow end of the swimming pool. Upon your arrival, the patient is still in the water, floating on his back with the aid of a friend holding him at the top of the water.
   A) Should you and your crew jump into the water to assist?
   B) Should the patient be removed from the pool prior to placing him on a spine board?
   C) The patient has no sensation below the nipples. What did he probably do to himself?
   D) How should you treat this patient?

KEY TERMS MATCHING

Assess your knowledge of the chapter key terms by matching the terms on the left to the definitions on the right.

______ 1. Battle's Sign

______ 2. Cerebrospinal Fluid (CSF)

______ 3. Closed Head Injury

______ 4. Compression Injury

______ 5. Concussion

______ 6. Dementia

______ 7. Glasgow Coma Scale (GCS)

______ 8. Open Head Injury

______ 9. Paresthesia (pair-as-THEEZ-e-uh)

(A) Temporary disruption of normal brain function usually caused by blunt trauma to the head

(B) A loss of cognitive and intellectual functions caused by a variety of disorders

(C) Fluid that fills the ventricles and cavities of the brain and surrounds the spinal cord

(D) A tool for assessing a patient's level of responsiveness

(E) Bruising behind the ears or mastoid process due to basilar skull fracture

(F) A severe traumatic head injury in which the skull is fractured

(G) Spinal cord injury caused when a strong force is transmitted up or down the length of the body.

(H) Abnormal sensations of tingling, numbness, burning, coldness, pain, or tightness in the extremities

(I) Trauma to the head in which the skull remains intact; scalp may or may not be lacerated

LABELING DIAGRAM

Write in the correct terms in the blanks in the diagram.

THE SPINAL COLUMN

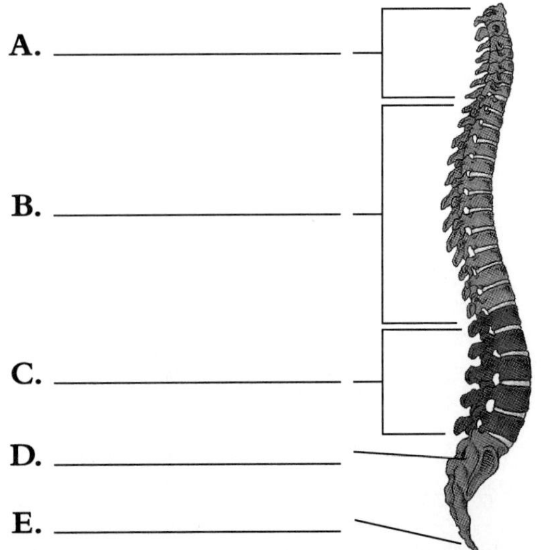

SKILLS CHECKLISTS

Check your knowledge of important EMT-B skills by marking off each step in the following skills sheets.

SPINAL IMMOBILIZATION: SUPINE PATIENT

- [ ] Take BSI precautions.
- [ ] Direct assistant to place head in neutral, in-line position and to maintain manual stabilization until the patient is completely immobilized.
- [ ] Assess distal pulses, motor ability, and sensory response (PMS).
- [ ] Apply a properly sized rigid extrication collar.
- [ ] Position immobilization device appropriately.
- [ ] Move patient onto device without compromising integrity of spine. Apply padding to voids between torso and board as needed.
- [ ] Immobilize patient's torso to device.
- [ ] Evaluate and pad behind patient's head as necessary.
- [ ] Pad and immobilize patient's head.
- [ ] Secure patient's arms and legs to board.
- [ ] Reassess distal PMS.

SPINAL IMMOBILIZATION: SEATED PATIENT

- [ ] Take BSI precautions.
- [ ] Direct assistant to manually stabilize head in neutral, in-line position.
- [ ] Assess distal pulses, motor ability, and sensory response (PMS).
- [ ] Apply a properly sized rigid extrication collar.
- [ ] Position immobilization device behind the patient.
- [ ] Secure device to the patient's torso.
- [ ] Evaluate and pad behind head as needed.
- [ ] Secure patient's head to device.
- [ ] Evaluate and adjust straps.
- [ ] Secure wrists and legs.

☐ Reassess distal PMS.

☐ Transfer patient to long backboard.

RAPID EXTRICATION

Step 1: Perform an initial assessment.

☐ Rescuer A: Maintain manual stabilization of patient's head and neck.

☐ Rescuer B: Conduct initial assessment of patient and determine need for rapid extrication based on patient status. Assess pulses, motor ability, and sensory response (PMS) in four extremities.

Step 2: Apply a cervical collar.

☐ Rescuer B: Apply a properly sized cervical collar.

☐ Rescuer A: Continue to maintain manual stabilization before, during, and after application of collar.

Step 3: Lift patient and position the long backboard.

☐ Rescuer B: Hold patient's armpit, and join hands with Rescuer C under patient's thighs.

☐ Rescuer A: Call for a lift, while maintaining manual stabilization.

☐ Rescuers B: Lift patient approx. two inches off seat with Rescuer C.

☐ Bystander (or 4th Rescuer): Insert long backboard under patient on seat.

Step 4: Begin to position patient for extrication.

☐ Rescuer B: Reach across patient's chest and support by both armpits.

☐ Rescuer A: While maintaining manual stabilization, call for one-fourth turn, so patient is moved perpendicular to steering wheel, ready to exit car head first.

☐ Rescuer C: Free patient's lower legs from any obstructions.

☐ Rescuer B: Begin to turn patient's back toward door until Rescuer A says "stop turn."

☐ Rescuer A: Turn patient. Call for "stop turn" just before being unable to hold patient's head anymore.

☐ Rescuer C: Begin to turn patient's back toward door, freeing legs, then sliding up to thighs until Rescuer A says "stop."

Step 5: Complete another one-fourth turn.

- [ ] Rescuer B: Stop move and wait for Rescuer C. Then take over manual stabilization of head and neck from Rescuer A.
- [ ] Rescuer A: Maintain head/neck stabilization until Rescuer B takes over, allowing him or her to either exit car and work from outside or reach over seat from inside if there is room or roof has been removed.
- [ ] Rescuer C: Move hands from thighs to patient's armpits. Then replace Rescuer B.
- [ ] Complete another one-fourth turn.

Step 6: Lower patient onto the long backboard.

- [ ] Rescuer B: Lower patient onto long backboard.
- [ ] Rescuer A: Call for move to lower patient's torso into a supine position on the long backboard.
- [ ] Rescuer C: Lower patient onto long backboard.
- [ ] Bystander (or 4th Rescuer): Stabilize the board.

Step 7: Position patient on the backboard.

- [ ] Rescuer B: Slide patient as a unit.
- [ ] Rescuer A: Call for move to slide patient toward head end of backboard. Once in position, tell partners to "stop." Slide chest as a unit.
- [ ] Rescuer C: Slide pelvis as a unit until Rescuer A says "stop."
- [ ] Bystander (or 4th Rescuer): Stabilize head end of long backboard.

Step 8: Secure patient to the backboard.

- [ ] Crew carefully straps patient's torso first, head last, and then moves backboard to stretcher.
- [ ] Reassess PMS.

WATER RESCUE: POTENTIAL SPINE INJURY

- [ ] Take BSI precautions.
- [ ] Conduct an initial assessment.
- [ ] Splint head and neck with arms.
- [ ] Roll patient over into supine position.
- [ ] Assess airway and breathing. (Note: If patient is not breathing, remove him or her from water on a backboard as soon as possible.)

- [ ] Provide manual stabilization of head/neck.
- [ ] Assess pulses, motor ability, and sensory response (PMS) in four extremities.
- [ ] Slide backboard under patient.
- [ ] Apply a properly sized rigid extrication collar.
- [ ] Tie down torso, then head/neck with straps.
- [ ] Float board to edge of the water.
- [ ] Remove patient from water with as much assistance as needed.
- [ ] Obtain baseline vital signs.
- [ ] Conduct focused history and physical exam.
- [ ] Reassess PMS in four extremities.
- [ ] Apply oxygen and prepare to transport.

(reprinted from *Pocket Reference for The EMT-B and First Responder* by Bob Elling, Prentice Hall, 1999)

D.O.T. OBJECTIVES CHECKLIST

Use the following list of knowledge objectives to check what you've learned. Check off only those objectives that you feel you completely understand and have mastered. For any objectives not checked, go back and review that section of the text chapter. Textbook page references have been provided to help you review the text material.

- [ ] State the components of the nervous system. *(p. 632)*
- [ ] List the functions of the central nervous system. *(p. 632)*
- [ ] Define the structure of the skeletal system as it relates to the nervous system. *(p. 632)*
- [ ] Relate mechanism of injury to potential injuries of the head and spine. *(p. 633)*
- [ ] Describe the implications of not properly caring for potential spine injuries. *(p. 632)*
- [ ] State the signs and symptoms of a potential spine injury. *(p. 635)*
- [ ] Describe the method of determining if a responsive patient may have a spine injury. *(p. 637)*

- [ ] Relate the airway emergency medical care techniques to the patient with a suspected spine injury. *(p. 638)*
- [ ] Describe how to stabilize the cervical spine. *(p. 645)*
- [ ] Discuss indications for sizing and using a cervical spine immobilization device. *(p. 646)*
- [ ] Establish the relationship between airway management and the patient with head and spine injuries. *(p. 643)*
- [ ] Describe a method for sizing a cervical spine immobilization device. *(p. 646)*
- [ ] Describe how to log roll a patient with a suspected spine injury. *(p. 650)*
- [ ] Describe how to secure a patient to a long spine board. *(p. 650)*
- [ ] List instances when a short spine board should be used. *(p. 647)*
- [ ] Describe how to immobilize a patient using a short spine board. *(p. 647)*
- [ ] Describe the indications for the use of rapid extrication. *(p. 654)*
- [ ] List steps in performing rapid extrication. *(p. 654)*
- [ ] State the circumstances when a helmet should be left on the patient. *(p. 656)*
- [ ] Discuss the circumstances when a helmet should be removed. *(p. 656)*
- [ ] Identify different types of helmets. *(p. 656)*
- [ ] Describe the unique characteristics of sports helmets. *(p. 656)*
- [ ] Explain the preferred methods to remove a helmet. *(p. 656)*
- [ ] Discuss alternative methods for removal of a helmet. *(p. 656)*
- [ ] Describe how the patient's head is stabilized to remove the helmet. *(p. 656)*
- [ ] Differentiate how the head is stabilized with a helmet compared to without a helmet. *(p. 656)*

CHAPTER 23

Infants and Children

CHAPTER 23 SUMMARY

Children are very different from adults. The EMT-Basic should be open and honest when caring for children. Approach them at their level and be aware of the concerns of children in each age group. Fear is a motivating factor in many children's behavior. Expect to see that newborn through school-aged children may have difficulty communicating, especially when acutely ill or injured.

A child's airway is smaller and anatomically different from an adult's. The airway passages are smaller and more easily obstructed. Children compensate very well for a short time, then they decompensate very quickly.

From the door, your general impression of a child is very important. A child who looks sick usually is, and a child who is very attentive to your entering the room may not be as ill. When forming your general impression, watch how the child interacts with parents and the environment. Listen and be attentive to the quality of the child's cry or speech. Note how the child responds to your presence.

Cardiac arrest in children is usually caused secondary to a respiratory arrest. Be very attentive to any respiratory distress as it often leads to a downward spiral to respiratory compromise and then failure and ultimately respiratory arrest.

Respiratory emergencies, seizures, alterations in mental status, poisonings, and trauma are frequent causes of EMS calls for children. Evaluate and manage the child's airway and breathing carefully.

Sudden Infant Death Syndrome (SIDS) is the sudden death of an infant during the first year of life. The causes are not clearly understood. The EMT-Basic should try to resuscitate suspected SIDS patients unless rigor mortis is present. Always follow your local protocols and Medical Director's advice in this area. A large part of your role is to provide emotional support for the parents of a SIDS patient.

Trauma is the number one cause of death in infants and children. Blunt injury is more common than penetrating. Children can sustain serious internal injuries but show few external signs because their protective bone structure is very pliable. Care of the pediatric trauma patient should focus on managing the airway and breathing, and providing rapid transport.

Child abuse and neglect are serious problems in today's society. Be aware of the signs and symptoms of abuse and neglect. Learn the specific reporting requirements of your state. When caring for children when abuse is suspected, focus on providing emergency care. Do not accuse the parents as they may not be the perpetrators and could disapprove of you providing care to their child. Document carefully, and provide objective information to the emergency department physician who in all states is a mandated reporter of child abuse.

Because of advances in technology, many children with special needs are being cared for at home. Children may have feeding tubes, tracheostomy tubes, home ventilators, central IV lines, or shunts. Use the parents as resources for managing these patients. They will often know more about the equipment than you do.

Treating a child involves treating the entire family. The best way to avoid conflict with parents of an injured or ill child is to involve them in the child's care and let them sense a measure of control over the situation.

REVIEW QUESTIONS

Please circle the best answer for each question.

1. The majority of pediatric injuries are severe trauma emergencies.
   A) True **B)** False
   [Reference text page 672]

2. Children in the 1-to-3-year-old age group are referred to as:
   A) newborns. **B)** infants. **C)** toddlers. **D)** preschoolers.
   [Reference text page 673]

3. Which of the following is not a "golden rule" when dealing with children?
   A) It is OK to lie to a child, especially if he or she asks, "Will it hurt?"
   B) Tell the child that any child can hear and understand everything that is said.
   C) Tell the child everything you are going to do before doing it.
   D) Involve the parents in the child's care as much as possible.
   [Reference text page 673]

4. Infants are sensitive to stimulation around the face so you should examine the head last.
   A) True **B)** False
   [Reference text page 674]

5. The easiest place to count the heart rate in an infant is at the:
   A) femoral artery. **B)** brachial artery.
   C) chest with a stethoscope. **D)** radial artery.
   [Reference text page 674]

6. Although a child's anatomy is different from an adult's, physiological functions are the same.
   A) True **B)** False
   [Reference text page 672]

7. In general, toddlers do not like:
   A) to be touched. **B)** to be separated from their parents.
   C) to have clothing removed. **D)** all of the above.
   [Reference text page 674]

8. If a child resists having an oxygen mask on his or her face, the EMT-Basic should:
   A) insist the parent hold the mask in place.
   B) consider the use of "blow by" oxygen.
   C) not use oxygen.
   D) turn up the liter flow so it feels like a fan.
   [Reference text pages 681-82]

9. When assessing a toddler, each of these strategies is helpful EXCEPT:
A) allow the child to hold a security object.
B) remove clothing, examine the child, then replace the clothes.
C) speak in a soothing voice and maintain a relaxed facial expression.
D) examine the child from head to toe.
[Reference text page 675]

10. A toddler may believe his or her injury was a punishment.
A) True **B)** False
[Reference text page 674]

11. Preschoolers have a sense of body integrity. They also are afraid of:
A) pain. **B)** shame.
C) permanent injury. **D)** all of the above.
[Reference text page 675]

12. Infants' tongues are so small that blockage of the airway is rarely a concern.
A) True **B)** False
[Reference text page 677]

13. Because the mouth and nose of a child are ________ than in adults, they are more easily obstructed.
A) longer **B)** smaller **C)** wider **D)** larger
[Reference text pages 677-78]

14. When examining a school-aged child:
A) do not worry about explaining complex concepts.
B) do not worry about rushing to cover bleeding injuries.
C) ask your questions to the child not the parents.
D) do not worry about the child's modesty.
[Reference text page 676]

15. It is usually fairly easy to get an adolescent to reveal information about drug use or sexual history.
A) True **B)** False
[Reference text page 676]

16. Since the cartilage in the chest wall is softer, a child or an infant depends more on the ________ for breathing.
A) rib muscles **B)** diaphragm
C) mouth **D)** shoulder muscles
[Reference text pages 240, 696]

17. A child's tongue takes up ________ space in the pharynx compared to an adult's.
A) more
B) less
C) the same amount of
D) half as much
[Reference text page 677]

18. When a child becomes unconscious, the oral muscles relax, which may obstruct the airway.
A) True
B) False
[Reference text page 678]

19. A common strategy for conducting a hands-on physical exam of a conscious younger child patient is:
A) the head-to-trunk-to-toe approach.
B) the toe-to-trunk-to-head approach.
C) to use the parent to touch the child approach.
D) the same procedure as used on an adult patient.
[Reference text pages 674-75]

20. A child in early respiratory ________ may become exhausted and suddenly decompensate into respiratory failure or respiratory arrest.
A) arrest
B) failure
C) absence
D) distress
[Reference text page 686]

21. Blockage of air movement due to swallowing a foreign object is called:
A) respiratory distress.
B) ventilation compromise.
C) airway obstruction.
D) airway restriction.
[Reference text page 687]

22. Artificial ventilation should be provided as soon as practical in which of the following situations?
A) Severe respiratory distress
B) Cyanosis, despite supplemental oxygen by non-rebreather mask
C) Decompensated respiratory failure
D) All of the above
[Reference text page 679]

23. When your patient is an unconscious child with an obstructed airway, a variation of the Heimlich maneuver can be done with the child in the prone position.
A) True
B) False
[Reference text page 797]

24. If a child resists placement of all types of oxygen delivery masks, the EMT-Basic can use a nasal cannula to administer oxygen at ________ lpm.
A) 2
B) 4
C) 6
D) 8
[Reference text page 682]

25. Examples of abnormal breath sounds found in children are:
A) stridor. **B)** wheezing. **C)** unequal sounds. **D)** all of the above.
[Reference text page 684]

26. Normal capillary refill time should be greater than two seconds in a child.
A) True **B)** False
[Reference text page 684]

27. Increased breathing effort in a child is indicated by any of the following EXCEPT:
A) stridor. **B)** grunting.
C) nasal flaring. **D)** all of the above.
[Reference text page 686]

28. In a pediatric trauma case, secure the airway using the jaw-thrust maneuver combined with spinal immobilization.
A) True **B)** False
[Reference text page 697]

29. The management of a seizure in a child includes:
A) assuring airway patency.
B) suctioning as needed.
C) administering high-flow oxygen by non-rebreather mask.
D) all of the above.
[Reference text page 689]

30. A febrile seizure is usually caused by:
A) a rapid rise in body temperature.
B) a slow steady rise in body temperature.
C) a preexisting seizure history.
D) epilepsy or hypoglycemia.
[Reference text pages 689-90]

31. Which of the following signs would not be present in a child with dehydration?
A) Crying without tears **B)** Sunken eyes
C) Strong, slow pulse **D)** Rash
[Reference text page 691]

32. Usually, children do not have the same disease processes as adults have.
A) True **B)** False
[Reference text page 686]

33. When a child exhibits injuries inconsistent with the MOI, fresh burns, lacerations or bruises in a pattern, or human bite marks, the EMT-Basic should consider:
A) child abuse. **B)** poisoning.
C) SIDS. **D)** none of the above.
[Reference text page 698]

34. Low blood sugar in children can cause altered mental status and seizures.
A) True **B)** False
[Reference text page 689]

35. The administration of ________ should be considered when poisoning is suspected.
A) syrup of ipecac **B)** activated charcoal
C) castor oil **D)** milk and water
[Reference text page 690]

36. Death by drowning usually occurs when the vocal part of the larynx, or the ________ , comes in contact with water and closes, obstructing the airway.
A) pharynx **B)** epiglottis **C)** glottis **D)** trachea
[Reference text page 692]

37. When resuscitating a child taken from a body of water, the EMT-Basic should be especially aggressive if:
A) the water was cold.
B) the child was submerged over 30 minutes.
C) the water was insect-ridden.
D) none of the above occurred.
[Reference text page 692]

38. Sudden Infant Death Syndrome, or SIDS, is commonly known as ________ death.
A) slow **B)** final **C)** crib **D)** fetal
[Reference text page 693]

CD-ROM LINK: *Review the* Child's Trauma *video in Chapter 23 of the MedEMT CD-ROM.*

39. Compared to an adult, trauma to a child's chest is:
A) more likely to cause fractured ribs.
B) more likely to cause internal injury.
C) more likely to cause vomiting.
D) all of the above.
[Reference text page 696]

40. Which of the following circumstances should cause you to consider the possibility of child abuse?
A) The child has several injuries in various stages of healing.
B) The child appears fearful of the EMS personnel.
C) The parent tries to console the child, but the child remains upset.
D) The child is not interested in going to the hospital.
[Reference text page 698]

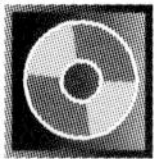

CD-ROM LINK: *Review the* Mechanism of Injury—Pedestrian Accident *video in Chapter 23 of the MedEMT CD-ROM.*

41. Common injuries in a child who was riding a bike and struck by a car include:
A) head. **B)** spinal. **C)** abdominal. **D)** all of the above.
[Reference text page 694]

42. Examples of medical support equipment used in the home include:
A) tracheostomy tubes and artificial ventilators.
B) central intravenous lines.
C) gastrostomy tubes and shunts.
D) all of the above.
[Reference text page 700]

43. The most common cause of obstruction in tracheostomy tubes is accumulation of mucus.
A) True **B)** False
[Reference text page 701]

44. Before, between, and after suctioning a tracheostomy tube, it is recommended that a child be hyperoxygenated.
A) True **B)** False
[Reference text page 701]

45. A device that drains excess fluid from the brain to the abdomen is called a:
A) suction unit. **B)** shunt.
C) hickman catheter. **D)** gastrostomy tube.
[Reference text page 704]

46. A Critical Incident Stress Debriefing (CISD) may be:
A) a voluntary program, offered to EMS providers who need support.
B) triggered automatically after a call involving a critically injured child.
C) an important part of maintaining an EMT-Basic's well-being.
D) all of the above.
[Reference text page 705]

CASE STUDIES

Use a separate piece of paper to answer the case study questions. Number your answers with the case study number and question letter (1A, 1B, etc.).

GENERAL PEDIATRIC ASSESSMENT

1. You are dispatched to a downtown apartment complex with an initial complaint of an unknown medical emergency involving a child. The father of the child meets you in the lobby, carrying the 6-week-old infant. The father states he was feeding the child as usual, but the baby suddenly choked on the formula.
   A) How do you conduct the assessment of such a young child?
   B) As you approach, the child is fidgeting in the man's arms. The infant's skin is pink and appears dry. The respiratory rate is around 50 breaths per minute. The child has a hoarse, dry cough. The child begins to cry loudly, interrupted by frequent coughs. In your assessment, you note that the child appears very warm. You determine that this is a medical call and not a life-threatening illness. What questions might be appropriate to ask, aside from SAMPLE?
   C) What findings would make the EMT-Basic suspect a serious illness?

SEIZURES

2. You are dispatched to a child seizure call at the local high school. When you arrive, the principal directs you to the library, where you find a 14-year-old male lying supine under a table. The patient appears unresponsive.
   A) What is your immediate concern about consent?
   B) As you approach the patient, another violent, full-body seizure begins. What are your immediate actions?
   C) What aspects of the seizure should the EMT-Basic take note of?
   D) If a patient history is available, what information is important?

PEDIATRIC TRAUMA

3. Your agency is asked to respond to a motor vehicle collision late one afternoon. When you arrive, you find an unconscious 8-year-old boy lying supine on the pavement. Witnesses indicate that the boy was riding a bicycle on the wrong side of the road and was struck head-on by a car. There is a moderate amount of damage to the vehicle, which was traveling about 35 miles per hour. A bicycle helmet appears to be stuck in the windshield.
   A) What injuries are common to this type of accident?
   B) Based on the mechanism of injury, what are your primary suspicions?
   C) As you perform the initial assessment, you observe significant amounts of blood in the airway. The patient is breathing spontaneously and has a very rapid pulse. What are your treatment priorities for this patient?

4. You are dispatched to a minor motor vehicle collision in the middle of the business district. Your scene assessment notes minor damage to both vehicles. Vehicle A is occupied only by a driver, who refuses treatment. Vehicle B is occupied by a mother and her 3-year-old daughter. The mother refuses treatment, but insists that you transport her daughter for evaluation. The little girl is restrained in her safety seat, calmly observing everything.
   A) What is an appropriate way of assessing this patient?
   B) The little girl indicates that her "head and tummy hurt." Based on these complaints, transport to the emergency department is indicated. Is it appropriate to immobilize a child of this age? If so, how?

NEAR-DROWNING

5. You respond to a call for a child who fell in a pool. Upon your arrival, the child is floating facedown in the swimming pool. The person who called is afraid of water and did not go in after the child. You call for additional assistance immediately and begin to kick off your shoes and empty your pockets.
   A) Should you enter the water?
   B) How should the child be removed from the pool, and what care is appropriate in the pool?
   C) Once removed from the pool, the child is taking gasping breaths and begins to vomit. What should you do?
   D) Are there any other resources that would be helpful in this situation?

KEY TERMS MATCHING

Assess your knowledge of the chapter key terms by matching the terms on the left to the definitions on the right.

_____ **1.** Adolescent

_____ **2.** Capillary Refill Time

_____ **3.** Early Respiratory Distress

_____ **4.** Febrile (FEE-brile)

_____ **5.** Hydrocephalus (high-dro-SEF-il-is)

_____ **6.** Preschooler

_____ **7.** School-Aged

_____ **8.** Sudden Infant Death Syndrome (SIDS)

_____ **9.** Toddler

(A) Excessive fluid accumulation inside the brain

(B) Having a fever

(C) Child who is 3 to 6 years old

(D) Respiratory problem in which patient can compensate for decreased oxygenation or circulation by increasing breathing rate and effort

(E) Child who is 12 to 18 years old

(F) Time required for the capillary beds to refill with blood after blanching; used for assessing perfusion in infants and children

(G) Crib death; cause unknown

(H) Child from 1 to 3 years old

(I) Child who is 6 to 12 years old

LABELING DIAGRAM

Complete the table by filling in the characteristics of a well child and a sick child in their respective blank columns.

GENERAL IMPRESSION: INFANTS AND CHILDREN

Characteristic	Well Child	Sick Child
Emotional State	A. ______________	G. ______________
Quality of Crying	B. ______________	H. ______________
Activity	C. ______________	I. ______________
Responsiveness	D. ______________	J. ______________
Skin Color	E. ______________	K. ______________
Skin Tone and Body Position	F. ______________	L. ______________

SKILLS CHECKLISTS

Check your knowledge of important EMT-B skills by marking off each step in the following skills sheets.

INFANT FBAO—CONSCIOUS PATIENT

☐ Take BSI precautions.

☐ Confirm complete airway obstruction.

☐ Check for serious breathing difficulty, ineffective cough, weak cry.

☐ Give up to 5 back blows and 5 chest thrusts.

☐ Repeat back blows and chest thrusts until obstruction is cleared.

INFANT FBAO—PATIENT BECOMES UNCONSCIOUS

- [ ] If second rescuer is available, have him or her activate EMS system.
- [ ] Perform a tongue-jaw lift, and if you see object, perform a finger sweep to remove it.
- [ ] Open airway and try to ventilate. If still obstructed, reposition head and try to ventilate again.
- [ ] Give up to 5 back blows and 5 chest thrusts.
- [ ] Repeat last three steps until obstruction is cleared.
- [ ] If airway obstruction is not relieved after about one minute, activate EMS system.

NOTE: If patient is breathing or resumes effective breathing, place in recovery position.

INFANT FBAO—UNCONSCIOUS PATIENT

- [ ] Take BSI precautions.
- [ ] Establish unresponsiveness. If second rescuer is available, have him or her activate EMS system.
- [ ] Open airway and try to ventilate. If still obstructed, reposition head and try to ventilate again.
- [ ] Give up to 5 back blows and 5 chest thrusts.
- [ ] Perform a tongue-jaw lift, and if you see object, perform a finger sweep to remove it.
- [ ] Repeat last three steps until obstruction is cleared.
- [ ] If airway obstruction is not relieved after about one minute, activate the EMS system.

NOTE: If patient is breathing or resumes effective breathing, place in recovery position.

INFANT CPR—ONE-RESCUER

- [ ] Take BSI precautions.
- [ ] Establish unresponsiveness.
- [ ] If second rescuer is available, have him or her activate EMS system.
- [ ] Open airway (head-tilt/chin-lift or jaw-thrust).

- [ ] Check breathing (look, listen, feel).
- [ ] Give two slow breaths (1 to 1 1/2 seconds per breath), watch chest rise, allow for exhalation between breaths.
- [ ] Check brachial pulse.
- [ ] If breathing is absent but pulse is present, provide rescue breathing (one breath every 3 seconds at about 20 breaths per minute).
- [ ] If no pulse, give cycles of 5 chest compressions (at a rate of at least 100 per minute) followed by one slow breath.
- [ ] After about one minute of rescue support, check pulse. If rescuer is alone, activate EMS system.
- [ ] If no pulse, continue 5:1 cycles.

NOTE: If patient is breathing or resumes effective breathing, place in recovery position.

CHILD FBAO—CONSCIOUS PATIENT

- [ ] Ask "Are you choking?"
- [ ] Give abdominal thrusts.
- [ ] Repeat thrusts until effective or patient becomes unconscious.

CHILD FBAO—PATIENT BECOMES UNCONSCIOUS

- [ ] If second rescuer is available, have him or her activate EMS system.
- [ ] Perform a tongue-jaw lift, and if you see object, perform a finger sweep to remove it.
- [ ] Open airway and try to ventilate. If still obstructed, reposition head and try to ventilate again.
- [ ] Give up to 5 abdominal thrusts.
- [ ] Repeat last three steps until obstruction is cleared.
- [ ] If airway obstruction is not relieved after about one minute, activate EMS system.

NOTE: If patient is breathing or resumes effective breathing, place in recovery position.

CHILD FBAO—UNCONSCIOUS PATIENT

- [ ] Take BSI precautions.
- [ ] Establish unresponsiveness. If second rescuer is available, have him or her activate EMS system.
- [ ] Open airway and try to ventilate. If still obstructed, reposition head and try to ventilate again.
- [ ] Give up to 5 abdominal thrusts.
- [ ] Perform a tongue-jaw lift, and if you see object, perform finger sweep to remove it.
- [ ] Repeat last three steps until obstruction is cleared.
- [ ] If airway obstruction is not relieved after about one minute, activate EMS system.

NOTE: If patient is breathing or resumes effective breathing, place in recovery position.

CHILD CPR—ONE RESCUER

- [ ] Take BSI precautions.
- [ ] Establish unresponsiveness.
- [ ] If second rescuer is available, have him or her activate EMS system.
- [ ] Open airway (head-tilt/chin-lift or jaw-thrust).
- [ ] Check breathing (look, listen, feel).
- [ ] Give two slow breaths (1 to 1 1/2 seconds per breath), watch chest rise, allow for exhalation between breaths.
- [ ] Check carotid pulse. If breathing is absent but pulse is present, provide rescue breathing (one breath every 3 seconds at about 20 breaths per minute).
- [ ] If no pulse, give 5 chest compressions (at a rate of 100 per minute), open airway, and provide one slow breath. Repeat this cycle.
- [ ] After about one minute of rescue support, check pulse. If rescuer is alone, activate EMS system. If no pulse, continue 5:1 cycles.

NOTE: If patient is breathing or resumes effective breathing, place in recovery position.

CHILD SAFETY SEAT IMMOBILIZATION: ASSESSMENT

- [ ] Take BSI precautions.
- [ ] Rescuer A: Get in position behind patient. Apply manual in-line stabilization of head and neck. Maintain manual stabilization throughout procedure.
- [ ] Based on initial assessment and patient's status, determine if patient should be immobilized in seat (#74) or rapidly extricated (#75).
- [ ] Rescuer B: Perform an assessment of pulses, motor ability, and sensory response (PMS) in all four extremities before immobilization.

IMMOBILIZING PATIENT IN A CHILD SAFETY SEAT

- [ ] Take BSI precautions.
- [ ] Rescuer A: Stabilize child safety seat in an upright position. Maintain manual stabilization of head and neck throughout procedure until patient is completely immobilized.
- [ ] Rescuer B: Prepare equipment. Apply rigid extrication collar, or improvise a collar with rolled hand towel for newborn or infant.
- [ ] Place a small blanket or bath towel on child's lap. Either strap or use wide tape to secure pelvis and chest area to seat.
- [ ] Carry patient and seat to ambulance and strap them onto stretcher with stretcher head raised.
- [ ] Place a towel roll on both sides of head to fill voids. Tape forehead in place. Then place tape across collar or maxilla. Avoid taping chin, which would place pressure on child's neck and close airway.
- [ ] Reassess PMS.

RAPID EXTRICATION FROM A CHILD SAFETY SEAT

- [ ] Take BSI precautions.
- [ ] Rescuer A: Stabilize child safety seat in upright position. Maintain manual stabilization of head and neck throughout procedure until patient is completely immobilized.
- [ ] Rescuer B: Prepare equipment. Loosen or cut seat straps and raise front guard.

- [ ] Apply rigid extrication collar, or improvise with rolled hand towel in newborn/infant.
- [ ] Place child safety seat on center of long backboard and slowly tilt it back into a supine position, being careful not to allow patient to slide out of chair. If patient has a large head, it is helpful to place a towel under area where shoulders will end up on board.
- [ ] Rescuer A: Call for a coordinated long axis move onto board.
- [ ] Rescuer B: Grasp chest and axilla with each hand and do a coordinated long axis move onto board. Make sure child is positioned at end of board and not in middle.
- [ ] Place a rolled blanket on each side of patient.
- [ ] Strap pelvis and upper chest to board. Do not strap abdomen down. Tape lower legs to board with wide tape.
- [ ] Place a towel roll on both sides of head to fill voids. Tape forehead in place. Then place tape across collar or maxilla. Do not tape across chin to avoid pressure on patient's neck.
- [ ] Reassess PMS.

(reprinted from *Pocket Reference for The EMT-B and First Responder* by Bob Elling, Prentice Hall, 1999)

D.O.T. OBJECTIVES CHECKLIST

Use the following list of knowledge objectives to check what you've learned. Check off only those objectives that you feel you completely understand and have mastered. For any objectives not checked, go back and review that section of the text chapter. Textbook page references have been provided to help you review the text material.

- [ ] Identify the developmental considerations for the following age groups: infants, toddlers, pre-school, school age, adolescent. *(p. 672)*
- [ ] Describe differences in anatomy and physiology of the infant, child and adult patient. *(p. 677)*
- [ ] Differentiate the response of the ill or injured infant or child (age specific) from that of an adult. *(p. 672)*
- [ ] Indicate various causes of respiratory emergencies. *(p. 687)*

- [ ] Differentiate between respiratory distress and respiratory failure. *(p. 686)*
- [ ] List the steps in the management of foreign body airway obstruction. *(p. 687)*
- [ ] Summarize emergency medical care strategies for respiratory distress and respiratory failure. *(p. 687)*
- [ ] Identify the signs and symptoms of shock (hypoperfusion) in the infant and child patient. *(p. 691)*
- [ ] Describe the methods of determining end organ perfusion in the infant and child patient. *(p. 683)*
- [ ] State the usual cause of cardiac arrest in infants and children versus adults. *(p. 686)*
- [ ] List the common causes of seizures in the infant and child patient. *(p. 689)*
- [ ] Describe the management of seizures in the infant and child patient. *(p. 689)*
- [ ] Differentiate between the injury patterns in adults, infants, and children. *(p. 694)*
- [ ] Discuss the field management of the infant and child trauma patient. *(p. 697)*
- [ ] Summarize the indicators of possible child abuse and neglect. *(p. 697)*
- [ ] Describe the medical legal responsibilities in suspected child abuse. *(p. 699)*
- [ ] Recognize need for EMT-Basic debriefing following a difficult infant or child transport. *(p. 704)*

CHAPTER 24

Operations

CHAPTER 24 SUMMARY

Every EMS call has specific stages, beginning with preparation and ending with post-run activities. Learn your responsibilities in each stage. Carefully plan for the next stage as you handle each call. Safety is the highest concern at any call. As the EMT-Basic, you are responsible for your own safety, the safety of your crew, the patient, and bystanders.

Air medical services are an excellent resource for managing critically ill or injured patients. They provide advanced care and rapid transport to definitive care. Safety is always your first priority when dealing with air medical services.

Your role may include rescuing the patient. Patient care takes priority over rescue unless delayed movement will endanger the life of the patient or rescuers. Rescue workers and EMT-Basics must work closely together so that each step they take is in the interest of time and the patient.

When trying to gain access to the patient, remember to:

- *Try simple things first, such as unlocking doors, rolling down windows, and opening doors.*
- *Always consider the path of least resistance if it is safe.*
- *Have sufficient personnel to rescue the patient safely.*
- *Protect the patient from hazards created during the rescue, such as covering patients with an aluminized blanket when glass is being broken.*
- *Use available resources in your community for special rescue situations.*

Hazardous materials (HAZ-MAT) are transported by air, land, rail, and water. Safety is your primary concern in an incident that may involve HAZ-MAT. Never enter a hazardous materials scene without proper training and protective equipment. Always park your vehicle upwind and uphill of a hazardous material scene. Secure the scene to keep bystanders away. As you approach the scene of any incident, look for evidence of hazardous materials. Shipping containers, placards, container labels, and shipping papers provide information. Use resources such as CHEMTREC (800-424-9300) for additional information if necessary.

Incident management (command) systems (IMS or ICS) help to control and coordinate emergency resources during events. Sectors or divisions (such as triage, treatment, transport, safety, staging, public information, rescue) are established to support EMS operations. The incident commander assigns responsibilities to individuals based on a preestablished plan.

Mass casualty incidents (MCI) place a great demand on resources. The goal is to provide the greatest good for the most people possible. Patients are triaged based on their priority for treatment. This is determined by the initial assessment or an abbreviated assessment. After triage, patients are treated and transported based on priority, available resources, and destination hospital.

REVIEW QUESTIONS

Please circle the best answer for each question.

1. EMT-Basics function primarily in the ________ environment.
   A) prehospital **B)** outdoor **C)** indoor **D)** foreign
   [Reference text page 714]

2. All supplies should be restocked, cleaned, or maintained after each run.
   A) True **B)** False
   [Reference text page 724]

3. If you receive information from the dispatch center that is unclear or seems wrong, you should:
   A) repeat the information received from the dispatcher.
   B) request the dispatcher to repeat or restate the information.
   C) write down the information.
   D) do all of the above.
   [Reference text page 719]

4. The minimum staffing for an ambulance should be one EMT-Basic in the patient compartment.
   A) True **B)** False
   [Reference text page 715]

5. At a minimum, an ambulance must carry:
   A) suction equipment. **B)** oxygen equipment.
   C) splinting supplies. **D)** all of the above.
   [Reference text page 716]

6. If the patient's family wants to follow the ambulance in their private car, they should be instructed in all of the following EXCEPT:
   A) directions to the receiving facility.
   B) follow very closely behind the ambulance.
   C) they must obey traffic lights while driving to the hospital.
   D) your crew will provide the best possible care during transport.
   [Reference text page 723]

CD-ROM LINK: *Review the* Paramedic in the Ambulance *video in Chapter 24 of the MedEMT CD-ROM.*

7. The written PCR can be dropped off at the hospital later in the day after you complete it back at your station.
   A) True **B)** False
   [Reference text page 723]

8. Before returning to your station, prepare for the next call. This should include:
A) cleaning and disinfecting the ambulance.
B) cleaning and disinfecting the equipment.
C) restocking disposable supplies.
D) all of the above.
[Reference text page 724]

9. When is it important to make full use of your time by assessing equipment, clarifying information, and predetermining responsibilities?
A) At the scene **B)** En route **C)** After the call **D)** None of the above
[Reference text page 720]

10. While en route, the ambulance operator must be especially careful when entering a/n:
A) highway. **B)** parkway. **C)** intersection. **D)** parking lot.
[Reference text page 730]

CD ROM LINK: *Review the* Paramedic in the Emergency Room *video in Chapter 24 of the MedEMT CD-ROM.*

11. The CDC has identified four levels of decontamination. Which of the following levels should be used for the inside surfaces of the ambulance after a bloody call?
A) Sterilization **B)** High-level disinfection
C) Disinfection **D)** Cleaning
[Reference text pages 725-26]

12. Removal of germs, bacteria, or other potentially infectious materials is called:
A) sterilization. **B)** high-level disinfection.
C) disinfection. **D)** cleaning.
[Reference text page 726]

13. Wiping the surface with a common disinfectant that is not capable of killing tuberculosis bacterium is called:
A) sterilization. **B)** high-level disinfection.
C) disinfection. **D)** cleaning.
[Reference text page 726]

14. Emergency vehicle driving regulations usually allow you to do all of the following with an emergency response vehicle EXCEPT:
A) disregard "no turn" signs for right or left turns.
B) drive past a stopped school bus with its flashing red lights.
C) exceed the posted speed limit.
D) drive through red lights when it is safe to proceed.
[Reference text page 727]

15. Most states that have laws that govern the operation of ambulances often include provisions about:
A) speed limit regulations.
B) vehicle parking and standing.
C) use of visual warning devices.
D) all of the above.
[Reference text page 727]

16. Before taking any of the exemptions in most state's vehicle and traffic laws, there is usually a requirement that the call be known to be a true emergency.
A) True
B) False
[Reference text page 728]

17. Safe driving practices would include all of the following EXCEPT:
A) selecting an appropriate route.
B) driving with due regard for the safety of others.
C) using lights to go through all the red lights as fast as possible.
D) using a spotter when backing up.
[Reference text page 729]

18. Elements that contribute to unsafe emergency vehicle operation include:
A) using the headlights all the time.
B) paying attention to the weather and road conditions.
C) multiple emergency vehicle response.
D) insisting all passengers use seat belts.
[Reference text page 729]

19. If you must use an escort vehicle, follow at least 500 feet behind.
A) True
B) False
[Reference text page 730]

20. It is a safe practice to park approximately 50 feet from the motor vehicle collision upon arriving.
A) True
B) False
[Reference text page 731]

21. Aeromedical services should be considered at calls when:
A) a vehicle rollover involved unrestrained patients.
B) a pedestrian was struck by a car at a speed of greater than 10 mph.
C) an adult has fallen greater than 20 feet.
D) all of the above have occurred.
[Reference text pages 732-33]

22. The minimum acceptable area for a landing zone is 150 feet by 150 feet.
A) True
B) False
[Reference text page 735]

23. Extrication may be needed at which of the following situations?
A) Trench collapse
B) Motor vehicle crashes
C) Structural collapses
D) All of the above
[Reference text page 736]

24. The three fundamental components of extrication are equipment, patient management, and:
A) safety.
B) rapid response.
C) immediate access.
D) multiple tools.
[Reference text page 737]

25. Providing a passageway for patient access and removal is called:
A) extrication.
B) disentanglement.
C) entrapment.
D) extension.
[Reference text page 736]

26. The EMT-Basic should assess the stability of each vehicle before moving too close to it.
A) True
B) False
[Reference text page 738]

27. For extrication, the appropriate PPE would include:
A) impact-resistant helmet.
B) latex gloves.
C) eyeshields.
D) gowns and gloves.
[Reference text page 739]

28. The patient should be covered throughout the extrication.
A) True
B) False
[Reference text page 739]

29. The boundary established around the patient at an extrication scene is called the:
A) hot zone.
B) cold zone.
C) inner circle.
D) kill zone.
[Reference text page 739]

30. A rescue that does not require sophisticated equipment is called a:
A) complex access.
B) simple access.
C) basic extrication.
D) disentanglement.
[Reference text page 743]

31. A substance that is potentially harmful or that presents an unreasonable risk for injury, health problems, or significant property damage if not properly controlled is called a:
A) biohazard.
B) toxic waste.
C) hazardous material.
D) dangerous cargo.
[Reference text page 745]

32. Which of the following senses is unreliable and unsafe to use during a hazardous material response?
A) Sight
B) Sound
C) Smell
D) It is best not to rely on any one sense in a hazardous material response.
[Reference text page 746]

33. A U.S. D.O.T. placard that is designed to warn of a flammable product would be:
A) red. **B)** yellow. **C)** green. **D)** orange.
[Reference text page 747]

34. A U.S. D.O.T. placard that is designed to warm of a poison product would be:
A) red. **B)** white. **C)** orange. **D)** blue.
[Reference text page 747]

35. A U.S. D.O.T. placard that is designed to warm of an explosive product would be:
A) white. **B)** yellow. **C)** green. **D)** orange.
[Reference text page 747]

36. A placard that is white and black represents a ________ material.
A) corrosive **B)** flammable **C)** oxidizer **D)** radioactive
[Reference text page 747]

37. On the NFPA 704 placard, the blue section designates the ________ hazard.
A) fire **B)** health **C)** bio **D)** reactivity
[Reference text page 748]

38. If you need to call CHEMTREC, be prepared with:
A) identification number of the material. **B)** location of the emergency.
C) shipper or manufacturer. **D)** all of the above.
[Reference text page 750]

39. The term *triage* refers to:
A) a special nonadhesive bandage used for treating head injuries.
B) a method of sorting ill or injured patients according to severity of injury.
C) a piece of equipment used to extricate patients from vehicle pileups.
D) none of the above.
[Reference text pages 752-53]

40. After transferring care of the patient to the receiving personnel and completing all written reports, you are ready to return to quarters.
A) True **B)** False
[Reference text page 723]

41. Upon arriving at the receiving facility, the EMT-Basics should not speak to attending physicians unless they are asked a question.
A) True **B)** False
[Reference text page 723]

42. No matter how many exemptions to traffic laws are allowed, the emergency vehicle operator must always operate the ambulance with due regard for:
A) his or her own safety. **B)** the rules of the road.
C) the safety of all others. **D)** none of the above.
[Reference text page 728]

43. When selecting the route to the hospital, consider potential hazards, such as detours, time of day and the weather.
A) True **B)** False
[Reference text pages 730-31]

44. Once the team has decided to call for aeromedical services, you must prepare a/n ________ on level ground.
A) litter basket. **B)** evacuation harness.
C) spinal immobilization. **D)** landing zone.
[Reference text page 734]

45. As soon as the helicopter lands, move in to load the patient without delay.
A) True **B)** False
[Reference text page 734]

46. The area where the helicopter rotor blades pull upwards is usually the safest location to wait for the arrival of an emergency helicopter.
A) True **B)** False
[Reference text page 734]

47. A rescue unit that carries dive equipment is a ________ unit.
A) light-duty **B)** medium-duty **C)** heavy-duty **D)** none of the above
[Reference text page 742]

48. Light-duty units carry all of the following EXCEPT:
A) patient care supplies. **B)** simple hand tools.
C) basic hydraulic tools. **D)** low pressure bags.
[Reference text page 740]

49. Who are usually the first patients to be extricated?
A) Those who are most entrapped **B)** Those who are least entrapped
C) Those who are walking around **D)** None of the above
[Reference text page 742]

50. As a non-rescue EMT-Basic, your first priority is always patient care, unless delay would endanger the life of a rescuer or patient.
A) True **B)** False
[Reference text page 737]

CASE STUDIES

Use a separate piece of paper to answer the case study questions. Number your answers with the case study number and question letter (1A, 1B, etc.).

EQUIPMENT

1. Several crews have used the ambulance since your last rotation. Unfortunately, you are not always sure that all the off-going crews have restocked the unit according to the mandatory equipment list. Your supervisor is aware of the situation and gives your unit a few extra minutes to check out the unit before going available with dispatch.
A) What medical supplies frequently need replacing on the ambulance?

PHASES OF AN AMBULANCE CALL

2. The ambulance company has adopted an oral interview as part of their hiring process. You have always been a little nervous about interviews and right now is no different. The panel is mainly asking field care and protocol questions. Just as the interview is finishing, the local medical director asks you to list the typical phases of an ambulance call.
A) What are the typical phases of an ambulance call?

3. The station alarm is a sound you will never get out of your head. In this small town, it usually signals the beginning of what almost always ends up being a significant EMS response. People just don't use EMS in your area unless things are really bad. You are operating without much thought or effort as you throw on your turnouts and slip on your boots. But, as the diesel motor roars to life, you realize you must pay close attention to your actions, even though it is 3 A.M.
A) Describe the steps you should complete prior to leaving the station and responding to an emergency call.

4. Dispatch traffic suggests that several people are down in what sounds like a drive-by shooting behind one of the local high schools. School security guards advise EMS dispatch that four young males and one female are shot, and bystanders are performing CPR on the female patient. En route, dispatch advises that three additional units have been requested from a nearby town and the trauma center helicopter has been dispatched to the scene. Your three-member crew seems unusually quiet and overwhelmed by the radio traffic.
A) Describe what you might you do while responding to this scene to help take full advantage of the time you will have once you arrive on scene.

As you arrive on scene, the entrance is a narrow alleyway with a dead end. The security guards have parked their patrol cars to light the scene, and have blocked off your only exit from the scene once you proceed up close. Both guards are performing CPR on a patient several feet away and you can hear several other responding emergency vehicles off in the distance.

B) What are some of the considerations an ambulance operator would have in approaching this scene?

5. You are responding to a tractor rollover accident on a farm just outside the city limits. The tractor operator was very fortunate, and his only apparent injuries are a left leg mid-shaft femur fracture and a broken wrist. Medical direction has requested the patient be transported to the local emergency department with an estimated time of arrival of 20 minutes. The patient has been properly packaged and all appropriate interventions have begun.
   A) Assuming you are the EMT-Basic in charge of patient care, what are the steps in your emergency treatment while en route to the receiving facility?
   B) While en route, the patient's level of consciousness begins to deteriorate. His blood pressure begins to fall, and his heart rate increases. In addition to checking all earlier interventions, what steps should the EMT-Basic take?

VEHICLE ESCORTS

6. The EMS agency and local prison staff have just published a draft policy outlining the steps required when arriving and transporting prisoners from the prison facility. You and your partner notice that the new policy includes both a prison escort and a chase car. You are concerned about the safety of this new policy and the fact that nothing is mentioned about how each unit will operate or communicate during the escorts. The Medical Director agrees with your concerns and requests that you investigate the proper standards for escorts and emergency vehicles.
   A) Describe some of the basic safety precautions that should be followed during cases where an escort is required.

SCENE AND PATIENT SAFETY

7. A local convalescent facility has requested an EMS response for a man down. As you round the corner, you see activity in your peripheral vision just south of the facility. You slow down and confirm that several people are surrounding a person lying on the ground. They wave you over, confirming they are the reporting party. As you exit the ambulance, you notice a wheelchair that looks mangled. A bystander tells you they think the man was run over by a large four-wheel-drive truck.
   A) List some of the procedures or precautions you should take prior to patient contact.
   B) What kinds of scene safety questions should you be asking yourself as you arrive on scene?

8. A nearby manufacturing facility covers about 20 square blocks. Over 3,000 people work inside the plant each day. As the emergency response coordinator, you have noticed a recent increase in the number of serious falls. During your weekly safety meeting, you help your emergency response crew to appreciate the importance of proper spine immobilization after a fall. You have asked the group to suggests some questions they might ask themselves when deciding whether to move a patient or wait for EMS.
   A) What types of questions can a provider ask to determine if movement is indicated?

DECONTAMINATION

9. You are returning from a particularly intense EMS response, and upon evaluating the condition of the ambulance, you decide you've never seen such a mess. You and your partner must have touched and opened just about everything in the patient compartment.

A) As the person in charge of preparing the unit for the next response, what must you do prior to becoming available for your next call?

10. A memo from the commanding officer's desk is short and to the point. Recent reports have been lodged of crews not adequately cleaning the patient compartment of their helicopters after EMS responses. Random inspections are to begin immediately. The memo also makes mention of the four levels of decontamination. It has been such a long time since you took the helicopter orientation class that you cannot remember each of the levels and their corresponding decontamination requirements.

A) Describe the four levels of decontamination as identified by the CDC.

DRIVING SAFETY

11. Part of your preemployment review is an evaluation of your ability to safely operate an emergency vehicle. The instructor has just given you a passing grade on the driving segment of the course and requests that you now answer a few essay questions. You have been studying the state manual and feel pretty confident in your abilities. The questions are as follows:

A) What legal standard will be used during litigation to evaluate your operation of an emergency vehicle?

B) Assume the operator is operating the unit in a safe manner. What aspects of motor vehicle operation only apply to the operation of an emergency vehicle?

12. Responding to a call, you are traveling along a crowded freeway. You notice a small sports car that has begun following behind you as traffic clears to the right shoulder. The operator is much too close, and has on several occasions even had to slam on his brakes to avoid rear ending your ambulance. You have about ten minutes left in your response.

A) What might you do to reduce your risks in this situation?

AEROMEDICAL SERVICES

13. The regional trauma center has just purchased a new helicopter, and the director of the aero-medical program is talking with your class about the medical benefits gained from the use of a medical helicopter. The statistics are impressive, and the medical rationale is logical. During a break, several of your classmates are interested in learning more about requesting the service of a helicopter. When the class reconvenes, your instructor calls on each study group to give one reason or justification for requesting such service.

A) List some of the conditions or situations that may justify the request for an aero medical response.

B) At the conclusion of the lecture, the aeromedical program director asks you to prepare a landing zone for the helicopter. What steps are involved in preparing a landing zone?

INCIDENT MANAGEMENT SYSTEMS

14. As is sometimes the case, your last response seems in retrospect to have been poorly organized. As you think back on it, you realize that the scene became less and less manageable as more EMS personnel arrived. You were particularly discouraged by frequent requests for your EMT-Basic crew to perform tasks they are not trained to perform. In a post-event discussion, the incident commander asks you and your team to help identify the exact roles of a non-rescue EMT-Basic.

A) Describe the specific role of an EMT-Basic functioning in a non-rescue role.

B) During the same discussion, the group would like to hear the steps required of the EMT-Basic when assuming a rescuer role. Describe the change of focus for the EMT-Basic when providing basic rescue services.

15. The local amusement park and EMS system were overwhelmed when the new multimillion dollar tunnel ride suffered a complete collapse. First reports suggest that inside the mountain of twisted steel and concrete are several dozen patients needing care. You have been requested to respond as part of the regional response plan. As you exit your unit, the staging area supervisor asks you to utilize all appropriate personal protective equipment in preparation for extrication services.

A) What general types of PPE would be required for this response?

16. The early morning tones usually suggest either a natural death or an auto involving commuters. You don't expect to be dispatched to a multi-vehicle crash involving several semi-tractor trailers and approximately 20 passenger vehicles, but it has happened. En route, dispatch advises that several of the big rigs are on fire and initial reports from bystanders indicate multiple fatalities. As you approach the rural highway intersection, you observe the fires, the smell of burning tires, and the fact that you are the first to arrive on scene.

A) What should your first actions be, since you are the first arriving EMS unit?

B) Describe the basic purpose of Incident Management Systems.

EXTRICATION

17. Your EMT-Basic class has been a wonderful experience. Your instructor is a skilled and exciting public speaker, and has excellent insight into the world of the EMT-Basic. As the presentation proceeds, you are called upon to identify the three fundamental components of extrication and some specifics of the local EMS system's hazardous materials response plan.

A) What are the three fundamental components or considerations surrounding extrication?

18. The volunteer fire department arrived on the scene of an automobile accident several minutes prior to your unit. They have begun using power tools to rescue three trapped and injured teenagers. Estimates are that their vehicle left the roadway at 60 mph and struck a large concrete pillar 20 feet below the roadway. It looks like it will be several more minutes before you can make safe patient contact. A local news reporter is riding along with your crew and asks you to explain the difference between extrication and disentanglement.

A) Describe the difference between extrication and disentanglement.

19. Recently, several patients have been significantly injured along a bad stretch of highway just south of the county line. Officers of the sheriff's department are almost always the first to arrive on scene and subsequently advise medical dispatch of the situation. In some recent incidents, the responding crews have asked the officers what type of rescue vehicle is most appropriate. The officers are willing to help out, but need basic orientation on the different types of rescue units the fire department has available. Every available officer from the sheriff's office is at the firehouse this morning, and you will conduct a vehicle orientation.

A) Describe the different types of rescue units and their specific capabilities.

20. A drilling rig has been almost completely buried in a rockslide, along with six workers. Directly after the rock slide, the drilling company's extrication team began working with local heavy rescue experts to locate the exact spot where the workers could be found. After three hours, you and your partner are advised that two patients have been located and require immediate medical attention. The two patients are still trapped, and it will be several more hours before they are disentangled. Two cave-in specialists have been assigned to provide for your safety and assist you with patient care.

A) Describe some of the basic steps and guidelines the EMT-Basic can take to help ensure a safe and efficient extrication process.

HAZARDOUS MATERIALS

21. As the EMT-Basic crew on duty, you are responding to a call from the sheriff's office for three men down. En route, dispatch advises that a major ammonia leak has been detected, and that the hazardous materials team from the nearby chemical plant has been activated. You can see the lights of the sheriff's cruiser but are unable to see any patients thus far.

A) Describe the general safety steps necessary when approaching a possible hazardous materials scene.

22. The metal plating operation in an older section of town has requested assistance for a job-related injury. The employee is complaining of a severe burn on his right hand and a large rash covering his chest and abdomen. He denies any complaint of shortness of breath. The patient is sitting on a chair in a large open area. There are several large tanks full of boiling liquids nearby. You notice several people working around these tanks, all wearing thick leather gloves and aprons. You are unable to locate anyone who speaks English well enough to help determine the exact nature of the patient's injuries. There are several 55-gallon drums stacked against the walls, and one drum appears to have fallen and spilled its contents. The patient states the fallen drum was the cause of his injuries. You and your partner are unfamiliar with the symbols and so you decide to load the patient onto the gurney and begin transport to the regional trauma center.

A) Are these actions appropriate under the circumstances?

B) Identify the various methods available to your crew to help identify the potentially hazardous materials on scene.

23. Recent news reports of major hazardous materials shipments via the local railroad system have prompted many community members to question the training and preparation of the local EMS system. While on lunch break at the local diner, several people ask you and your partner to identify the training your department receives. Confidently, you briefly explain the different types of hazardous materials training.

A) Identify and describe the levels of hazardous materials training.

KEY TERMS MATCHING

Assess your knowledge of the chapter key terms by matching the terms on the left to the definitions on the right.

_____ **1.** Complex access

_____ **2.** Disinfection

_____ **3.** Hazardous Material (HAZ-MAT)

_____ **4.** HAZ-MAT Team

_____ **5.** Incident Management System (IMS)

_____ **6.** Multiple Casualty Incident (MCI)

_____ **7.** Self-Contained Breathing Apparatus (SCBA)

_____ **8.** Simple Access

(A) A system designed to control, direct, and coordinate emergency responders and resources in case of a disaster

(B) Response that can involve a few serious injuries or several hundred patients; can place great demands on a local EMS system

(C) Equipment that provides clean air to a rescuer and protects him or her from hazardous vapors

(D) A rescue that does not require sophisticated equipment

(E) A rescue requiring specialized skills and equipment

(F) Removal of germs, bacteria, or other potentially infectious materials [high-level disinfection; used for instruments that have come in contact with mucous membranes and involving a process of hot-water pasteurization (176° to 212° F)].

(G) Substance that is potentially harmful or that presents an unreasonable risk for injury, health problems, or significant property damage if not properly controlled

(H) Personnel specially trained to manage emergencies involving hazardous materials

SKILLS CHECKLISTS

Check your knowledge of important EMT-B skills by marking off each step in the following skills sheets.

AIRBORNE INFECTION PROCEDURES

(such as TB)

- [ ] You have transported a patient who is infected with a life-threatening airborne disease but you are not aware that the patient is infected.
- [ ] After the medical facility diagnoses the disease in the patient, they must notify your designated officer (DO) within 48 hours.
- [ ] Your DO then notifies you that you have been exposed.
- [ ] Your employer arranges for you to be evaluated and followed up by a doctor or appropriate other health care professional.

BLOODBORNE INFECTION

(such as HIV or HBV)

- [ ] You have come into contact with blood and body fluids of a patient, and you wonder if that patient is infected with a life-threatening disease such as HIV or HBV.
- [ ] You seek immediate medical attention and document the incident for worker's compensation.
- [ ] You ask your designated officer (DO) to determine if you have been exposed to an infectious disease.
- [ ] Your DO must gather information and, if warranted, consults the medical facility to which the patient was transported.
- [ ] The medical facility must gather information and report findings to your DO within 48 hours.
- [ ] Your DO notifies you of the findings.
- [ ] Your employer arranges for you to be evaluated and followed up by a doctor or appropriate other health care professional.

TRANSFERRING THE PATIENT

- [ ] Transfer patient as soon as possible. In a routine admission or when an illness or injury is not life-threatening, first check to see what is to be done with patient.
- [ ] A rescuer should remain with patient until transfer is complete.
- [ ] Assist emergency department staff as required.
- [ ] Give a complete verbal report of patient's condition and treatment administered.
- [ ] Complete your prehospital care report and turn a copy over to hospital staff.
- [ ] Transfer patient's personal effects.
- [ ] Obtain your release from hospital, if required in your region.

ACTIONS TO BE TAKEN AT THE HOSPITAL

- [ ] Take BSI precautions.
- [ ] Clean ambulance interior as required by your service exposure control plan.
- [ ] Replace respiratory equipment as required.
- [ ] Replace disposable items according to local policies.
- [ ] Exchange equipment according to local policies.
- [ ] Make up ambulance stretcher.

TERMINATION OF ACTIVITIES IN QUARTERS

- [ ] Place contaminated linens in biohazard container and non-contaminated linens in regular hamper.
- [ ] Remove and clean patient care equipment as required.
- [ ] Clean and sanitize respiratory equipment as needed.
- [ ] Clean and sanitize ambulance interior as required. Use germicide on devices and surfaces that were in contact with blood and body fluids.
- [ ] Wash thoroughly and change soiled clothing.
- [ ] Replace expendable supplies and equipment as required.

CLEANING AND DISINFECTING EQUIPMENT

- [ ] Use *low-level disinfectant*—one approved by the EPA, such as Lysol, to clean and kill germs on ambulance floors and walls.
- [ ] Use *intermediate-level disinfectant*—such as a mixture of 1:100 bleach-to-water to clean and kill germs on equipment.
- [ ] Use *high-level disinfectant*—such as Cidex Plus, to destroy all forms of microbial life except high numbers of bacterial spores.

NOTE: Sterilization is required to destroy all possible sources of infection on equipment that will be used invasively.

ESTABLISHING COMMAND AT AN MCI

- [ ] Perform a scene size-up.
- [ ] Locate police and fire officers and establish a unified command post.
- [ ] Don EMS command vest.
- [ ] Notify EMS dispatcher:
    - [ ] Declaring an MCI.
    - [ ] Extent of incident.
    - [ ] Ongoing or contained.
    - [ ] Approximate number of patients.
    - [ ] Location of command post.
    - [ ] Request number of BLS/ALS units.
- [ ] Designate a triage officer.
- [ ] Designate a staging officer:
    - [ ] Location for staging sector.
    - [ ] Notify dispatcher to have all additional ambulances respond to staging.
- [ ] Request dispatcher roll call hospitals for bed availability.
- [ ] Designate treatment officer and location for this sector (as needed).
- [ ] Designate transportation officer and location for this sector (as needed).
    - [ ] Consider need for aeromedical evacuation and appropriate landing zone nearby scene.

- [ ] Consider usefulness of a school bus to transport walking wounded (low-priority) patients. Make sure everyone on bus is medically examined and that medical personnel also ride bus.

- [ ] Consider need for extrication sector (if not already established).
- [ ] Consider need for a safety officer (as needed).
- [ ] Consider need for a follow-up CISD and rehab of personnel.
- [ ] Keep dispatcher and other service chiefs in close contact throughout incident.
- [ ] Along with police and fire officers, consider need for a public information officer to work with arriving media.

(reprinted from *Pocket Reference for The EMT-B and First Responder* by Bob Elling, Prentice Hall, 1999)

D.O.T. OBJECTIVES CHECKLIST

Use the following list of knowledge objectives to check what you've learned. Check off only those objectives that you feel you completely understand and have mastered. For any objectives not checked, go back and review that section of the text chapter. Textbook page references have been provided to help you review the text material.

- [ ] Discuss the medical and nonmedical equipment needed to respond to a call. *(p. 715)*
- [ ] List the phases of an ambulance call. *(p. 714)*
- [ ] Describe the general provisions of state laws relating to the operation of the ambulance and privileges in any or all of the following categories: speed, warning lights, sirens, right-of-way, parking, turning. *(p. 727)*
- [ ] List contributing factors to unsafe driving conditions. *(p. 728)*
- [ ] Describe the considerations that should be given to: request for escorts, following an escort vehicle, intersections. *(p. 729)*
- [ ] Discuss "Due Regard For Safety of All Others" while operating an emergency vehicle. *(p. 728)*
- [ ] State what information is essential in order to respond to a call. *(p. 719)*
- [ ] Discuss various situations that may affect response to a call. *(p. 730)*

- [ ] Differentiate between the various methods of moving a patient to the unit based upon injury or illness. *(p. 721)*
- [ ] Apply the components of the essential patient information in a written report. *(p. 723)*
- [ ] Summarize the importance of preparing the unit for the next response. *(p. 725)*
- [ ] Identify what is essential for completion of a call. *(p. 724)*
- [ ] Distinguish among the terms cleaning, disinfection, high-level disinfection, and sterilization. *(p. 725)*
- [ ] Describe how to clean or disinfect items following patient care. *(p. 725)*
- [ ] Describe the purpose of extrication. *(p. 736)*
- [ ] Discuss the role of the EMT-Basic in extrication. *(p. 737)*
- [ ] Identify what equipment for personal safety is required for the EMT-Basic. *(p. 738)*
- [ ] Define the fundamental components of extrication. *(p. 736)*
- [ ] State the steps that should be taken to protect the patient during extrication. *(p. 738)*
- [ ] Evaluate various methods of gaining access to the patient. *(p. 742)*
- [ ] Distinguish between simple and complex access. *(p. 742)*
- [ ] Explain the EMT-Basic's role during a call involving hazardous materials. *(p. 745)*
- [ ] Describe what the EMT-Basic should do if there is reason to believe that there is a hazard at the scene. *(p. 746)*
- [ ] Describe the actions that an EMT-Basic should take to ensure bystander safety. *(p. 745)*
- [ ] State the role the EMT-Basic should perform until appropriately trained personnel arrive at the scene of a hazardous materials situation. *(p. 745)*

- [ ] Break down the steps to approaching a hazardous situation. *(p. 746)*
- [ ] Discuss the various environmental hazards that affect EMS. *(p. 745)*
- [ ] Describe the criteria for a multiple-casualty situation. *(p. 752)*
- [ ] Evaluate the role of the EMT-Basic in the multiple-casualty situation. *(p. 752)*
- [ ] Summarize the components of basic triage. *(p. 752)*
- [ ] Define the role of the EMT-Basic in a disaster operation. *(p. 750)*
- [ ] Describe basic concepts of incident management. *(p. 750)*
- [ ] Explain the methods for preventing contamination of self, equipment, and facilities. *(p. 748)*
- [ ] Review the local mass casualty incident plan. *(p. 752)*

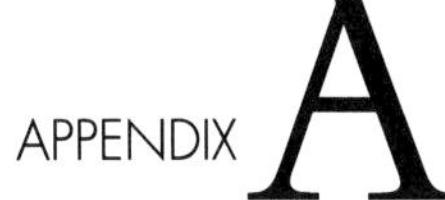

Advanced Airway Management

APPENDIX A SUMMARY

As an EMT-Basic, your Medical Director will need to make a decision, in concert with the acceptable standards of the region and state in which your service is located, on the need for training in the advanced airway management module of the EMT-Basic course. When the latest version of the curriculum was written, this module was included as an optional module of training with the understanding that some states and regions may allow their EMT-Basics to utilize the skill in this module. Still other states and regions may have adequate access to ALS providers, such as EMT-Intermediates and Paramedics, so that the Medical Directors do not feel there is a need to train the EMT-Basic in the advanced airway module.

The topics included in this module of training include the following:

- *A review of the anatomy and physiology of the adult and pediatric airway*
- *A review of the equipment used for intubation*
- *The nasogastric tube insertion in a pediatric patient*
- *Adult and pediatric orotracheal intubation*
- *Orotracheal suctioning*

REVIEW QUESTIONS

Please circle the best answer for each question.

1. The cartilage has not yet developed its full rigidity in infants and children.
   A) True **B)** False
   [Reference text page 763]

2. The soft chest wall causes infant and children to do which of the following?
   A) Rely more heavily on the diaphragm
   B) Use their chest muscles more to breathe
   C) Breathe at a faster rate than an adult
   D) None of the above
   [Reference text page 763]

3. The narrowest part of a child's airway is the:
   A) glottic opening. **B)** oropharynx. **C)** cricoid cartilage. **D)** hyoid bone.
   [Reference text page 763]

4. The OPA helps maintain a patent airway; it is used on ________ patients ________
   A) unresponsive; without a gag reflex. **B)** responsive; with a gag reflex.
   C) all; with or without a gag reflex. **D)** none of the above.
   [Reference text page 764]

5. Gurgling sounds suggest that the patient needs immediate suctioning of liquid secretions.
   A) True **B)** False
   [Reference text page 764]

6. A tube inserted into the nasal passage can be used for:
   A) decompression of the stomach. **B)** decompression of the proximal bowel.
   C) gastric lavage. **D)** all of the above.
   [Reference text page 764]

7. Gastric distention can be a problem with a patient of any age.
   A) True **B)** False
   [Reference text page 764]

8. The ________ tube can be used for a route for administration of medications and nutrition.
   A) OPA **B)** NG **C)** ET **D)** NPA
   [Reference text page 765]

9. The nasogastric tube size typically used for toddlers and preschoolers is ________ French.
A) 8.0 **B)** 10.0 **C)** 12.0 **D)** 14.0
[Reference text page 765]

10. In order to insert an NG tube, you should have:
A) a 20-mL syringe. **B)** a suction unit and connecting tube.
C) an emesis basin. **D)** all of the above.
[Reference text page 765]

11. Orotracheal intubation is the most effective means of controlling the airway in an apneic patient.
A) True **B)** False
[Reference text page 767]

12. Which of the following is NOT an indication for orotracheal intubation?
A) Patients who are unable to protect their own airways
B) Patients who are responsive to painful stimuli
C) Patients with no gag reflex or coughing
D) Inability to ventilate the apneic patient
[Reference text page 767]

13. Complications associated with advanced airway management include all of the following EXCEPT:
A) hypoxia from prolonged attempts at intubation.
B) vomiting or dry regurgitation from stimulation of a partially active gag reflex.
C) increasing heart rate from vagus nerve stimulation.
D) accidental extubation during movement and transport.
[Reference text page 768]

14. An instrument with a light and interchangeable blades, used for holding the tongue out of the way for intubation is called a/n:
A) stethoscope. **B)** endoscope. **C)** oroscope. **D)** laryngoscope.
[Reference text page 769]

15. Because of anatomical differences, the curved blade is preferred for infants and children.
A) True **B)** False
[Reference text page 769]

16. The proper size endotracheal tube used to intubate an average-size male patient is:
A) 6.5 **B)** 7.5. **C)** 8.5. **D)** 9.5.
[Reference text page 769]

17. The endotracheal tube size most frequently used for an average-size adult female is:
A) 6.5. **B)** 7.5. **C)** 8.5. **D)** 9.5.
[Reference text page 771]

18. Which of the following ET tube sizes would be uncuffed?
A) 5 **B)** 6 **C)** 7 **D)** 8
[Reference text page 771]

19. The standard adult ET tube when inserted should be approximately ________ cm at the patient's teeth.
A) 18 **B)** 22
C) 26 **D)** none of the above
[Reference text page 772]

20. It is suggested that a ________ be used to provide stiffness and shape to the ET tube.
A) syringe **B)** balloon **C)** stylet **D)** lyringoscope
[Reference text page 772]

21. For intubation attempts on a medical patient, it is suggested that a towel be placed behind the patient's shoulders or head.
A) True **B)** False
[Reference text page 773]

22. Pressure applied over the cricoid cartilage is called ________ maneuver.
A) Berman's **B)** larynx **C)** Sellick's **D)** Heimlich's
[Reference text page 773]

23. If you hear gurgling over the epigastrium when checking the tube placement, this usually indicates a misplaced tube.
A) True **B)** False
[Reference text page 777]

24. To be assured that the ET tube is inserted in the correct location, the EMT-Basic should:
A) observe it pass through the vocal cords.
B) use an esophageal intubation detector device.
C) use an end tidal CO-2 monitor.
D) do all of the above.
[Reference text page 777]

25. A method of estimating the size of the ET tube is to:
A) use half the child's age.
B) use the diameter of the patient's smallest finger.
C) use the patient's age divided by four.
D) do any of the above
[Reference text page 781]

KEY TERMS MATCHING

Assess your knowledge of the chapter key terms by matching the terms on the left to the definitions on the right.

_______ **1.** Barotrauma

_______ **2.** Endotracheal intubation (en-do-TRAY-ke-ul)

_______ **3.** Laryngoscope

_______ **4.** Nasogastric (NG) Tube

_______ **5.** Orotracheal Intubation

_______ **6.** Right Mainstem Intubation

_______ **7.** Sellick's Maneuver

_______ **8.** Vagus Nerve

(A) Tenth cranial nerve; controls smooth muscles of the lungs, heart, and abdominal viscera

(B) Advanced airway technique involving insertion of a tube through the mouth and into the trachea; also endotracheal intubation

(C) Placement of an endotracheal tube beyond the carina and into the right mainstem bronchus; results in ventilation of the right lung only

(D) Pressure applied directly over the cricoid cartilage; also cricoid pressure

(E) Tube inserted into the nasal passage for decompression of the stomach or proximal bowel or for gastric lavage

(F) Ruptured lung resulting from overaggressive ventilations

(G) Advanced airway technique involving insertion of a tube through the mouth and into the trachea; also orotracheal intubation

(H) An instrument with a light and interchangeable blades, used for holding the tongue out of the way for intubation

LABELING DIAGRAM

Label the anatomical structures of the respiratory system.

THE RESPIRATORY SYSTEM

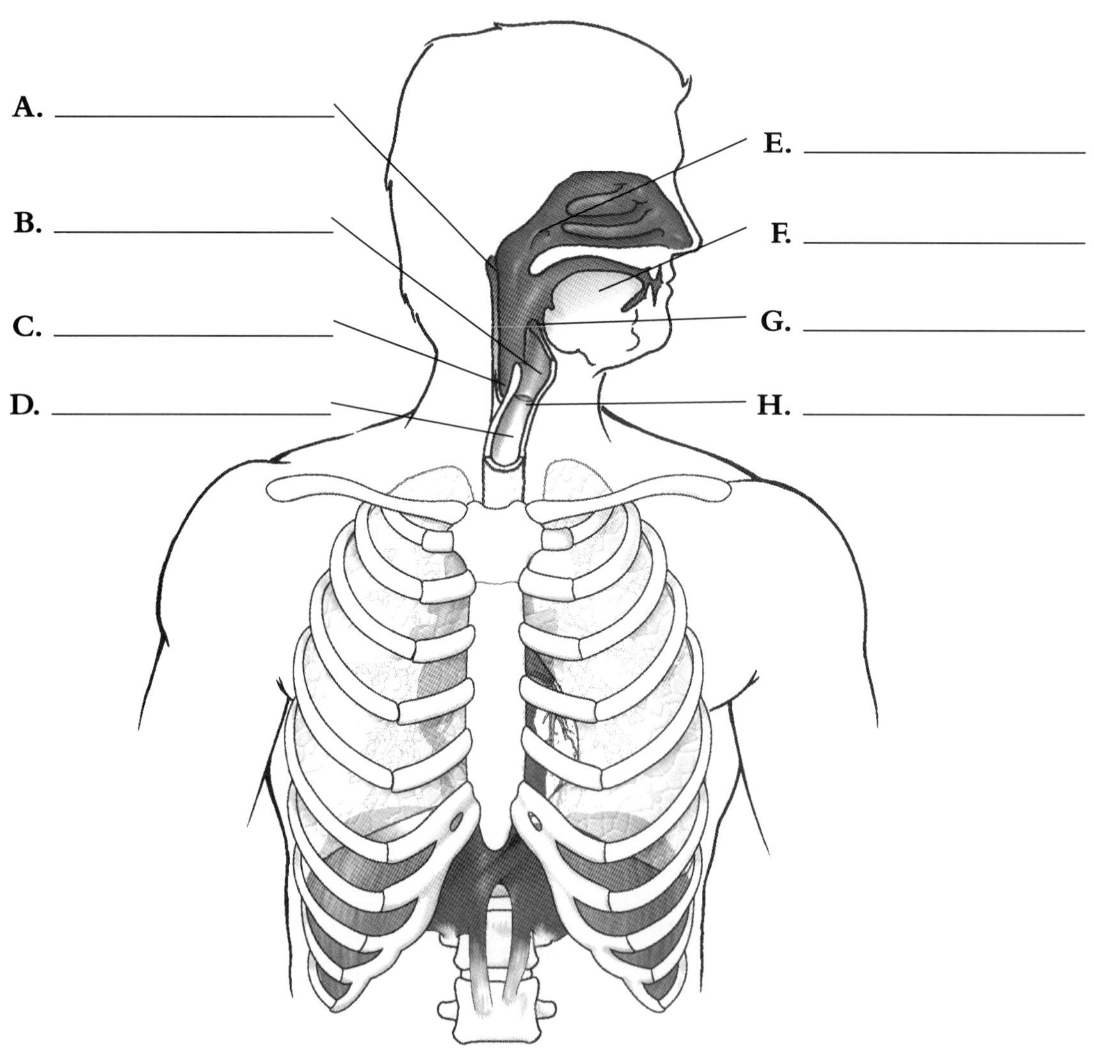

SKILLS CHECKLISTS

Check your knowledge of important EMT-B skills by marking off each step in the following skills sheets.

INSERTION OF THE EOA®

- [ ] Take BSI precautions.
- [ ] Position yourself at the patient's head.
- [ ] Assemble equipment:
    - [ ] An EOA® tube with proper mask.
    - [ ] A water-soluble lubricant.
    - [ ] BVM with reservoir.
    - [ ] Stethoscope.
    - [ ] Suction unit and rigid Yankauer tip.
    - [ ] A few 4 × 4 gauze pads.
    - [ ] A 35 cc syringe.
    - [ ] Gloves, mask, and protective eyewear.
- [ ] Have another rescuer hyperventilate the patient with a BVM.
- [ ] Lubricate the tip of tube with water-soluble gel.
- [ ] Stop resuscitation momentarily and lift the jaw and tongue straight upward without hyperextending neck. This is best accomplished with neck in neutral or slightly flexed position.
- [ ] Pass tube following the pharyngeal curvature until mask is seated against the face.
- [ ] Give one ventilation with the BVM, and watch for the chest to rise.
- [ ] Inflate the cuff using the 35 cc syringe. (Be certain tube is in esophagus.)
- [ ] Use stethoscope to listen to both lung fields. Listen for sounds of air moving in the lungs, and listen over epigastrium for absence of air moving.
- [ ] Ventilate patient using BVM or a flow-restricted, oxygen-powered ventilation device.
- [ ] Maintain a good mask seal at all times.

ET INTUBATION AND MANAGEMENT

- [ ] Take BSI precautions.
- [ ] Open airway manually.
- [ ] Elevate tongue and insert airway adjunct (oropharyngeal or nasopharyngeal airway).
- [ ] Ventilate patient immediately using a BVM device unattached to oxygen.
- [ ] Hyperventilate patient with room air.
- [ ] Attach oxygen reservoir to BVM.
- [ ] Attach BVM to high-flow oxygen.
- [ ] Ventilate patient at proper volume and rate.
- [ ] Direct assistant to hyperventilate patient.
- [ ] Identify and select proper equipment for intubation.
- [ ] Check equipment (cuffs for leaks, laryngoscope batteries, and bulb for tightness).
- [ ] Position head properly.
- [ ] Insert laryngoscope blade with left hand while displacing tongue.
- [ ] Elevate mandible with laryngoscope.
- [ ] Insert the ET and advance it to proper depth (until cuff is past vocal cords).
- [ ] Inflate cuff to proper pressure (5 cc to 10 cc of air) and disconnect syringe.
- [ ] Continue to hold onto the ET until it is secured in place.
- [ ] Direct ventilation of the patient.
- [ ] Confirm proper placement by auscultation bilaterally and over epigastrium.*
- [ ] Secure the ET.

***NOTE:** Some medical directors also require the use of an esophageal intubation detector device, pulse oximeter or colormetric end-tidal CO_2 device to confirm tube placement.

INSERTION OF THE NASOGASTRIC TUBE

- [ ] Take BSI precautions.
- [ ] Prepare and assemble the equipment.

- [ ] Oxygenate the patient.
- [ ] Measure tube from tip of nose, over ear, to below xiphoid process.
- [ ] Lubricate end of tube, and pass tube gently downward along nasal floor to stomach.
- [ ] To confirm correct placement, auscultate over epigastrium. Listen for bubbling while injecting 10 to 20 cc air into tube.
- [ ] Use suction to aspirate stomach contents.
- [ ] Secure tube in place.

(reprinted from *Pocket Reference for The EMT-B and First Responder* by Bob Elling, Prentice Hall, 1999)

D.O.T. OBJECTIVES CHECKLIST

Use the following list of knowledge objectives to check what you've learned. Check off only those objectives that you feel you completely understand and have mastered. For any objectives not checked, go back and review that section of the text chapter. Textbook page references have been provided to help you review the text material.

- [ ] Identify and describe the airway anatomy in the infant, child, and the adult. *(p. 763)*
- [ ] Differentiate between the airway anatomy in the infant, child, and the adult. *(p. 763)*
- [ ] Explain the pathophysiology of airway compromise. *(p. 763)*
- [ ] Describe the proper use of airway adjuncts. *(p. 764)*
- [ ] Review the use of oxygen therapy in airway management. *(p. 764)*
- [ ] Describe the indications, contraindications, and technique for insertion of nasal gastric tubes. *(p. 764)*
- [ ] Describe how to perform the Sellick maneuver (cricoid pressure). *(p. 773)*
- [ ] Describe the indications for advanced airway management. *(p. 766)*
- [ ] List the equipment required for orotracheal intubation. *(p. 768)*

- [ ] Describe the proper use of the curved blade for orotracheal intubation. *(p. 769)*
- [ ] Describe the proper use of the straight blade for orotracheal intubation. *(p. 769)*
- [ ] State the reasons for and proper use of the stylet in orotracheal intubation. *(p. 772)*
- [ ] Describe the methods of choosing the appropriate size endotracheal tube in an adult patient. *(p. 770)*
- [ ] State the formula for sizing an infant or a child endotracheal tube. *(p. 781)*
- [ ] List complications associated with advanced airway management. *(p. 766)*
- [ ] Define the various alternative methods for sizing the infant and child endotracheal tube. *(p. 781)*
- [ ] Describe the skill of orotracheal intubation in the adult patient. *(p. 775)*
- [ ] Describe the skill of orotracheal intubation in the infant and child patient. *(p. 783)*
- [ ] Describe the skill of confirming endotracheal tube placement in the adult, infant, and child patient. *(p. 775)*
- [ ] State the consequence of and the need to recognize unintentional esophageal intubation. *(p. 775)*
- [ ] Describe the skill of securing the endotracheal tube in the adult, infant, and child patient. *(p. 775)*

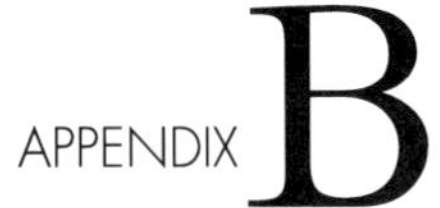

National Registry Skill Sheets

The National Registry of Emergency Medical Technicians is an organization founded in 1970, one of whose goals is to establish nationwide professional standards for EMTs. Many state EMS systems use examinations developed by the National Registry to establish certification of EMTs.

The National Registry has prepared a certification examination correlated to the 1994 Department of Transportation Emergency Medical Technician-Basic: National Standard Curriculum. The examination includes both a written portion and a practical portion that consists of a series of performance-based skill stations.

To assist students in preparing for the skill stations that are part of the EMT-Basic examination, as well as to establish guidelines and parameters for those who will evaluate students' performance at the skill stations, the National Registry has developed a series of skill sheets. Each skill sheet contains a set of directions, the skill criteria, and the critical criteria that if not met by the student result in immediate failure of the station.

In studying for the National Registry examination, you should use these skills sheets in conjunction with the material presented in the textbook and not as the sole means of learning the individual skills. The skill sheets will aid you in organizing the steps necessary to perform each skill and in identifying the criteria that will be used to evaluate your performance. You can use these sheets to evaluate your own performance when practicing these skills and preparing for your practical skills evaluation.

Note: Three skill sheets regarding advanced airway management are included. The use of these skills will vary based on your medical director, training program, and local protocol.

Organization of the National Registry Examination

The practical examination consists of six stations, five mandatory stations and one random basic skill station, consisting of both skill-based and scenario-based testing. The random skill station is conducted so the candidate is totally unaware of the skill to be tested until he or she arrives at the test site.

The candidate will be tested individually in each station and will be expected to direct the actions of any assistant EMTs who may be present in the station. The candidate should pass or fail the examination based solely on his or her actions and decisions.

On the next page is a list of the stations and their established time limits. The maximum time is determined by the number and difficulty of tasks to be completed.

INSTRUCTIONS TO THE CANDIDATE

PATIENT ASSESSMENT/MANAGEMENT—TRAUMA

This station is designed to test your ability to perform a patient assessment of a victim of multi-system trauma and voice-treat all conditions and injuries discovered. You must conduct your assessment as you would in the field, including communicating with your patient. You may remove the patient's clothing down to shorts or swimsuit if you feel it is necessary. As you conduct your assessment, you should state everything you are assessing. Clinical information not obtainable by visual or physical inspection, for example, blood pressure, will be given to you after you demonstrate how you would normally gain that information. You may assume that you have two EMTs working with you and that they are correctly carrying out the verbal treatments you indicate. You have ten (10) minutes to complete this skill station. Do you have any questions?

PATIENT ASSESSMENT/MANAGEMENT—MEDICAL

This station is designed to test your ability to perform a patient assessment of a victim with a chief complaint of a medical nature and voice-treat all conditions and injuries discovered. You must conduct your assessment as you would in the field, including communicating with your patient. As you conduct your assessment, you should state everything you are assessing. Clinical information not obtainable by visual or physical inspection, for example, blood pressure, will be given to you after you demonstrate how you would normally gain that information. You may assume that you have two EMTs working with you and that they are correctly carrying out the verbal treatments you indicate. You have ten (10) minutes to complete this skill station. Do you have any questions?

CARDIAC ARREST MANAGEMENT/AED

This station is designed to test your ability to manage a prehospital cardiac arrest by integrating CPR skills, defibrillation, airway adjuncts, and patient/scene management skills. There will be an EMT assistant in this station. The EMT assistant will only do as you instruct him. As you arrive on the scene, you will encounter a patient in cardiac arrest. A First Responder will be present performing single rescuer CPR. You must immediately establish control of the scene and begin resuscitation of the patient with an automated external defibrillator. At the appropriate time, you must control the airway and ventilate the victim using adjunctive equipment. You may not delegate this action to the EMT assistant. You may use any of the supplies available in this room. You have fifteen (15) minutes to complete this skill station. Do you have any questions?

AIRWAY, OXYGEN, VENTILATION SKILLS BAG-VALVE-MASK APNEIC PATIENT WITH PULSE

This station is designed to test your ability to ventilate a patient using a bag-valve mask. As you enter the station, you will find an apneic patient with a palpable central pulse. There are no bystanders and artificial ventilation has not been initiated. The only patient intervention required is airway management and ventilatory support using a bag-valve mask. You must initially ventilate the patient for a minimum of 30 seconds. You will be evaluated on the appropriateness of ventilator volumes. I will inform you that a second rescuer has arrived and will instruct you that you must control the airway and the mask seal while the second rescuer provides ventilation. You may use only the equipment available in this room. You have ten (10) minutes to complete this procedure. Do you have any questions?

SPINAL IMMOBILIZATION—SUPINE PATIENT

This station is designed to test your ability to provide spinal immobilization on a patient using a long spine immobilization device. You arrive on the scene with an EMT assistant. The assistant EMT has completed the scene size-up as well as the initial and focused assessments. As you begin the station, there are no airway, breathing, or circulatory problems. You are required to treat the specific, isolated problem of an unstable spine using a long spine immobilization device. When moving the patient to the device, you should use the help of the assistant EMT and the evaluator. The assistant EMT should control the head and cervical spine of the patient while you and the evaluator move the patient to the immobilization device. You are responsible for the direction and subsequent action of the EMT assistant. You may use any equipment available in this room. You have ten (10) minutes to complete this procedure. Do you have any questions?

Station 1:	Patient Assessment/Management—Trauma	10 min
Station 2:	Patient Assessment/Management—Medical	10 min
Station 3:	Cardiac Arrest Management/AED	15 min
Station 4:	Bag-Valve-Mask Apneic Patient	10 min
Station 5:	Spinal Immobilization Station	
	Spinal Immobilization—Supine Patient	10 min
	Spinal Immobilization—Seated Patient	10 min
Station 6:	Random Basic Skill Verification	
	Long Bone Injury	5 min
	Joint Injury	5 min
	Traction Splint	10 min
	Bleeding Control/Shock Management	10 min
	Upper Airway Adjuncts and Suction	5 min
	Mouth-to-Mask with Supplemental Oxygen	5 min
	Supplemental Oxygen Administration	5 min

SPINAL IMMOBILIZATION—SEATED PATIENT

This station is designed to test your ability to provide spinal immobilization on a patient using a half spine immobilization device. You arrive on the scene with an EMT assistant. The assistant EMT has completed the scene size-up, initial and focused assessments. As you begin the station, there are no airway, breathing, or circulatory problems. You are required to treat the specific, isolated problem of an unstable spine using a half spine immobilization device. Continued assessment of airway, breathing, and central circulation is not necessary. You are responsible for the direction and subsequent actions of the EMT assistant.

Transferring the patient to the long spine board should be accomplished verbally. You may use any equipment available in this room. You have ten (10) minutes to complete this procedure. Do you have any questions?

IMMOBILIZATION—LONG BONE INJURY

This station is designed to test your ability to properly immobilize a closed, non-angulated long bone injury. You are required to treat only the specific, isolated injury. The scene size-up and initial assessment have been completed and during the focused assessment a closed, non-angulated injury of the ________ (radius, ulna, tibia, fibula) was detected. Ongoing assessment of the patient's airway, breathing, and central circulation is not necessary. You may use any equipment available in this room. You have five (5) minutes to complete this procedure. Do you have any questions?

IMMOBILIZATION—JOINT INJURY

This station is designed to test your ability to properly immobilize a non-complicated shoulder injury. You are required to treat only the specific, isolated injury. The scene size-up and initial assessment have been accomplished on the victim and during the focused assessment a shoulder injury was detected. Ongoing assessment of the patient's airway, breathing, and central circulation is not necessary. You may use any equipment available in this room. You have five (5) minutes to complete this procedure. Do you have any questions?

IMMOBILIZATION—TRACTION SPLINTING

This station is designed to test your ability to properly immobilize a mid-shaft femur injury with a traction splint. You will have an EMT assistant to help you in the application of the device by applying manual traction when directed to do so. You are required to treat only the specific, isolated injury. The scene size-up and initial assessment have been accomplished on the victim, and during the focused assessment a mid-shaft femur deformity was detected. Ongoing assessment of the patient's airway, breathing, and central circulation is not necessary. You may use any equipment available in this room. You have ten (10) minutes to complete this procedure. Do you have any questions?

BLEEDING CONTROL/SHOCK MANAGEMENT

This station is designed to test your ability to control hemorrhage. This is a scenario-based testing station. As you progress through the scenario, you will be offered various signs and symptoms appropriate for the patient's condition. You will be required to manage the patient based on these signs and symptoms. A scenario will be read aloud to you, and you will be given an opportunity to ask clarifying questions about the scenario; however, you will not receive answers to any questions about the actual steps of the procedures to be performed. You may use any of the supplies and equipment available in this room. You have ten (10) minutes to complete this skill station. Do you have any questions?

AIRWAY, OXYGEN, VENTILATION SKILLS UPPER AIRWAY ADJUNCTS AND SUCTION

This station is designed to test your ability to properly measure, insert, and remove an oropharyngeal and a nasopharyngeal airway as well as suction a patient's upper airway. This is an isolated skills test comprised of three separate skills. You may use any equipment available in this room. You have five (5) minutes to complete this skill station. Do you have any questions?

AIRWAY, OXYGEN, VENTILATION SKILLS MOUTH-TO-MASK WITH SUPPLEMENTAL OXYGEN

This station is designed to test your ability to ventilate a patient with supplemental oxygen using a mouth-to-mask technique. This is an isolated skills test. You may assume that mouth-to-mouth ventilation is in progress and that the patient has a central pulse. The only patient management required is ventilatory support using a mouth-to-mask technique with supplemental oxygen. You must ventilate the patient for at least 30 seconds. You will be evaluated on the appropriateness of ventilatory volumes. You may use any equipment available in this room. You have five (5) minutes to complete this skill station. Do you have any questions?

AIRWAY, OXYGEN, VENTILATION SKILLS SUPPLEMENTAL OXYGEN ADMINISTRATION

This station is designed to test your ability to correctly assemble the equipment needed to administer supplemental oxygen in the prehospital setting. This is an isolated skills test. You will be required to assemble an oxygen tank and regulator and administer oxygen to a patient using a non-rebreather mask. At this point, you will be instructed to discontinue oxygen administration by the non-rebreather mask because the patient cannot tolerate the mask and start oxygen administration using a nasal cannula. Once you have initiated oxygen administration using a nasal cannula, you will be instructed to discontinue oxygen administration completely. You may use only the equipment available in this room. You have five (5) minutes to complete this skill station. Do you have any questions?

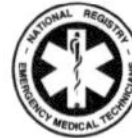

PATIENT ASSESSMENT/MANAGEMENT—TRAUMA

		Points Possible	Points Awarded
Takes or verbalizes body substance isolation precautions		1	
SCENE SIZE-UP			
Determines the scene is safe		1	
Determines the mechanism of injury		1	
Determines the number of patients		1	
Requests additional help if necessary		1	
Considers stabilization of spine		1	
INITIAL ASSESSMENT			
Verbalizes general impression of patient		1	
Determines responsiveness		1	
Determines chief complaint/apparent life threats		1	
Assesses airway and breathing	Assessment	1	
	Initiates appropriate oxygen therapy	1	
	Assures adequate ventilation	1	
	Injury management	1	
Assesses circulation	Assesses for and controls major bleeding	1	
	Assesses pulse	1	
	Assesses skin (color, temperature, and condition)	1	
Identifies priority patients/makes transport decision		1	
FOCUSED HISTORY AND PHYSICAL EXAM/RAPID TRAUMA ASSESSMENT			
Selects appropriate assessment (focused or rapid assessment)		1	
Obtains or directs assistant to obtain baseline vital signs		1	
Obtains SAMPLE history		1	
DETAILED PHYSICAL EXAMINATION			
Assesses the head	Inspects and palpates the scalp and ears	1	
	Assesses the eyes	1	
	Assesses the facial area including oral and nasal area	1	
Assesses the neck	Inspects and palpates the neck	1	
	Assesses for JVD	1	
	Assesses for tracheal deviation	1	
Assesses the chest	Inspects	1	
	Palpates	1	
	Auscultates the chest	1	
Assesses the abdomen/pelvis	Assesses the abdomen	1	
	Assesses the pelvis	1	
	Verbalizes assessment of genitalia/perineum as needed	1	
Assesses the extremities	1 point for each extremity includes inspection, palpation, and assessment of pulses, sensory and motor activity	4	
Assesses the posterior	Assesses thorax	1	
	Assesses lumbar	1	
Manages secondary injuries and wounds appropriately **1 point for appropriate management of secondary injury/wound**		1	
Verbalizes reassessment of the vital signs		1	
	TOTAL:	40	

CRITICAL CRITERIA

___ Did not take or verbalize body substance isolation precautions
___ Did not assess for spinal protection
___ Did not provide for spinal protection when indicated
___ Did not provide high concentration of oxygen
___ Did not find or manage problems associated with airway, breathing, hemorrhage, or shock (hypoperfusion)
___ Did not differentiate patients needing transportation versus continued on scene assessment
___ Did other detailed physical examination before assessing airway, breathing, and circulation
___ Did not transport patient within ten (10) minute time limit

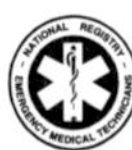

PATIENT ASSESSMENT/MANAGEMENT—MEDICAL

		Points Possible	Points Awarded
Takes or verbalizes body substance isolation precautions		1	
SCENE SIZE-UP			
Determines the scene is safe		1	
Determines the mechanism of injury/nature of illness		1	
Determines the number of patients		1	
Requests additional help if necessary		1	
Considers stabilization of spine		1	
INITIAL ASSESSMENT			
Verbalizes general impression of patient		1	
Determines responsiveness/level of consciousness		1	
Determines chief complaint/apparent life threats		1	
Assesses airway and breathing	Assessment Initiates appropriate oxygen therapy Assures adequate ventilation	1 1 1	
Assesses circulation	Assesses/controls major bleeding Assesses pulse Assesses skin (color, temperature, and condition)	1 1 1	
Identifies priority patients/makes transport decision		1	
FOCUSED HISTORY AND PHYSICAL EXAM/RAPID ASSESSMENT			
Signs and Symptoms (Assesses history of present illness)		4	

Respiratory	Cardiac	Altered Mental Status	Allergic Reaction	Poisoning/ Overdose	Environmental Emergency	Obstetrics	Behavioral
•Onset? •Provokes? •Quality? •Radiates? •Severity? •Time? •Interventions?	•Onset? •Provokes? •Quality? •Radiates? •Severity? •Time? •Interventions?	•Description of the episode •Onset? •Duration? •Associated symptoms? •Evidence of trauma? •Interventions? •Seizures? •Fever?	•History of allergies? •What were you exposed to? •How were you exposed? •Effects? •Progression? •Interventions?	•Substance? •When did you ingest/become exposed? •How much did you ingest? •Over what time period? •Interventions? •Estimated weight? •Effects?	•Source? •Environment? •Duration? •Loss of consciousness? •Effects— General or local?	•Are you pregnant? •How long have you been pregnant? •Pain or contractions? •Bleeding or discharge? •Do you feel the need to push? •Last menstrual period? •Crowning?	•How do you feel? •Determine suicidal tendencies •Is the patient a threat to self or others? •Is there a medical problem? •Interventions?

	Points Possible	Points Awarded
Allergies	1	
Medications	1	
Past pertinent history	1	
Last oral intake	1	
Events leading to present illness (rule out trauma)	1	
Performs focused physical examination Assesses affected body part/system or, if indicated, completes rapid assessment	1	
VITALS (Obtains baseline vital signs)	1	
INTERVENTIONS Obtains medical direction or verbalizes standing order for medication interventions and verbalizes proper additional intervention/treatment	1	
TRANSPORT (Re-evaluates transport decision)	1	
Verbalizes the consideration for completing a detailed physical examination	1	
Ongoing ASSESSMENT (verbalized)		
Repeats initial assessment	1	
Repeats vital signs	1	
Repeats focused assessment regarding patient complaint or injuries	1	
Checks interventions	1	
TOTAL:	34	

CRITICAL CRITERIA

___ Did not take or verbalize body substance isolation precautions if necessary
___ Did not determine scene safety
___ Did not obtain medical direction or verbalize standing orders for medication interventions
___ Did not provide high concentration of oxygen
___ Did not evaluate and find conditions of airway, breathing, circulation
___ Did not find or manage problems associated with airway, breathing, hemorrhage, or shock (hypoperfusion)
___ Did not differentiate patients needing transportation versus continued assessment at the scene
___ Did detailed or focused history/physical examination before assessing airway, breathing, and circulation
___ Did not ask questions about the present illness
___ Administered a dangerous or inappropriate intervention

CARDIAC ARREST MANAGEMENT/AED

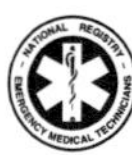

	Points Possible	Points Awarded
ASSESSMENT		
Takes or verbalizes body substance isolation precautions	1	
Briefly questions rescuer about arrest events	1	
Directs rescuer to stop CPR	1	
Verifies absence of spontaneous pulse *(skill station examiner states "no pulse")*	1	
Turns on defibrillator power	1	
Attaches automated defibrillator to patient	1	
Ensures all individuals are standing clear of the patient	1	
Initiates analysis of rhythm	1	
Delivers shock (up to three successive shocks)	1	
Verifies absence of spontaneous pulse *(skill station examiner states "no pulse")*	1	
TRANSITION		
Directs resumption of CPR	1	
Gathers additional information on arrest event	1	
Confirms effectiveness of CPR (ventilation and compressions)	1	
INTEGRATION		
Directs insertion of a simple airway adjunct (oropharyngeal/nasopharyngeal)	1	
Directs ventilation of patient	1	
Assures high concentration of oxygen connected to the ventilatory adjunct	1	
Assures CPR continues without unnecessary/prolonged interruption	1	
Re-evaluates patient/CPR in approximately one minute	1	
Repeats defibrillator sequence	1	
TRANSPORTATION		
Verbalizes transportation of patient	1	
TOTAL:	20	

CRITICAL CRITERIA

___ Did not take or verbalize body substance isolation precautions
___ Did not evaluate the need for immediate use of the AED
___ Did not direct initiation/resumption of ventilation/compressions at appropriate times
___ Did not assure all individuals were clear of patient before delivering each shock
___ Did not operate the AED properly (inability to deliver shock)

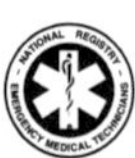

BAG-VALVE-MASK
APNEIC PATIENT

	Points Possible	Points Awarded
Takes or verbalizes body substance isolation precautions	1	
Voices opening the airway	1	
Voices inserting an airway adjunct	1	
Selects appropriate size mask	1	
Creates a proper mask-to-face seal	1	
Ventilates patient at no less than 800 ml volume ***(The examiner must witness for at least 30 seconds)***	1	
Connects reservoir and oxygen	1	
Adjusts liter flow to 15 liters/minute or greater	1	
The examiner indicates the arrival of second EMT. The second EMT is instructed to ventilate the patient while the candidate controls the mask and the airway.		
Voices re-opening the airway	1	
Creates a proper mask-to-face seal	1	
Instructs assistant to resume ventilation at proper volume per breath ***(The examiner must witness for at least 30 seconds)***	1	
TOTAL:	11	

CRITICAL CRITERIA

___ Did not take or verbalize body substance isolation precautions
___ Did not immediately ventilate the patient
___ Interrupted ventilations for more than 20 seconds
___ Did not provide high concentration of oxygen
___ Did not provide or direct assistant to provide proper volume/breath
(more than 2 ventilations per minute are below 800 ml)
___ Did not allow adequate exhalation

SPINAL IMMOBILIZATION
SUPINE PATIENT

	Points Possible	Points Awarded
Takes or verbalizes body substance isolation precautions	1	
Directs assistant to place/maintain head in neutral in-line position	1	
Directs assistant to maintain manual immobilization of the head	1	
Assesses motor, sensory, and distal circulation in extremities	1	
Applies appropriate size extrication collar	1	
Positions the immobilization device appropriately	1	
Directs movement of the patient onto device without compromising the integrity of the spine	1	
Applies padding to voids between the torso and the board as necessary	1	
Immobilizes the patient's torso to the device	1	
Evaluates the pads behind the patient's head as necessary	1	
Immobilizes the patient's head to the device	1	
Secures the patient's legs to the device	1	
Secures the patient's arms to the device	1	
Reassesses motor, sensory, and distal circulation in extremities	1	
TOTAL:	14	

CRITICAL CRITERIA

___ Did not immediately direct or take manual immobilization of the head
___ Released or ordered release of manual immobilization before it was maintained mechanically
___ Patient manipulated or moved excessively, causing potential spinal compromise
___ Patient moves excessively up, down, left, or right on the device
___ Head immobilization allows for excessive movement
___ Upon completion of immobilization, head is not in the neutral in-line position
___ Did not reassess motor, sensory, and distal circulation after immobilization to the device
___ Immobilized head to the board before securing torso

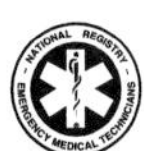

SPINAL IMMOBILIZATION SEATED PATIENT

	Points Possible	Points Awarded
Takes or verbalizes body substance isolation precautions	1	
Directs assistant to place/maintain head in neutral in-line position	1	
Directs assistant to maintain manual immobilization of the head	1	
Reassesses motor, sensory, and distal circulation in extremities	1	
Applies appropriate size extrication collar	1	
Positions the immobilization device behind the patient	1	
Secures the device to the patient's torso	1	
Evaluates torso fixation and adjusts as necessary	1	
Evaluates and pads behind the patient's head as necessary	1	
Secures the patient's head to the device	1	
Verbalizes moving the patient to a long board	1	
Reassesses motor, sensory, and distal circulation in extremities	1	
TOTAL:	12	

CRITICAL CRITERIA

___ Did not immediately direct or take manual immobilization of the head
___ Released or ordered release of manual immobilization before it was maintained mechanically
___ Patient manipulated or moved excessively, causing potential spinal compromise
___ Device moves excessively up, down, left, or right on patient's torso
___ Head immobilization allows for excessive movement
___ Torso fixation inhibits chest rise, resulting in respiratory compromise
___ Upon completion of immobilization, head is not in the neutral position
___ Did not reassess motor, sensory, and distal circulation after voicing immobilization to the long board
___ Immobilized head to the board before securing the torso

IMMOBILIZATION SKILLS
LONG BONE

	Points Possible	Points Awarded
Takes or verbalizes body substance isolation precautions	1	
Directs application of manual stabilization	1	
Assesses motor, sensory, and distal circulation	1	
NOTE: The examiner acknowledges present and normal.		
Measures splint	1	
Applies splint	1	
Immobilizes the joint above the injury site	1	
Immobilizes the joint below the injury site	1	
Secures the entire injured extremity	1	
Immobilizes hand/foot in the position of function	1	
Reassesses motor, sensory, and distal circulation	1	
NOTE: The examiner acknowledges present and normal.		
TOTAL:	10	

CRITICAL CRITERIA

___ Grossly moves injured extremity
___ Did not immobilize adjacent joints
___ Did not assess motor, sensory, and distal circulation before and after splinting

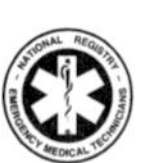

IMMOBILIZATION SKILLS
JOINT INJURY

	Points Possible	Points Awarded
Takes or verbalizes body substance isolation precautions	1	
Directs application of manual stabilization of the injury	1	
Assesses motor, sensory, and distal circulation	1	
NOTE: The examiner acknowledges present and normal.		
Selects proper splinting material	1	
Immobilizes the site of the injury	1	
Immobilizes bone above injured joint	1	
Immobilizes bone below injured joint	1	
Reassesses motor, sensory, and distal circulation	1	
NOTE: The examiner acknowledges present and normal.		
TOTAL:	8	

CRITICAL CRITERIA

___ Did not support the joint so that the joint did not bear distal weight
___ Did not immobilize bone above and below injured joint
___ Did not reassess motor, sensory, and distal circulation before and after splinting

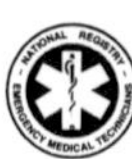

IMMOBILIZATION SKILLS
TRACTION SPLINTING

	Points Possible	Points Awarded
Takes or verbalizes body substance isolation precautions	1	
Directs application of manual stabilization of the injured leg	1	
Directs the application of manual traction	1	
Assesses motor, sensory, and distal circulation	1	
NOTE: *The examiner acknowledges present and normal.*		
Prepares/adjusts splint to the proper length	1	
Positions the splint on the injured leg	1	
Applies the proximal securing device (e.g., ischial strap)	1	
Applies the distal securing device (e.g., ankle hitch)	1	
Applies mechanical traction	1	
Positions/secures the support straps	1	
Re-evaluates the proximal/distal securing devices	1	
Reassesses motor, sensory, and distal circulation	1	
NOTE: *The examiner acknowledges present and normal.*		
NOTE: *The examiner must ask candidate how he/she would prepare the patient for transportation.*		
Verbalizes securing the torso to the long board to immobilize the hip	1	
Verbalizes securing the splint to the long board to prevent movement of the splint	1	
TOTAL:	14	

CRITICAL CRITERIA

___ Loss of traction at any point after it is assumed
___ Did not reassess motor, sensory, and distal circulation before and after splinting
___ The foot is excessively rotated or extended after splinting
___ Did not secure the ischial strap before taking traction
___ Final immobilization failed to support the femur or prevent rotation of the injured leg
___ Secured leg to splint before applying mechanical traction

NOTE: **If the Sager splint or Kendrick Traction Device is used without elevating the patient's leg, application of manual traction is not necessary. The candidate should be awarded 1 point as if manual traction were applied.**

NOTE: **If the leg is elevated at all, manual traction must be applied before elevating the leg. The ankle hitch may be applied before elevating the leg and used to provide manual traction.**

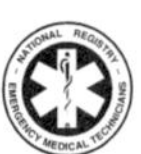

BLEEDING CONTROL/SHOCK MANAGEMENT

	Points Possible	Points Awarded
Takes or verbalizes body substance isolation precautions	1	
Applies direct pressure to the wound	1	
Elevates the extremity	1	
NOTE: The examiner must now inform the candidate that the wound continues to bleed.		
Applies an additional dressing to the wound	1	
NOTE: The examiner must now inform the candidate that the wound still continues to bleed. The second dressing does not control the bleeding.		
Locates and applies pressure to appropriate arterial pressure point	1	
NOTE: The examiner must now inform the candidate that the bleeding is controlled.		
Bandages the wound	1	
NOTE: The examiner must now inform the candidate that the patient is showing signs and symptoms indicative of hypoperfusion.		
Properly positions the patient	1	
Applies high-concentration oxygen	1	
Initiates steps to prevent heat loss from the patient	1	
Indicates need for immediate transportation	1	
TOTAL:	10	

CRITICAL CRITERIA

___ Did not take or verbalize body substance isolation precautions
___ Did not apply high concentration of oxygen
___ Applied tourniquet before attempting other methods of bleeding control
___ Did not control hemorrhage in a timely manner
___ Did not indicate a need for immediate transportation

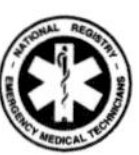

AIRWAY, OXYGEN, AND VENTILATION SKILLS
UPPER AIRWAY ADJUNCTS AND SUCTION

OROPHARYNGEAL AIRWAY

	Points Possible	Points Awarded
Takes or verbalizes body substance isolation precautions	1	
Selects appropriate size airway	1	
Measures airway	1	
Inserts airway without pushing the tongue posteriorly	1	
NOTE: The examiner must advise the candidate that the patient is gagging and becoming conscious.		
Removes oropharyngeal airway	1	

SUCTION

NOTE: The examiner must advise the candidate to suction the patient's oropharynx/nasopharynx.		
Turns on/prepares suction device	1	
Assures presence of mechanical suction	1	
Inserts suction tip without suction	1	
Applies suction to the oropharynx/nasopharynx	1	

NASOPHARYNGEAL AIRWAY

NOTE: The examiner must advise the candidate to insert a nasopharyngeal airway.		
Selects appropriate airway	1	
Measures airway	1	
Verbalizes lubrication of the nasal airway	1	
Fully inserts the airway with the bevel facing toward the septum	1	
TOTAL:	13	

CRITICAL CRITERIA

___ Did not take or verbalize body substance isolation precautions
___ Did not obtain a patent airway with the oropharyngeal airway
___ Did not obtain a patent airway with the nasopharyngeal airway
___ Did not demonstrate an acceptable suction technique
___ Inserted any adjunct in a manner dangerous to the patient

MOUTH-TO-MASK WITH SUPPLEMENTAL OXYGEN

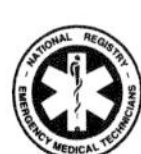

	Points Possible	Points Awarded
Takes or verbalizes body substance isolation precautions	1	
Connects one-way valve to mask	1	
Opens patient's airway or confirms patient's airway is open (manually or with adjunct)	1	
Establishes and maintains a proper mask to face seal	1	
Ventilates the patient at the proper volume and rate *(800–1200 ml per breath/10–20 breaths per minute)*	1	
Connects mask to high-concentration oxygen	1	
Adjusts flow rate to 15 liters/minute or greater	1	
Continues ventilation at proper volume and rate *(800–1200 ml per breath/10–20 breaths per minute)*	1	
NOTE: The examiner must witness ventilations for at least 30 seconds.		
TOTAL:	8	

CRITICAL CRITERIA

___ Did not take or verbalize body substance isolation precautions
___ Did not adjust liter flow to 15 L/min or greater
___ Did not provide proper volume per breath
(more than 2 ventilations per minute are below 800 ml)
___ Did not ventilate the patient at 10–20 breaths per minute
___ Did not allow for complete exhalation

OXYGEN ADMINISTRATION

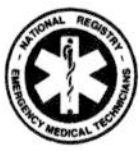

	Points Possible	Points Awarded
Takes or verbalizes body substance isolation precautions	1	
Assembles regulator to tank	1	
Opens tank	1	
Checks for leaks	1	
Checks tank pressure	1	
Attaches nonrebreather mask	1	
Prefills reservoir	1	
Adjusts liter flow to 12 liters/minute or greater	1	
Applies and adjusts mask to the patient's face	1	
NOTE: The examiner must advise the candidate that the patient is not tolerating the nonrebreather mask. Medical direction has ordered you to apply a nasal cannula to the patient.		
Attaches nasal cannula to oxygen	1	
Adjusts liter flow to 6 liters/minute or less	1	
Applies nasal cannula to the patient	1	
NOTE: The examiner must advise the candidate to discontinue oxygen therapy.		
Removes the nasal cannula	1	
Shuts off the regulator	1	
Relieves the pressure within the regulator	1	
TOTAL:	15	

CRITICAL CRITERIA

___ Did not take or verbalize body substance isolation precautions
___ Did not assemble the tank and regulator without leaks
___ Did not prefill the reservoir bag
___ Did not adjust the device to the correct liter flow for the nonrebreather mask (12 L/min or greater)
___ Did not adjust the device to the correct liter flow for the nasal cannula (up to 6 L/min)

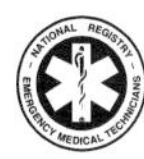

VENTILATORY MANAGEMENT
ENDOTRACHEAL INTUBATION

NOTE: If a candidate elects to initially ventilate with a BVM attached to a reservoir and oxygen, full credit must be awarded for steps denoted by "**" if the first ventilation is delivered within the initial 30 seconds

		Points Possible	Points Awarded
Takes or verbalizes body substance isolation precautions		1	
Opens airway manually		1	
Elevates tongue and inserts simple airway adjunct (oropharyngeal or nasopharyngeal airway)		1	
NOTE: The examiner now informs the candidate no gag reflex is present and the patient accepts the adjunct.			
**Ventilates the patient immediately using a BVM device unattached to oxygen		1	
**Hyperventilates the patient with room air		1	
NOTE: The examiner now informs the candidate that ventilation is being performed without difficulty.			
Attaches the oxygen reservoir to the BVM		1	
Attaches BVM to high-flow oxygen		1	
Ventilates the patient at the proper volume and rate *(800–1200 ml per breath/10–20 breaths per minute)*		1	
NOTE: After 30 seconds, the examiner auscultates and reports breath sounds are present and equal bilaterally and medical direction has ordered intubation. The examiner must now take over ventilation.			
Directs assistant to hyperventilate patient		1	
Identifies/selects proper equipment for intubation		1	
Checks equipment	Checks for cuff leaks Checks laryngoscope operation and bulb tightness	1 1	
NOTE: The examiner must remove the OPA and move out of the way when the candidate is prepared to intubate.			
Positions the head properly		1	
Inserts the laryngoscope blade while displacing the tongue		1	
Elevates the mandible with the laryngoscope		1	
Introduces the ET tube and advances it to the proper depth		1	
Inflates the cuff to the proper pressure		1	
Disconnects the syringe from the cuff inlet port		1	
Directs ventilation of the patient		1	
Confirms proper placement by auscultation bilaterally and over the epigastrium		1	
NOTE: The examiner must ask, "If you had proper placement, what would you expect to hear?"			
Secures the ET tube *(may be verbalized)*		1	
	TOTAL:	21	

CRITICAL CRITERIA

___ Did not take or verbalize body substance isolation precautions
___ Did not initiate ventilations within 30 seconds after applying gloves or interrupts ventilations for greater than 30 seconds at any time
___ Did not voice or provide high oxygen concentrations (15 L/min or greater)
___ Did not ventilate patient at a rate of at least 10/minute
___ Did not provide adequate volume per breath (maximum of 2 errors/minute permissible)
___ Did not hyperventilate the patient prior to intubation
___ Did not successfully intubate within 3 attempts
___ Used the patient's teeth as a fulcrum
___ Did not assure proper tube placement by auscultation bilaterally and over the epigastrium
___ If used, the stylette extended beyond the end of the ET tube
___ Inserted any adjunct in a manner that would be dangerous to the patient
___ Did not disconnect syringe from cuff inlet port

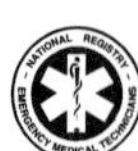

VENTILATORY MANAGEMENT
DUAL LUMEN AIRWAY DEVICE (PTL OR COMBI-TUBE) INSERTION FOLLOWING AN UNSUCCESSFUL ENDOTRACHEAL INTUBATION ATTEMPT

		Points Possible	Points Awarded
Continues body substance isolation precautions		1	
Confirms the patient is being properly ventilated with high-percentage oxygen		1	
Directs assistant to hyperventilate the patient		1	
Checks/prepares airway device		1	
Lubricates distal tip of the device *(may be verbalized)*		1	
Removes the oropharyngeal airway		1	
Positions the head properly		1	
Performs a tongue-jaw lift		1	
Inserts airway device to proper depth		1	
COMBI-TUBE	PTL		
Inflates pharyngeal cuff and removes syringe	Secures strap	1	
Inflates distal cuff and removes syringe	Blows into tube #1 to inflate both cuffs	1	
Ventilates through proper first lumen		1	
Confirms placement by observing chest rise and auscultating over the epigastrium and bilaterally over the chest		1	
NOTE: The examiner states: "You do not see rise and fall of the chest and hear sounds only over the epigastrium."			
Ventilates through the alternate lumen		1	
Confirms placement by observing chest rise and auscultating over the epigastrium and bilaterally over the chest		1	
NOTE: The examiner confirms adequate chest rise, bilateral breath sounds, and absent sounds over the epigastrium.			
Secures tube at appropriate step in sequence		1	
	TOTAL:	16	

CRITICAL CRITERIA

___ Did not take or verbalize body substance isolation precautions
___ Interrupted ventilation for greater than 30 seconds
___ Did not direct hyperventilation of the patient prior to placement of the device
___ Did not assure proper placement of the device
___ Did not successfully ventilate patient
___ Did not provide high-flow oxygen (15 L/min or greater)
___ Inserted any adjunct in a manner that would be dangerous to the patient

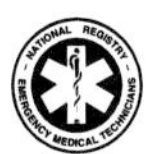

VENTILATORY MANAGEMENT
ESOPHAGEAL OBTURATOR AIRWAY INSERTION FOLLOWING AN UNSUCCESSFUL ENDOTRACHEAL INTUBATION ATTEMPT

	Points Possible	Points Awarded
Continues body substance isolation precautions	1	
Confirms the patient is being properly ventilated	1	
Directs assistant to hyperventilate the patient	1	
Identifies/selects proper equipment	1	
Assembles airway	1	
Tests cuff	1	
Inflates mask	1	
Lubricates tube *(may be verbalized)*	1	
Removes the oropharyngeal airway	1	
Positions head properly with neck in the neutral or slightly flexed position	1	
Grasps and elevates tongue and mandible	1	
Inserts tube in the same direction as the curvature of the pharynx	1	
Advances tube until the mask is sealed against the face	1	
Ventilates the patient while maintaining a tight mask seal	1	
Confirms placement by observing chest rise and auscultating over the epigastrium and bilaterally over the chest	1	
NOTE: The examiner confirms adequate chest rise, bilateral breath sounds, and absent sounds over the epigastrium.		
Inflates the cuff to the proper pressure	1	
Disconnects the syringe	1	
Continues ventilation of the patient	1	
TOTAL:	18	

CRITICAL CRITERIA

___ Did not take or verbalize body substance isolation precautions
___ Interrupted ventilation for more than 30 seconds
___ Did not direct hyperventilation of the patient prior to placement of the device
___ Did not assure proper placement of the device
___ Did not successfully ventilate the patient
___ Did not provide high-flow oxygen (15 L/min or greater)
___ Inserted any adjunct in a manner that would be dangerous to the patient

MEDREVIEW ANSWERS

CHAPTER 1
Introduction to Emergency Medical Care

Review Questions

1. C	9. D	17. B	25. C	33. B
2. D	10. B	18. C	26. A	34. D
3. A	11. C	19. B	27. D	35. A
4. B	12. B	20. B	28. B	36. A
5. A	13. C	21. A	29. C	37. A
6. B	14. B	22. B	30. D	38. A
7. D	15. D	23. B	31. A	39. A
8. D	16. B	24. D	32. C	40. B

Case Studies

Access to the EMS System

1A. Office or administrative numbers are traditional telephone numbers requiring that callers remember or identify a seven- or ten-digit number. Such numbers may not be answered twenty-four hours a day, and may be specific to an individual agency. Universal access numbers or emergency access numbers are designed so that anyone experiencing an emergency can reach help without delay. The universal access number, 911, can be used to obtain help in most areas of the United States without the caller having to remember a seven-digit number.

1B. There are many handout items available to promote an access number; common examples are stickers for telephone handsets or cradles, refrigerator magnets, and "panic buttons," which dial a pre-defined number when pressed. Other strategies to promote the "citizen access" component of the system can include:

- Tours of your dispatch facility
- Having a dispatcher meet and talk with community organizations
- Conduct role plays with groups simulating a call to the access number

Levels of EMS Training

2A. Actually, all providers are similar in the types of care they provide. They focus on assessing patients and providing emergency medical care. First Responders are trained to provide lifesaving care until the arrival of an ambulance. EMT-Basics are trained to provide care during the transport of a patient to the hospital. In most states, you must be at least an EMT-Basic before you can be in charge of patient care on an ambulance.

2B. EMT-Intermediates and EMT-Paramedics are essential for providing care for critically ill or injured patients. Both can perform invasive procedures, such as establishing intravenous lines and inserting endotracheal tubes. Paramedics provide the highest level of care available outside the hospital, and are extensively trained to monitor cardiac rhythms, administer medications, and perform certain other advanced procedures. The type of care each level of provider can provide is determined by the physician who oversees each individual agency.

3A. Extended members of the EMS system in unusual situations could include:

- Tow truck companies
- Earth moving companies
- Food and beverage services
- Heavy equipment and crane operators
- Equipment rental companies
- Construction companies
- Engineering organizations
- Flood control
- Environmental agencies
- Armed services
- Aircraft companies
- Satellite and communication organizations
- Rehabilitation services
- Community, state or private colleges and universities

4A. Emergency Medical Dispatching is a program designed to educate telecommunicators on how to instruct callers to provide medical care until EMS arrives. EMD training prepares personnel on how to calmly assist callers in performing first aid until EMS arrives.

4B. Callers can anticipate a telecommunicator trained to calm them, ask pertinent medical questions, and provide basic medical assistance to aid the bystander with lifesaving care.

4C. The presence of an EMD means that in most cases, some care will have been given to the patient prior to the arrival of EMS. Callers may provide lifesaving interventions for patients, even though the caller may not be certified in first aid or CPR. With the additional information collected by the EMD, EMS resources can also be allocated more efficiently.

Roles and Responsibilities of the EMT-Basic

5A. An EMT-Basic should be in good physical condition, exhibit emotional stability, practice appropriate personal hygiene, and carry a positive attitude. EMT-Basics must look and act professional.

5B. Every EMT-Basic should actively participate in refresher training as well as other EMS-related continuing education. Subscribing to EMS journals and attending educational conferences are excellent ways to keep current on skills and concepts.

5C. The patient's needs are an EMT-Basic's main priority outside of safety. Some choose to think of the patient as if he or she was a family member or close personal friend. The golden rules of "do unto others as you would have them do unto you" and "do no harm" are also guiding principles for many EMT-Basics.

Quality Improvement

6A. QI helps any system or organization quickly identify the strengths and weaknesses of current processes. At the ambulance company, a QI program can help reduce potential liability, improve response times, cut down on repair expenses, etc.

6B. QI in the communications standard could be implemented to increase the quality of information obtained from the caller, and subsequently provided to responding units. QI efforts can improve the quality of care provided over the phone. In the human resources management standard, QI may help improve the quality of the new employee, the interview process, the explanation of company benefits, the selection of partnerships in the field, and the quality of the continuing education secured by each employee.

6C. The EMT-Basic can make sure his or her documentation is clear and concise. He or she can also participate in QI committees and attend non-EMS conferences to learn more about the improving performance and quality improvement. The EMT-Basic can also participate by identifying areas where problems exist, or where things could be done "better" and reporting those to the QI supervisor, committee, or manager.

Medical Direction

7A. Because the mill site is remote, written protocols and communications will be especially important to the care of persons becoming ill or injured. The medical emergency team is probably operating under the licensure of the physician, therefore, the physician has a significant interest in the care at the site.

7B. Local EMS agencies must design and implement policies and procedures in the event that direct medical control is lost or unavailable. In many regions of the country, standing orders are written that allow the EMT-Basic to function without immediate direct medical control under these circumstances.

7C. The physician may require specific training or continuing education based on the hazards found at the mill. It would also be appropriate for the physician to review patient care reports to improve the quality of care provided at the site.

Duties of the EMT-Basic

8A. The student should include the following in their list:

- Personal, crew, bystander and patient safety
- Early recognition and treatment of life-threatening conditions
- Proper packaging and safe transport to appropriate facilities
- Clear and concise medical documentation of all EMS response
- Continuous activity with continuing medical education

Key Terms Matching

1. Assessment: (C) Evaluation of a situation or patient; the information is used to determine priorities for management

2. Emergency Medical Dispatchers (EMDs): (A) Specially trained personnel who answer calls for help, gather essential information, and when indicated, provide prearrival instructions over the phone until EMS personnel arrive

3. Emergency Medical Services Systems (EMSS) Act: (F) The 1973 Congressional Act that provided federal dollars to begin EMS systems throughout the United States

4. EMT-Basic (EMT-B): (K) Personnel trained in prehospital techniques including assessment and primary care for the ill or injured patient

5. EMT-Intermediate (EMT-I): (I) An advanced EMT trained in intravenous lines, airway techniques, manual defibrillation, and administration of some medications

6. EMT-Paramedic (EMT-P): (B) The most highly

trained EMT personnel; paramedics perform invasive field care

7. First Responder: (H) One whose training emphasizes immediate care and scene control prior to the arrival of additional EMS services
8. Protocols: (J) Medical orders designed by a physician for a given list of procedures or medications; protocols will vary among localities
9. Quality Improvement (QI): (G) Component of an EMS system that identifies the program's strengths and weaknesses and guarantees that the public receives the highest caliber of prehospital care
10. Standing Orders: (E) Preexisting written plans for treatment of specific complaints interventions or medications allowed by protocol without direct contact with medical direction.
11. Trauma Centers: (D) Regional facilities having specialized physicians and equipment necessary for treating trauma injuries

CHAPTER 2
The Well-Being of the EMT-Basic

Review Questions

1. A	9. A	17. B	25. B	33. B
2. A	10. B	18. D	26. C	34. A
3. A	11. B	19. D	27. A	35. B
4. B	12. A	20. B	28. A	36. D
5. A	13. B	21. B	29. B	37. A
6. C	14. B	22. B	30. A	38. A
7. B	15. D	23. B	31. A	39. A
8. D	16. A	24. D	32. B	40. C

Case Studies

Emotional Aspects of Emergency Care

1A. The best way to determine if Steven is experiencing one of the steps in the grieving process is simply to listen carefully to what he is saying. In this difficult situation, it may be helpful to remember that anger is a normal reaction for some patients when faced with the reality of their own impending or unexpected death.

1B. Progression through the stages of grief is not always a linear process. An angry patient may revert back to denial, perhaps saying, "There must be a mistake, I couldn't be sick." A patient in the bargaining stage might use words like, "If I am going to die, just let me run the next city marathon." The dying patient may move to a stage where the reality of death sets in and he becomes sad or depressed. He might use words such as, "I am going to die, and think of all the things I haven't done yet." In the final stage of a normal grieving process, the patient accepts his fate, feeling, "Death isn't such a bad thing; being sick forever would be a bad thing."

2A. Some common signs and symptoms of stress include:

Irritability

Lack of concentration

Anxiety

Exhaustion

Guilt

Loss of appetite

Isolation from family and friends

Lack of interest in sexual activities

Substance abuse

Depression

2B. Different methods exist to help control, manage, or reduce stress. Some ideas include:

Healthy diet

No smoking

Regular exercise

Rest

Change in work schedule or work location

Better balance among work, family, and recreation

A formal request for a station change

2C. In circumstances where the stress is too much, you should first seek information regarding the organization's employee assistance program. Check local listings for professional resources that may be able and capable of helping an EMT-Basic. In many areas of the country, the EMS agency supports one or more groups that are specially trained in handling EMS stress. Always remember that professional assistance can help keep things in perspective.

3A. Critical Incident Stress Debriefing is a process used within 72 hours of a critical or high-stress event to help EMS professionals communicate openly and frankly about their emotions. The primary purpose of CISD is to allow public safety workers an opportunity to constructively deal with the stresses of their jobs. A formal CISD team may facilitate the process. Mental health professionals may offer guidelines or suggestions for effectively dealing with the stress inherent with the job.

3B. Any comprehensive CISD team should include at least the following components: pre-incident education programs and literature availability, on scene and one-on-one support, long-term support pathways, and follow-up programs.

4A. Body substance isolation (BSI) and standard precautions are practices and procedures designed to protect EMS providers and others from direct contact with a patient's body fluids. The nature of EMS places responders in constant danger of contact with potentially infectious body fluids. Through the use of engineering controls, work practices, and personal protective equipment, the risks to an EMS provider are minimized.

4B. According to the latest guidelines published by the Department of Transportation and the Centers for Disease Control and Prevention, gloves are the only BSI equipment necessary for taking a patient's blood pressure.

5A. The report from the health department seems to indicate several active cases of tuberculosis in your area. If that is the case, then a NIOSH-approved respirator may be mandatory to prevent transmission of airborne disease particles. NIOSH has certified both high-efficiency particulate air (HEPA) respirators and those bearing the N95 designation. While the memo highlights a current problem, remember to remain diligent with BSI precautions with every patient.

5B. Most areas have access to an occupational safety and health agency. The federal Occupational Safety and Health Administration and corresponding state authorities have numerous resources regarding workplace regulations and BSI. Your local health department and the Centers for Disease Control and Prevention, are other excellent resources. Remember that regulations do no good if people do not follow the guidelines and practice standard precautions in the field.

Scene Safety

6A. This scene should be considered unsafe. Consequently, your EMS crew should exit the scene and stand by until law enforcement can control the scene.

Safety Precautions in Advance

7A. Commonly transmitted contagious diseases requiring immunization include: tetanus, hepatitis B, mumps, measles and rubella, chicken pox, and influenza.

7B. You can gather immunization records from parents, schools, or physicians. Childhood immunization records, along with any recent immunizations, are important to the EMT-Basic. Immunizations and records are an important part of any sound infection control or exposure control plan. You can be given boosters for some diseases if necessary.

Key Terms Matching

1. Body Substance Isolation (BSI): (G) Equipment and standards designed to prevent the spread of communicable diseases
2. Critical Incident Stress Debriefing (CISD): (D) A meeting held after a critical incident that encourages emergency care workers to discuss their feelings openly with trained mental health professionals and peer counselors.
3. High-efficiency particulate air (HEPA) respirator: (E) A specially filtered mask that is worn when caring for patients suspected or diagnosed with tuberculosis and other diseases caused by airborne pathogens
4. Pathogen: (B) Microorganism that causes disease
5. Personal Protective Equipment (PPE): (C) Equipment used by an emergency rescuer to protect against injury and infectious disease
6. Standard Precautions: (A) The first level of the Centers for Disease Control and Prevention's revised set of guidelines regarding isolation precautions established in 1996. Replaces BSI and universal precautions.
7. Stress: (F) Natural emotional or physical reaction to threatening or challenging situations

Labeling Diagram

A. yes
B. no
C. yes
D. yes
E. yes
F. yes
G. no
H. no
I. no
J. no

CHAPTER 3
Medical, Legal, and Ethical Issues

Review Questions

1. C	**9.** A	**17.** A	**25.** C	**33.** B
2. B	**10.** B	**18.** B	**26.** B	**34.** D
3. A	**11.** C	**19.** C	**27.** A	**35.** A
4. C	**12.** B	**20.** A	**28.** B	**36.** C
5. A	**13.** B	**21.** B	**29.** B	**37.** D
6. A	**14.** D	**22.** D	**30.** D	**38.** D
7. A	**15.** A	**23.** B	**31.** D	**39.** A
8. A	**16.** A	**24.** C	**32.** B	**40.** A

Case Studies

Scope of Practice

1A. A scope of practice defines the specific care and actions expected and allowed under law. It represents exactly the skills an EMT-Basic can use while treating a patient in the prehospital setting.

Ethics

2A. You have many options in this situation, but your ethical obligation is to report the crew to a higher authority. Typically, you might report this type of action to a supervisor, agency head, quality assurance person, or medical director. Inappropriate actions would be to confront the crew, or discuss the crew's actions with the patient. It is also unethical to discuss the case with anyone after reporting it for investigation.

3A. If the patient has not been subdued, appropriate action includes removing your partner from the scene, requesting assistance, and caring for your partner until help arrives. If the critically injured patient is also "down," then you should consider triaging the patients and treating accordingly.

4A. You should begin to treat the child based on the one parent's permission and request assistance from law enforcement or child protective services. Unless the child is a priority patient, transport should be avoided until assistance arrives. Based on your suspicions that the problem is related to child abuse, you are obligated to report this to the appropriate authorities.

Advance Directives

5A. The document represents an advance directive. These documents help an EMT-Basic determine the wishes of a dying patient. In most areas, the patient's physician must also sign the documents in order for them to be considered valid.

5B. In this scenario, most EMS protocols will allow an EMT-Basic to immediately stop any resuscitation efforts and then contact medical direction. You should also explain the EMS protocol covering cases like this to the family and others on scene.

5C. The durable power of attorney for health care is another type of advance directive commonly used for people who were able to make their health care wishes known at the time but who have since become incapacitated. Typically, the power of attorney is given to a family member or close friend. In some cases, a home health care professional may be the person given the responsibility for making health care choices.

6A. First, mention that you are stating your opinion and not offering legal advice or a legal opinion. Then identify the criteria for an advance directive to be considered valid in the prehospital environment. You may want to distribute copies of the local EMS protocol addressing DNR orders and other advance directives. Let them know that if a conflict does arise at the scene of an advance directive, an EMT-Basic is obligated to contact medical direction for advice.

6B. Advise them that it may be helpful to have several copies of a valid DNR order placed near the bed or area of the patient so that EMS responders can quickly recognize the DNR upon arrival and make the correct decisions. Also advise the family to discuss DNR orders with the patient's physician and attorney. Suggest having the telephone or pager number of the patient's physician readily available. In some cases, it may be appropriate to contact your local hospice group for information regarding dying at home.

Patient Consent

7A. As with any case, first make absolutely sure the scene is safe and that no dangers are present. It would be appropriate for you to complete an initial assessment. Efforts should be made to gain as much information as possible regarding the events leading up to this moment.

7B. Since the adolescent is unconscious and in a potentially life-threatening condition, you would be able to use implied consent as justification for beginning treatment. If a parent or legal guardian is on scene, you would obtain treatment consent through that person. In some areas, the school principal may have the power to make limited medical decisions for the student. Check your local protocol.

7C. You can begin treatment immediately based on implied consent. Efforts should be made to gain parental or guardian consent as quickly as possible. The school may be able to contact the parents and allow you to speak directly with them. In other cases, you might ask law enforcement to take custody of the patient to allow lifesaving treatment. As previously stated, school authorities may also have the ability to provide consent.

8A. The fact that this patient is conscious and alert means that you will be able to secure expressed consent or informed consent.

9A. Given this patient's mental status, you would be able to proceed under the implied consent criteria. If at any time the patient refused service, you would then be required to determine her ability to understand the consequences of refusal. Given her mental condition, it is unlikely that she could make a rational and informed decision, so she does not meet the criteria for informed or expressed consent.

9B. The primary difference between the two situations is the mental status of the patients. When attempting to gain consent, it is critical to evaluate the patient's ability to make an informed and rational decision. Any compromise to the patient's mental status must be considered and documented completely and precisely.

Assault and Battery

10A. Assault is defined as threatening or attempting to make physical contact without consent. No actual physical contact is necessary for assault to occur; it may result from a verbal expression of intent. Often, assault is determined to have existed once a battery has been committed.

10B. Battery is actual, intentional physical contact or touching of another person without his or her consent. Frequently, battery is combined with a charge of assault, particularly if threatening words were exchanged between the parties.

10C. The difference between assault and battery is actual physical contact between the individuals. In this rare instance, your response must be handled rapidly and delicately. Although you may disagree with the mother's beliefs, you generally do not have the legal authority to override her decision. Do not argue with her, which would make a difficult situation even worse. Contact medical direction for assistance. Get a response that you can document. You may want to immediately contact law enforcement for assistance. Depending on the state, they may or may not be able to intervene.

Abandonment or Negligence

11A. In this case, a strong argument could be made for a charge of patient abandonment. Given the fact that Tony has not taken his medications and has a medical complaint with a change in his level of consciousness, it would be appropriate to assess his condition and not base your opinion on his previous behavior. If unsure whether or not to transport, consult with medical direction.

11B. Medical abandonment is defined as the termination of care without the patient's consent and without making any provisions for continuing care at the same or higher level.

11C. Make absolutely sure the patient is competent and rationally able to decide against transport. Repeatedly offer him transport to the hospital. If the patient continues to refuse, have him sign a refusal of service form. Try to get several witnesses to sign the form, confirming the patient's level of consciousness. Completely and thoroughly document the incident.

11D. Negligence is defined as a failure to act as a reasonable, prudent person would under similar circumstances. An EMT-Basic would be responsible for providing care when a duty to act is present and for acting according to the standard of care and scope of practice. In this case, the failure to assess Tony's condition might constitute negligence.

Duty to Act

12A. This question depends on local or state regulations. In some states, a certified EMT-Basic is legally obligated to stop and render care when needed. In others areas, no duty to act exists unless the EMT-Basic is on duty (whether as paid staff or volunteer) and under a contractual obligation to respond.

12B. An EMT-Basic has an ethical obligation to render emergency care to the sick and injured. In this scenario, EMS is several minutes away and the patients need immediate assessment and possible treatment. Despite an ethical obligation, you may not be able to provide care if the scene is unsafe or personal protection would be compromised.

12C. A legal obligation is one placed by and governed by law. An ethical obligation is more of a moral issue. Reviewing the EMT-Basic Code of Ethics will help the EMT-Basic better understand the ethical obligation inherent in becoming a certified health care provider.

12D. A contractual duty to act exists when either a formal or implied contractual obligation to provide services exists. The most common type of contract is a written agreement by an EMS provider to provide a certain level of EMS service to a region. Under this agreement, employees of the provider, while on duty, are bound to follow that contractual obligation. Failure to provide service as required by contract can be grounds for a legal finding of breach of duty.

Potential Crime Scene/Evidence

13A. Immediately assess the safety of the scene. Have one team member secure the handgun for safety, without touching it if possible. (In many areas, the weapon may be covered with a box.) Ensure that law enforcement has been dispatched to the scene. If the scene is not safe, the EMS crew should leave their equipment and safely exit, returning only after the police have secured the scene. This scene should be considered a crime scene. A log should be kept with the names of all who enter and leave the scene. Keep bystanders away and ask family members to sit down and wait for the police to arrive.

13B. In situations involving stabbing, shooting, or other criminal acts, clothes can offer valuable information and evidence. When removing clothes, try not to cut directly through a bullet or knife hole. If possible, place all clothing in a paper bag; plastic bags destroy some types of evidence. Log the names of everyone who handled or took possession of the patient's clothing or other personal effects. Turn this log over to law enforcement when they arrive.

Special Reporting Situations

14A. Due to the circumstances in the home, you may be legally required or ethically bound to report the husband's condition to a social services agency or the police. Certainly, someone should be immediately notified to provide help for the husband. Record the names of people you contact at each step of the process.

15A. Most EMS systems have specific steps for documenting possible exposure to an infectious disease. Immediately contact the designated infectious control officer who will manage each step in the notification, treatment, and documentation process. In some EMS systems, you will be requested to return to the emergency department for initial testing and documentation. In other cases, a form is completed and sent to the hospital for follow-up. Follow your local protocol. In all cases, begin personal documentation of all exposures. Some diseases do not show any significant complications until some time later.

Key Terms Matching

1. Abandonment: (L) Termination of care without the patient's consent and without making any provisions for continuing care at the same or higher level
2. Advance Directive (M) A legal statement of a patient's wishes regarding his or her health care: used in the event the patient becomes unable to make decisions
3. Assault: (N) Threatening or attempting to inflict offensive physical contact: physical contact is not necessary
4. Battery: (K) Actual offensive physical contact or touching of another person without his or her consent: usually combined with a charge of assault, particularly if threatening words were exchanged between the parties
5. Confidentiality: (J) An obligation to protect the patient's privacy by not disclosing information to unauthorized individuals
6. Do Not Resuscitate (DNR) Orders: (I) Written physician's order directing health care providers to withhold lifesaving care from a patient in cardiac or respiratory arrest.
7. Durable Power of Attorney for Health Care (DPAC): (H) A type of advance directive that assigns another person to make medical decisions on the patient's behalf; used only if an individual becomes unable to make decisions
8. Duty to Act: (G) A contractual or legal obligation to care for any patient who requests services; does not apply if caring for the patient endangers the EMT-Basic's life
9. Expressed Consent: (F) Permission for treatment from a patient who is of legal age and is able to make rational decisions; expressed consent is given after the patient is informed of procedures involved in a treatment in a language he or she understands
10. Implied Consent: (E) Used for unconscious or mentally incompetent patients requiring emergency intervention; based on the assumption that the patient would give permission to treat life-threatening conditions
11. Medical Director: (D) Physician experienced and knowledgeable in all aspects of emergency care who delegates emergency medical practice to non-physician providers, such as EMT-Basics and other EMS personnel
12. Negligence: (A) Failure to act as a reasonable, prudent, similarly trained person would act under similar circumstances
13. Scope of Practice: (B) A description of the specific care and actions expected and allowed by law
14. Standard of Care: (C) The minimum acceptable level of care provided in an EMS system

CHAPTER 4
The Human Body

Review Questions

1. B	**29.** B	**57.** C	**85.** A
2. C	**30.** C	**58.** C	**86.** A
3. D	**31.** A	**59.** C	**87.** A
4. A	**32.** C	**60.** B	**88.** B
5. B	**33.** A	**61.** D	**89.** A
6. C	**34.** A	**62.** A	**90.** A
7. B	**35.** B	**63.** A	**91.** D
8. A	**36.** C	**64.** A	**92.** C
9. C	**37.** A	**65.** B	**93.** B
10. B	**38.** B	**66.** A	**94.** A
11. A	**39.** A	**67.** B	**95.** B
12. A	**40.** C	**68.** A	**96.** D
13. B	**41.** A	**69.** C	**97.** D
14. C	**42.** D	**70.** D	**98.** D
15. C	**43.** A	**71.** A	**99.** B
16. D	**44.** A	**72.** B	**100.** B
17. B	**45.** C	**73.** D	**101.** C
18. B	**46.** A	**74.** B	**102.** A
19. B	**47.** A	**75.** B	**103.** A
20. A	**48.** D	**76.** C	**104.** A
21. B	**49.** A	**77.** C	**105.** B
22. A	**50.** B	**78.** C	**106.** B
23. B	**51.** D	**79.** A	**107.** B
24. B	**52.** B	**80.** B	**108.** D
25. D	**53.** A	**81.** A	**109.** A
26. C	**54.** D	**82.** D	**110.** C
27. C	**55.** B	**83.** A	
28. B	**56.** B	**84.** B	

Case Study

1A. There is a large deformity in the area of the right femoral neck, distal to the greater trochanter. The leg is externally rotated and shortened by the injury.

1B. The femoral artery and vein, as well as the femur, are the primary areas of concern. There may also be damage to the pelvic girdle, the bladder, ureters, and uterus from the force of the fall.

Labeling Diagrams

Regions of the Human Skeleton

A. upper extremity
B. pelvis
C. skull
D. thorax
E. spinal column
F. lower extremity

The Human Skull

A. parietal bone
B. occipital bone
C. temporal bone
D. frontal bone
E. sphenoid bone
F. nasal bone
G. maxilla
H. zygomatic bone
I. mandible

The Upper Respiratory Tract

A. nose
B. mouth
C. soft palate
D. larynx
E. nasopharynx
F. oropharynx
G. epiglottis
H. esophagus
I. trachea

The Blood Flow Through the Heart

A. superior vena cava
B. right atrium
C. tricuspid valve
D. right ventricle
E. aorta
F. pulmonary trunk
G. left pulmonary vein
H. pulmonary valve
I. left atrium
J. mitral valve
K. aortic valve
L. left ventricle
M. myocardium

The Brain

A. medulla oblongata
B. cerebrum
C. cerebellum
D. spinal cord

Key Terms Matching

1. Abdominal cavity: (A49) The portion of the torso beneath the thorax and above the pelvis; contains the liver, gallbladder, stomach, pancreas, intestines, spleen, kidneys, and ureters
2. Acromion: (A45) The highest point of the shoulder
3. Anatomy: (A47) The study of the structures of the body and how they relate to one another
4. Anterior: (A46) Toward the front; front of the body; also called ventral
5. Aorta: (A48) The main trunk of the arterial system of the body; it leaves the heart from the upper surface of the left ventricle
6. Arteries: (A44) Blood vessels that carries blood away from the heart
7. Arterioles: (A43) Smaller vessels that branch off the arteries and lead to the capillaries
8. Atrium: (A42) One of two upper chambers of the heart
9. Ball-and-Socket Joint: (A40) Cup-shaped surface of a bone that joins with the ball-shaped head of a long bone
10. Bilateral: (A41) On both sides of the midline (right and left sides)
11. Blood Pressure: (A39) Force of the blood on the vessels; systolic pressure is the working pressure; diastolic pressure is the resting pressure
12. Brachial Artery: (A38) Major artery of the upper arm
13. Bronchi: (A37) The two major subdivisions of the trachea
14. Bronchioles: (A36) Subdivisions of the bronchi; terminate in the alveoli
15. Calcaneus: (A33) The heel bone
16. Capillaries: (A34) Tiny vessels that carry blood through the tissues; the network of capillaries in the tissues and organs is called the capillary bed
17. Cardiac Muscle: (A35) Involuntary muscle tissue of the heart that is usually not under conscious control
18. Carina: (A32) A triangular projection of the lowest tracheal cartilage; forms the division of the primary bronchi
19. Carotid Artery: (A31) Major artery in the neck
20. Carpals: (A30) The eight bones of the wrist
21. Central Nervous System: (A29) The brain and spinal cord
22. Cerebellum: (A28) Portion of the brain that coordinates voluntary muscular movements
23. Cerebrum: (A22) The largest part of the brain; consists of two hemispheres
24. Cervical, Cervical Vertebrae: (A26) First seven vertebrae; the neck
25. Circulation: (A25) Flow of blood from the heart through arteries to capillaries and returning to the heart through veins
26. Clavicle: (A24) Bone of the shoulder girdle that joins the sternum to the scapula; collarbone
27. Coccyx, Coccygeal Bones: (A23) The last four vertebrae; the tailbone
28. Contralateral: (A27) On the opposite side of the body
29. Coronary artery: (A21) Blood vessels that supply the heart with blood
30. Cranium: (A20) The skull
31. Cricoid Cartilage: (A19) Ring of cartilage that forms the bottom of the larynx and is an anatomical landmark
32. Dermis: (A18) Layer of skin located beneath the epidermis that supplies the skin with nutrients
33. Distal: (A14) Farthest from head or source; opposite of proximal
34. Dorsal: (A16) Pertaining to the back of the body; also called posterior
35. Dorsalis Pedis Artery: (A15) Artery located on the upper surface of the foot; can be used to assess blood supply distal to a leg injury
36. Endocrine System: (A17) Collection of ductless glands that internally secrete hormones into the bloodstream
37. Epidermis: (A11) Outermost layer of skin
38. Epiglottis: (A12) A leaf-shaped, lid-like structure attached to the top of the larynx; closes during swallowing, preventing food or liquid from entering the respiratory tract
39. Esophagus: (A13) Part of the gastrointestinal tract that joins the pharynx to the stomach
40. Face: (A10) Consists of orbits, nasal bone, maxilla, mandible, and zygomatic bones
41. Femur: (A9) The thigh bone
42. Femoral Artery: (A8) The major artery in the thigh
43. Fibula: (A7) The lateral and smaller bone of the lower leg
44. Fowler's Position: (A3) Supine position with the upper body elevated by a 45°–60° bend at the hips
45. Glottis: (A5) Space between the vocal cords; sound is produced when air passes through

opening, causing vocal cords to vibrate

46. Heart: (A4) Organ located in the thoracic cavity that receives blood from the veins and pumps it to the arteries
47. Hemoglobin : (A6) Protein in red blood cells responsible for oxygen transport
48. Hinge joint: (A2) Joint that allows movement in one plane, forward and backward
49. Hormones: (A1) Biologically active substances secreted by an endocrine gland; travel through the bloodstream to exert an influence on distant organs or body tissues
50. Humerus: (ZZZ) The upper arm bone
51. Hypoperfusion: (WWW) Shock; inadequate cardiac output causing a decrease in the delivery of oxygen and clearance of carbon dioxide
52. Iliac Crest: (XXX) Upper part of the pelvis
53. Inferior: (YYY) Below or beneath another structure
54. Involuntary Muscles: (VVV) Muscles that carry the automatic muscular functions of the body
55. Ischium: (UUU) One of the bones forming the pelvis
56. Joint: (TTT) A place where bones connect
57. Larynx: (SSS) Part of respiratory tract between the pharynx and the trachea, responsible for the production of voice; also called the voice box
58. Lateral: (RRR) Away from the midline, to the sides
59. Lateral Recumbent Position: (LLL) Lying on one side
60. Lumbar, Lumbar Vertebrae: (MMM) The five vertebrae forming the lower back
61. Lungs: (OOO) Respiratory organs that exchange oxygen, carbon dioxide, and water between the blood and the outside atmosphere
62. Malleolus: (NNN) The surface landmark of the ankle
63. Mandible: (PPP) The lower jaw bone
64. Manubrium: (QQQ) Superior portion of the sternum
65. Maxillae: (KKK) The two fused bones that form the upper jaw
66. Medial: (JJJ) Toward the middle of a body or region
67. Metacarpals: (III) The hand bones
68. Metatarsals: (HHH) Foot bones
69. Mid-axillary Line: (GGG) Imaginary line drawn vertically through the side of the body, extending from the middle of the armpit to the ankle, dividing the body into front and back sides
70. Mid-clavicular Line: (DDD) Imaginary line drawn through the middle of the clavicle (or collar bone), dividing the body into unequal right and left sides
71. Midline: (EEE) An imaginary vertical line that divides the body into equal right and left sides
72. Musculoskeletal system: (FFF) Consists of the muscular system and the skeletal system; human body functions through the actions and interactions of these systems
73. Nasal bone: (CCC) Bone of the nose
74. Nasopharynx : (YY) Part of pharynx above the level of the soft palate
75. Olecranon: (AAA) Elbow bone; tip of the elbow
76. Orbit: (ZZ): Eye socket
77. Oropharynx : (BBB) Part of pharynx between the soft palate and upper end of epiglottis
78. Palmar: (XX) Ventral surface of the hand; the palm of the hand
79. Patella: (TT) The kneecap
80. Pelvis: (VV) The massive cup-shaped ring of bone at the lower end of the trunk; formed by the hip bones
81. Perfusion: (UU) Microcirculation of blood within the organs and tissues, when oxygen and nutrients are delivered to the cells and their waste products are removed
82. Peripheral Nervous System: (WW) The sensory and motor nerves that extend from the spinal cord throughout the body
83. Phalanges: (SS) Small bones of the fingers and toes
84. Pharynx: (RR) The throat
85. Physiology: (QQ) The study of the normal functions of the human body
86. Plantar: (PP) Pertaining to the sole of the foot
87. Plasma: (MM) The serum, or fluid component, of blood
88. Platelets: (NN) Component of blood essential for clotting
89. Posterior: (OO) Toward the back of the body; also called dorsal
90. Prone: (LL) Lying on the stomach, face down
91. Proximal: (KK) Nearer to the head, trunk, or point of origin
92. Pubis: (JJ) Bony structure forming anterior part of hip bone

93. Pulmonary Artery: (GG) Originates in the right ventricle and enters the lungs where it branches off and follows the bronchi of the lungs
94. Radial Artery: (HH) Major artery of the forearm
95. Radius: (II) Bone forming the lateral side of the forearm
96. Red Blood Cells: (FF) Component of blood that contains hemoglobin; transport oxygen to the body's cells and remove carbon dioxide
97. Respiratory Rate: (EE) Breathing rate: measured in breaths per minute
98. Sacrum, Sacral Vertebrae: (AA) The five fused vertebrae that form the rigid part of the posterior side of the pelvis
99. Scapula: (CC) The shoulder blade
100. Skull: (BB) Cranium; the bones that comprise and protect the head
101. Spinal Column: (DD) Vertebral column; consists of the cervical, thoracic, and lumbar vertebrae
102. Standard Anatomical Position: (Z) Reference position in which the body is standing upright, facing the EMT with feet flat, arms at the side, palms forward
103. Sternum: (Y) Flat bone in the center of the anterior chest; the breastbone
104. Subcutaneous Layer: (V) The third layer of skin located under the dermis: attaches the skin to underlying structures.
105. Superior: (W) Above another structure
106. Supine (Position) (X) Lying on the back
107. Tarsal: (U) The ankle bone
108. Thorax: (T) Part of the body between the neck and abdomen
109. Tibia: (S) The shin bone
110. Torso: (N) The trunk of a body, not including the head or limbs
111. Trachea: (Q) The windpipe; main air passage, arising from larynx and dividing into bronchi
112. Trendelenburg Position: (P) The supine position inclined with the feet elevated about a foot above the head level
113. Ulna: (O) Bone forming the medial side of the forearm
114. Unilateral: (R) On one side of the body
115. Uvula: (M) The small structure that hangs from the roof of the mouth just in front of the oropharynx; made of connective tissue
116. Valves: (L) Structures within the heart and circulatory system that prevent backflow of blood
117. Veins: (K) Vessels carrying blood back to the heart
118. Vena Cava: (G) Inferior and superior; the final vein of the systemic circulation; it empties into the right atrium of the heart
119. Ventilation: (I) Exchange of air between lungs and ambient air
120. Ventral: (H) Front of the body; also called anterior
121. Ventricles: (J) The two lower chambers of the heart
122. Venules: (F) The smallest branches of the veins
123. Vertebrae: (E) Block-like bones that stack upon one another to form the spinal column
124. Voluntary muscles: (D) Muscles that are under conscious control
125. White Blood Cells: (C) Cells in the blood responsible for controlling disease conditions, such as infections caused by microorganisms
126. Xiphoid process: (A) The inferior tip of the sternum; it is prominent and easy to palpate
127. Zygomatic Bones: (B) The cheek bones

CHAPTER 5
Vital Signs and SAMPLE History

Review Questions

1. A	10. B	19. C	28. B	37. A
2. B	11. A	20. B	29. A	38. D
3. D	12. A	21. B	30. B	39. A
4. D	13. B	22. D	31. C	40. D
5. B	14. A	23. B	32. D	41. D
6. D	15. C	24. A	33. A	42. C
7. B	16. A	25. D	34. A	43. B
8. B	17. B	26. D	35. C	44. C
9. C	18. B	27. C	36. C	45. A

Case Studies

Chief Complaint

1A. The chief complaint is usually the main reason or problem that prompted a call to 911. A chief complaint is usually the patient's description of the problem or the problem identified based on information gathered on the scene (e.g., MVC, stabbing, or overdose) While a patient may have several problems, the chief complaint helps narrow this list to the one problem creating enough concern to request help.

1B. What made you call for help today? When did this problem begin? Has this ever happened before? What did the doctor tell you then? Are you currently taking any medications for this problem? How does today compare with previous episodes?

The Vital Signs

2A. Vital signs include respiratory rate and quality; pulse rate and quality; skin temperature, color, and condition; pupil size and reactivity; and blood pressure.

2B. As set of baseline vital signs establishes numbers for comparison to successive vital sign measurements. Changes in the values help provide a good idea of a patient's changing condition.

2C. Besides vital sign numbers, characteristics of the pulse, skin, and breathing are valuable pieces of information. The description of the breathing characteristics or quality should include mention of breathing effort (level of distress) and lung sounds. The pulse description should include the quality of the pulse (bounding, rapid, weak, or absent). The description of skin should include color, temperature, and condition.

3A. Your first priority in this unstable scene is your own safety and that of others. Once the scene becomes safe, you should approach and begin basic assessments on those complaining of trouble breathing.

3B. A single breath in an adult includes one cycle of inspiration and expiration. The normal breathing rate is 12 to 20 cycles per minute. Normal breathing is effortless and without pain. No extra sounds (e.g., gurgling) should be heard.

3C. Ask the patient to breathe normally while you count the number of respirations in 30 seconds. Multiply that number by 2 to find the rate per minute. You might want to distract the patient by palpating the radial pulse to ensure "normal breathing" while the rate is being counted.

3D. The four categories are normal, shallow, labored, and noisy.

4A. You can use either arm to obtain a baseline pulse measurement. However, it is also important to check that a pulse is present distal to the fracture site on the injured extremity. This should be done prior to applying the splint and after the splint is in place.

4B. The pulse volume and rhythm should also be recorded with a pulse measurement. Volume can be described as bounding or thready. Rhythm can be described as regular or irregular beating patterns.

5A. Normal (pink) color indicates adequate perfusion.

Pale skin indicates reduced red blood cell flow to the area.

Cyanotic skin indicates poor oxygenation of the blood cells and tissues.

Flushed color may represent a normal condition, exposure to heat, hormonal causes, or carbon monoxide poisoning.

Jaundiced skin may indicate cholecystitis, excessive levels of metabolites in the bloodstream, or liver failure.

5B. Normal skin temperature feels slightly warm relative to the back of your (normal temperature) hand.

5C. Skin temperature can usually be assessed by placing the back of your hand against the patient's skin and comparing temperatures. This can be done on the patient's forehead, armpit, or abdomen.

6A. Capillary refill time is measured by pressing on the skin or nail bed enough to blanch it, then releasing. The time it takes for the skin to return to the color of surrounding tissue is the capillary refill time. Normal time is less than two seconds.

6B. If capillary refill time exceeds two seconds, and the patient is demonstrating additional signs of cardiac compromise, you should assume that the patient is suffering from shock.

7A. Shine a small light into each pupil for a second or less. Watch for changes in pupil size and the speed of changes. While covering one eye against ambient light sources, quickly bring a penlight from the side of the eye directly over the pupil, hold for a second, then take the light source away. Repeat the procedure on the other eye. Make sure the patient is not looking directly at another light source.

7B. The three size classifications are:

Dilated (both pupils are larger than normal)

Constricted (both pupils are smaller than normal)

Unequal (one pupil is a significantly different size than the other pupil)

A pupil's reactivity is described as:

Reactive (normal muscle response to light source variations)

Sluggish (abnormally slow response to direct light sources)

Nonreactive (no muscle response to direct light sources)

8A. Blood pressure is the force that the blood exerts upon the walls of the vessels and organs of the body.

8B. Blood pressure consists of a systolic phase and a diastolic phase.

8C. The systolic sound is caused by the beating heart. As the left ventricle contracts, blood flows through the arteries. Compressing an artery with an inflated b.p. cuff creates turbulent blood flow and sound waves that bounce against the diaphragm of the stethoscope, resulting in a thumping sound. As the cuff is deflated, the artery expands to normal diameter, and blood flow becomes smooth (non-turbulent). The thumping sound disappears at this point, and we mark the diastolic pressure, the blood pressure when the heart is at rest.

8D. High blood pressure can cause the following conditions or abnormalities:

Blood clots

Stroke

Myocardial infarction

Aneurysm

Hemorrhage

9A. The steps to measure the patient's blood pressure using a blood pressure cuff and stethoscope are detailed in the "Blood Pressure by Auscultation" skill checklist in this chapter of the MedReview.

9B. The steps to measure the patient's blood pressure with only a cuff and no stethoscope are detailed in the "Blood Pressure by Palpation" skill checklist in this chapter of the MedReview.

9C. The average blood pressure ranges for infants, children, and adults are as follows: infant range is between 80/60 and 82/44, child range is between 82/44 and 110/64, and the adult average is 120/80.

SAMPLE History

10A. A medical history is information that describes or indicates former or current medical problems, surgery, or abnormal body functioning.

10B. **S** = signs and symptoms
A = allergies
M = medications taken
P = pertinent past medical history
L = last oral intake
E = events leading up to

10C. The OPQRST questions are used to elaborate on the chief complaint such as pain.

11A. To determine the severity of the patient's leg pain, try asking the patient to rate the pain on a scale of 1 to 10.

11B. During the "M" phase of the SAMPLE history assessment, be sure to ask if the patient is taking any medications and if they are prescribed to the patient and exactly for what reason they are prescribed.

Labeling Diagrams

SAMPLE History

S: **(F)** Signs and symptoms
A: **(D)** Allergies
M: **(E)** Medications
P: **(B)** Pertinent past medical history
L: **(A)** Last oral intake
E: **(C)** Events leading up to

OPQRST History

O: **(D)** Onset
P: **(E)** Provocation
Q: **(F)** Quality
R: **(A)** Radiation
S: **(B)** Severity
T: **(C)** Time

Pulse Locations

A. posterior tibial
B. carotid
C. brachial
D. radial
E. femoral
F. dorsalis pedis

Key Terms Matching

1. Auscultation: (BB) Listening for sounds with a stethoscope
2. Brachial Pulse: (AA) The flow of blood through the brachial artery, in the medial aspect of the upper arm
3. Bradycardia: (Z) Slow heart rate
4. Chief Complaint: (W): Patient's self-described worst or most serious concern
5. Conjunctiva: (X) Membrane lining the eyelids and the surface of the sclera of the eye
6. Cyanosis: (Y) Blue coloring of the skin; may indicate poor oxygen uptake or reduced perfusion
7. Diastolic Pressure: (V) The pressure exerted on the walls of the arteries when the heart is at rest;

when assessing blood pressure by auscultation, measured at point when the sound stops

8. Expiration: (U) Expelling air from the lungs (exhalation)
9. Femoral Pulse: (T) The flow of blood through the femoral artery in the upper thigh
10. Hypertension: (S) Abnormally high blood pressure
11. Inspiration: (R) Taking air into the lungs (inhalation)
12. Jaundice: (M) Yellow deposits in skin and whites of the eyes caused by increased bilirubin in the blood; indication of liver abnormality
13. Lens: (P) Refracting structure of the eye located directly behind the pupil
14. Oral Mucosa: (O) Pink membrane lining the inside of the mouth
15. Palpation: (N) Assessment by touch or feel
16. Pulse: (Q) Pressure caused by contraction of the heart; can be palpated where an artery lies close to an underlying bone; an indication of cardiac output
17. Pupil: (L) Circular opening in the iris that allows passage of light into the eye
18. Radial Pulse: (J) The flow of blood through the radial artery; palpated on the anterior lateral surface of the wrist, proximal to the thumb
19. Respiration: (K) Breathing; process through which air enters and leaves the lungs
20. SAMPLE History: (I) Mnemonic used to summarize a patient's relevant medical history (Signs/Symptoms, Allergies, Medications, Past history, Last oral intake, Events leading to injury or illness)
21. Sclera: (H) Outermost layer of the eyeball; whites of the eyes
22. Sign: (G) An observable indication of illness or injury
23. Sphygmomanometer: (F) Blood pressure cuff
24. Stridor: (E) Harsh, high-pitched sound during inspiration
25. Symptom: (A) Condition described by the patient that can't be observed
26. Systolic Pressure: (C) The pressure in the arterial system when the left ventricle contracts; first sound heard when assessing blood pressure by auscultation
27. Tachycardia: (B) An unusually rapid heart rate
28. Vital Signs: (D) Pulse rate and quality, breathing rate and quality, blood pressure, skin color, skin temperature, skin condition, pupil size and quality, and capillary refill in children

CHAPTER 6: *Lifting and Moving Patients*

Review Questions

1. C	8. A	15. A	22. B	29. A
2. A	9. B	16. B	23. A	30. A
3. A	10. C	17. B	24. A	31. B
4. B	11. D	18. D	25. D	32. B
5. D	12. B	19. C	26. B	33. B
6. B	13. A	20. A	27. C	34. C
7. B	14. C	21. D	28. A	35. A

Case Studies

Lifting Techniques

1A. Body mechanics are principles and applications that focus on efficient methods of body posture and lifting.

1B. During any lifting, follow these standard guidelines:

1) Focus on using the large muscles of your legs, hips, and buttocks during lifting, not the muscles of your back.
2) Contract your abdominal muscles.
3) Maintain proper body alignment.
4) Keep the weight of the object to be lifted as close to your body as possible.

1C. Safety guidelines for carrying include:

1) Consider the weight and size of the patient and the available resources prior to the lift. Call for additional help as required.
2) Know your own physical limitations and those of the lifting team.
3) Never twist your body when lifting, and keep your back in a locked position.
4) Your feet should remain flat, comfortably spaced, and turned slightly outward.
5) Assess and correct for any environmental obstructions or unsafe conditions prior to the lift.
6) Coordinate your moves and communicate clearly with other team members before and during a lift.
7) Never exceed the weight limitations of the equipment.
8) Keep the weight close to your body.
9) Flex at the hips and knees, not at the waist.
10) Do not hyperextend the back.

The guidelines for proper lifting are also appropriate during carrying.

2A. This answer depends on your judgment. If you believe that the patient requires immediate control of his airway, then an emergency move is called for. If you feel that he is in serious condition so that immediate transport is required, then an urgent move is warranted. An urgent move is also appropriate if you are concerned with potential hidden injuries that cannot be found in the patient's current position.

3A. The two most common nonurgent moves are the direct ground lift and the extremity lift.

3B. The steps for the direct ground lift include:

1) Position the stretcher as close to the patient as possible.
2) Two EMT-Basics position themselves alongside the patient with one knee down.
3) The EMT-Basic closest to the patient's head supports the head and neck.
4) The second EMT-Basic slides her arms under the patient's back and knees.
5) On a count from the EMT-Basic at the head, both EMT-Basics lift the patient onto their knees and towards their bodies.
6) On signal, the EMT-Basics stand in unison.
7) On signal, the EMT-Basics drop to one knee and gently roll the patient onto the stretcher.

The steps for the extremity lift include:

1) The EMT-Basic at the head slips his arms under the patient's arms and grasps the patient's opposite wrists.
2) The EMT-Basic at the legs slips her hands under the patient's knees.
3) Both EMT-Basics in unison lift to a crouching position.
4) Both EMT-Basics stand up together on a signal from the EMT-Basic at the head.

4A. Basic safety techniques include:

1) Avoid reaching across a distance of more than 15 or 20 inches in front of your body.
2) Keep your back locked into position.
3) Avoid reaching positions that require hyperextension.
4) Avoid positions where reaching will exceed one minute in duration.

4B. Keep your back straight, lean from the hips, and maintain proper body mechanics by utilizing shoulder muscles during a log roll.

4C. Answers should include:

1) It is always safer to push.
2) Keep the pull line through the center of your body.
3) Keep the weight close to your body.
4) Keep your back locked and elbows bent.
5) Keep your arms close to your sides.
6) Push from the area between your waist and shoulders.
7) Avoid pushing or pulling from over your head.

Patient Transport Equipment

5A. You might choose a long spine board or Stokes (wire basket). Since there is a possibility of spinal injury in this case, a scoop stretcher is not appropriate. If you suggest another acceptable method, include sufficient detail to justify your answer.

5B. Due to the mechanism of injury, there is potential for spinal injury. Besides the proper extrication and transport device, the patient must also have spinal immobilization using a rigid collar, short board, long spine board, padding, strapping, and head immobilization.

6A. Depending on local protocol, answers can include the long board, scoop stretcher, wire basket, portable stretcher, flexible stretcher, or stair chair. A creative student may even suggest the KED with its handles as a possible device. Make sure any suggestions are safe for both the patient and crew.

6B. Given the scenario as described, the stair chair seems most appropriate. This device is designed especially for transport down stairs and in other hard-to-maneuver locations. However, it is not designed to maintain any required spinal or cervical immobilization.

7A. Routine, although this situation will not be very routine due to his size.

7B. Get some additional help so you and your partner do not injure your backs.

7C. Collar and long backboard behind him and carefully tilt the chair back and slide him onto the board with lots of help.

Key Terms Matching

1. Body Mechanics: (R) Moving your body correctly while lifting and moving to prevent injury
2. Emergency Moves: (Q) Specific extrication or lifting and moving techniques used when immediate danger threatens the EMT or the patient
3. Flexible Stretcher: (J) Carrying device made of flexible materials with large carrying handles; used

for moving patients in narrow or confined spaces

4. Hyperextension: (O) Extension of a joint beyond its normal limit during movement
5. Long Backboard: (N) Device used for full spinal immobilization
6. Nonurgent (routine) Moves: (M) Lifting and moving patients when there is no immediate threat to life
7. Portable Stretcher: (H) Light, collapsible stretcher useful in small spaces
8. Power Grip: (L) Gripping items with palms and fingers in complete contact with the object; fingers bent at the same angle and hands ten inches apart
9. Power Lift: (K) A specialized lifting and moving technique that uses the large muscles of the legs to lift and carry the weight
10. Rapid Extrication: (P) Specialized techniques for quickly removing a patient from a vehicle without compromising the cervical spine
11. Recovery Position: (I) Standard transportation position for a patient without spinal injury; patient is rolled onto one side, usually the left
12. Scoop Stretcher: (G) Device used to move patients with no suspected spinal injuries from confined areas
13. Short Backboard: (F) Device for immobilizing the upper part of the spine when a long board cannot be used
14. Stair Chair: (B) Specialized device used for transportation of patients down stairs or through narrow spaces; may have wheels
15. Urgent Moves: (D) Techniques for moving a patient whose condition is life-threatening; cervical spine procedures are taken
16. Vest-Type Extrication Device: (C) A flexible device used to help immobilize the spine in confined spaces
17. Wheeled Stretcher: (E) Most commonly used ambulance stretcher; may be rolled on smooth surfaces; adjustable height
18. Wire Basket Stretcher (Stokes Litter): (A) Carrying device used for patient transport over rough or irregular terrain

CHAPTER 7
Airway Management

Review Questions

1. A	12. B	23. B	34. A	45. B
2. A	13. B	24. A	35. C	46. A
3. A	14. A	25. B	36. C	47. A
4. C	15. B	26. B	37. C	48. C
5. A	16. C	27. B	38. D	49. B
6. B	17. A	28. D	39. D	50. B
7. C	18. C	29. A	40. C	51. B
8. C	19. A	30. C	41. D	52. B
9. A	20. B	31. A	42. D	53. A
10. A	21. A	32. C	43. A	54. D
11. B	22. A	33. D	44. B	55. B

Case Studies

The Respiratory System

1A. The answer should include the nose, mouth, pharynx, epiglottis, larynx, and trachea.

1B. The blood could drain into either the trachea or esophagus if not cleared by the patient or the EMT-Basic. Blood in the trachea can affect the bronchi, bronchioles, and alveoli. Even small amounts of blood can impede air exchange in the alveoli and lead to respiratory compromise and potential respiratory failure. Blood in the esophagus can collect in the stomach, leading to nausea, vomiting, diarrhea, and abdominal pain.

Airway Management

2A. This patient requires high-flow oxygen via non-rebreather mask, or even assisted ventilations if tolerated.

3A. The patient currently has an open airway. Airway patency can be inferred because the patient is alert, oriented, and able to speak.

3B. Stabilize the cervical spine during assessment of the airway.

Provide high-flow oxygen via non-rebreather mask.

Use suction as required.

Rapid transport to a trauma center is indicated based on the mechanism of injury and respiratory distress.

Reassess the airway status at five-minute intervals or less.

3C. Snoring respirations frequently result from obstruction of the airway by the tongue.

3D. Open the airway using the jaw-thrust maneuver

while maintaining cervical spine control. If the patient has an intact gag reflex, a nasopharyngeal airway should be inserted. In the absence of a gag reflex, insertion of an oral airway is appropriate. Assist ventilations with a bag-valve mask, using supplemental oxygen. The rate of assistance should be one ventilation every three to five seconds. Begin transport as soon as possible.

4A. Basic components include a suction source, a collection container, tubing, and suction tips or catheters.

4B. The types available include mounted suction devices and portable suction devices (battery operated and hand operated).

4C. The catheter should only be inserted into the patient's airway as far as you can see. Otherwise, you risk stimulating the patient's gag reflex and causing additional airway compromise.

4D. Special attention must be paid to ensure that the catheter does not touch the back of the airway, which could cause slowing of the heart rate or soft tissue trauma. This stimulation usually occurs in the back third of the tongue.

5A. Body substance isolation precautions are extremely important. Use gloves, a mask, and eye protection at a minimum. If gowns are available, they should also be used.

5B. First, clear any visible nonliquid matter from the mouth, using finger sweeps. For small-diameter particles that cannot be suctioned with a rigid catheter, consider using the end of the connecting tube as a suction catheter. If the suction catheter is blocked, place the end into sterile saline or sterile water and apply suction. This will clear the catheter of obstructions.

6A. Nasopharyngeal airways are very useful for securing airways that cannot be managed using oral methods.

6B. Use a soft (French) suction catheter. Check all equipment and take appropriate BSI precautions. Measure the catheter as you would for an oropharyngeal airway, so that it will reach through the nose only as far as the base of the tongue. Insert the catheter (through a nasopharyngeal airway if necessary) without suction. When it is in place, apply suction and slowly withdraw the catheter. Limit suctioning to 15 seconds.

7A. The nasopharyngeal airway is preferred. Nasopharyngeal airways do not normally trigger a patient's gag reflex so are less likely to stimulate vomiting than an OPA. They can be used on patients with varying mental states. An EMT-Basic can adequately provide ventilation and suction through the NPA. And a nasal airway may be less traumatic than an oropharyngeal airway.

7B. The NPA is placed into the right or left nostril rather than into the oropharynx. Nasopharyngeal airways must be lubricated with a water-soluble product prior to insertion.

8A. Using proper BSI precautions (at least gloves), open the airway using the jaw-thrust maneuver. Extra care must be taken to ensure that little or no cervical spine movement occurs.

9A. Ability to deliver a tidal volume of 1600 mL

A self-refilling bag that is easily cleaned and sterilized or disposable

A non-jam valve that allows a maximum oxygen inlet flow of 15 lpm

No pop-off valve

Standardized 15/22 fittings

An oxygen inlet and reservoir to allow for high-flow oxygen

A true valve for non-rebreathing

Able to perform in all environmental conditions and temperature extremes

Available in infant, child, and adult sizes

9B. The signs of effective artificial ventilation include: the chest rises and falls with each ventilation, the ventilation rate is sufficient for the patient's age range, and the heart rate returns to normal limits.

10A. The device can deliver 100% oxygen at up to 40 lpm.

It vents excess gases to the atmosphere, or simply does not provide more oxygen.

An audible relief valve warns when pressures are exceeded.

It is weather-resistant.

The activating trigger allows the EMT-Basic to better maintain a seal between the mask and the patient's face.

10B. Use the fourth and fifth fingers to secure the mask to the jaw.

Connect the flow-restricted, oxygen-powered ventilation device to the mask.

Activate the trigger until the chest rises.

Relax the trigger and allow the patient to exhale passively.

Ventilate once every 5 seconds.

10C. As with any airway management, special consideration must be paid to reducing the amount of abdominal distention caused by the procedure. Gastric distention can seriously impede the delivery of lifesaving ventilations.

11A. Oxygen cylinders should be changed when the pressure drops below 500 psi, regardless of cylinder size. The last crew to use the cylinder could have replaced the empty bottle. Equipment checks at the beginning of each day or shift help prevent this type of occurrence. However, it is also important to remember that cylinders can occasionally leak.

11B. Both cylinders should always be secured, whether in the ambulance or horizontally on the stretcher. When changing the regulator, make sure to face the cylinder away from your body and others. Assure that there are no open flames in the area.

11C. The regulator should read between 2000 and 2200 psi. The pressure reading will change proportionally as the tank empties. (Note that this is true for any tank size.)

12A. For patients in respiratory distress or complaining of chest pain, the most appropriate delivery device is the non-rebreather mask with a 12 to 15 lpm flow rate.

12B. The non-rebreather mask should be used when a patient is:

In respiratory distress

Cyanotic, cool, or clammy

Experiencing shortness of breath that requires supplemental oxygen

Complaining of chest pain

In shock

Showing any form of altered mental status

Note that infants, children, and patients suffering from chronic obstructive pulmonary disease can receive high-flow oxygen for prehospital care.

12C. The nasal cannula is available.

12D. In general, any patient requiring oxygen should receive high-flow oxygen by non-rebreather mask. Try to coach the patient to continue using the non-rebreather mask. However, some patients cannot tolerate the mask and become uncooperative. In this case, apply a nasal cannula to the patient and use a flow rate of four to six liters per minute.

Special Considerations

13A. The primary change is that you must look, listen, and feel for breathing at the tracheostomy site rather than the mouth and nose. The tracheostomy should also be evaluated for patency and obstruction.

13B. Yes. A proper bag-valve-mask device should include a 15/22 fitting, which is standard on respiratory devices. This fitting will hook directly to the end of the tracheostomy tube, so the patient can be ventilated without difficulty. If the patient has an artificial nose on the tube, it should be removed to facilitate ventilation.

13C. It is appropriate to suction the tracheostomy tube. A French (soft) catheter should be used. Take care not to go beyond the distal end of the tracheostomy tube. No other changes are required to the suctioning procedure.

13D. Using an infant or child mask, you would place the mask directly over the stoma opening. If unable to ventilate, you would seal the stoma and provide ventilations through the patient's mouth and nose.

14A. Try to quickly replace the dental appliance. If it will not stay in place, then the appliance must be removed completely. If a dental appliance creates an airway obstruction, remove it.

Key Terms Matching

1. Agonal Respirations: (X) Occasional gasping breaths that may occur in the final stage of death
2. Airway Adjunct: (T) Device that helps keep the airway open by keeping the tongue away from the back of the throat
3. Alveoli: (V) Termination of the respiratory passages; the functional units of the lungs, across whose walls gas exchange occurs
4. Aspiration: (U) To draw foreign material, a foreign body, or fluid into the respiratory tract while inhaling
5. Bag-Valve-Mask Device: (W) An oxygen delivery device comprised of a self-inflating bag face mask, one-way valve, and oxygen reservoir
6. Diaphragm: (S) Primary muscle of breathing; forms the bottom portion of the thoracic cavity
7. Head-Tilt/Chin-Lift Maneuver: (R) The preferred method for opening and maintaining an airway in a patient without suspected neck injury
8. Hypoxia: (P) Deficiency of oxygen
9. Intercostal Muscles: (I) Muscles located between the ribs; involved in breathing
10. Jaw-Thrust Maneuver: (N) The preferred method for opening and maintaining an airway in a patient with suspected spinal injury
11. Laryngectomy: (M) Removal of the larynx
12. Nasal Cannula: (O) A tube inserted into the nose to deliver low-flow oxygen
13. Nasopharyngeal Airway: (K) A soft rubber airway

device inserted through the nose; designed to maintain an open airway by displacing the tongue off the pharynx

14. Non-Rebreather Mask: (J) High-flow oxygen delivery device characterized by an inflatable oxygen reservoir bag and a one-way valve that prevents exhaled air from being reinhaled
15. Oropharyngeal Airway: (L) A curved plastic device with a flange inserted in the patient's mouth; used to keep the tongue from blocking the pharynx
16. Patent: (H) Open; accessible
17. Retraction: (Q) Depressions in the neck, above the shoulder blades, between and below the ribs; indicates extensive muscle use during breathing due to respiratory distress
18. Rigid Suction Catheter: (G) Nonflexible catheter used to suction an unresponsive patient
19. Soft Suction Catheter: (F) A soft catheter used for suctioning the nasopharynx and in other situations where a rigid catheter cannot be used
20. Stoma: (A) A surgically created opening into a body cavity
21. Thoracic Cavity: (D) Body cavity enclosed by the sternum, ribs, and vertebral column
22. Tidal Volume: (C) The amount of air inhaled and exhaled in a single breath
23. Tracheostomy: (B) Surgical opening of the trachea
24. Tracheostomy Tube: (E) A specialized airway device for surgical placement into a tracheal stoma; used to maintain an airway passage

Labeling Diagrams

The Respiratory System

A. lung
B. pharynx
C. tongue
D. larynx
E. trachea
F. bronchus

Respiration Signs

A. normal
B. quiet
C. equal and symmetric
D. absent
E. rapid
F. stridor, crowing, or noisy
G. asymmetric &/ shallow
H. present

CHAPTER 8
Scene Size-Up and Initial Assessment

Review Questions

1. D	**8.** D	**15.** C	**22.** B	**29.** A
2. C	**9.** B	**16.** A	**23.** B	**30.** B
3. D	**10.** B	**17.** D	**24.** A	**31.** D
4. A	**11.** A	**18.** A	**25.** D	**32.** A
5. A	**12.** B	**19.** A	**26.** C	**33.** D
6. C	**13.** B	**20.** A	**27.** B	**34.** A
7. D	**14.** B	**21.** C	**28.** D	**35.** A

Case Studies

Scene Size-Up and Assessment

1A. Personal and scene safety is the foremost responsibility of an EMT-Basic. Safety responsibilities include safe operation of the emergency vehicles, body substance isolation precautions, as well as safety of the crew, patient, and bystanders.

1B. Your primary concern at this time is the potential for violence on the scene. The man is agitated and exhibiting abnormal behavior, has a traumatic injury, and the mechanism is unknown (assault, self-injury, etc.). These clues should warn the EMT-Basic that the scene is unsafe and law enforcement should be contacted for assistance.

2A. There are many threats to safety at accident and rescue scenes. Vehicle stability, downed electrical lines, broken glass or other materials, leaking fuel, fire, and traffic are some of the potential hazards.

2B. Determining the mechanism of injury is simply the process of determining what forces were involved in the incident. Determining these forces will provide clues to the type and extent of injuries that can be expected in the patient.

2C. Crash or rescue involving motor vehicles, aircraft or watercraft, hazardous materials spills, confined spaces and with low levels of oxygen, violent crime scenes, and fire scenes

2D. Yes, because the vehicle rolled over.

Other significant mechanisms are:

- Ejection from a vehicle
- Death of another passenger in the same vehicle
- Accidents at a high rate of speed
- Vehicle vs. pedestrian crash
- Motorcycle crash

- Falls of more than 20 feet
- Vehicle rollovers
- Blunt or penetrating trauma to the chest, head, or abdomen

Initial Assessment

3A. The primary function of the initial assessment is to identify and correct problems that are immediately life threatening.

3B. Components of the initial assessment include:
- Forming a general impression of the scene and patient
- Assessing the patient's mental status
- Assessing the patient's airway and assuring patency
- Assessing the adequacy of the patient's breathing, providing oxygen or assisted ventilations as necessary
- Assessing the circulation; initiating any corrective measures
- Determining the priority of the patient's condition

3C. Given the potential for exposure to body substances with the active bleeding, the student should respond with aggressive protection, including the following items: disposable gloves, protective eyewear, appropriate mask, and a gown (if possible).

4A. Two fractured femurs

4B. Serious head injury

4C. Critical or highest priority based on the MOI alone

Key Terms Matching

1. AVPU: (L) Memory aid used to help categorize a patient's level of unresponsiveness (A = Alert, V = Responds to Verbal stimuli, P = Responds to Pain, U = Unresponsive)
2. Blunt Trauma: (K) Injury caused by non-penetrating forces
3. Cavitation: (J) Tissue compression and cavity formation caused by the pressure of a projectile entering the body
4. General Impression: (F) The first step in initial assessment to quickly identify what is wrong and how serious it is; a time to use instinct and draw upon past experience
5. Initial Assessment: (H) Conducted after scene size-up in order to find and manage any life-threatening conditions
6. Interventions: (G) Procedures done in an effort to improve the patient's condition
7. Mechanism of Injury (MOI): (I) The forces involved or factors influencing an injury
8. Nature of Illness: (E) The type of condition or complaint a medical patient has
9. Penetrating Trauma: (B) An injury caused by an object that pierces the skin or other body structure
10. Scene Size-Up: (C) The process of determining scene safety, the nature of the problem, total number of patients, and need for additional resources
11. Trauma: (D) A serious injury to the body or a severe emotional shock
12. Triage: (A) The process of prioritizing patients to receive the appropriate level of care or transportation

Labeling Diagram

Critical Steps in Scene Size-Up

A. Do not proceed until the scene is safe.

B. Rapidly determine the mechanism of injury.

C. Determine the number of patients.

D. Call for assistance and begin triage.

E. Begin initial assessment.

CHAPTER 9
Patient Assessment

Review Questions

1. B	12. B	23. D	34. A	45. A
2. B	13. C	24. B	35. D	46. A
3. D	14. A	25. B	36. A	47. D
4. B	15. A	26. A	37. C	48. B
5. B	16. C	27. B	38. C	49. D
6. A	17. B	28. B	39. D	50. B
7. C	18. D	29. B	40. A	51. D
8. C	19. A	30. B	41. B	52. B
9. B	20. B	31. A	42. B	53. A
10. B	21. C	32. D	43. D	54. D
11. A	22. D	33. A	44. A	55. D

Case Studies

1A. The list can be large. Make sure the responses are appropriate and normal. A partial list includes:
- Ejection from a vehicle
- Death of another passenger in the same vehicle
- High-speed vehicle crash

- Vehicle vs. pedestrian crash
- Motorcycle crash
- Fall of more than 20 feet
- Penetrating injury to the head, chest, or abdomen
- Auto rollover
- Blunt trauma to the chest, head, or abdomen
- Multiple long-bone injuries

1B. Refer back to the flow chart or recreate the diagram. The steps should include the rapid trauma assessment, baseline vital signs, SAMPLE history, critical interventions, and a transport decision. (These are listed in order, although several of the steps can be completed simultaneously.)

1C. If no significant mechanism of injury is found, the patient should receive a focused trauma assessment, baseline vital signs, SAMPLE history, and a transport decision. (While these are listed in order, several steps can be completed simultaneously.)

2A. The boy would receive a rapid trauma assessment because he was exposed to significant force in ejection from the vehicle.

2B. In performing a rapid trauma assessment, the EMT-Basic evaluates the patient from head-to-toe for obvious injuries and may begin treatment simultaneously (e.g., immobilization, MAST). A focused history and physical exam evaluates only the areas involved in the patient's complaint.

2C. "DCAP-BTLS" refers to Deformities, Contusions, Abrasions, Penetrations, Burns, Tenderness, Lacerations, and Swelling. It is a mnemonic that is used to quickly recall soft-tissue injuries that may be found during a physical assessment.

2D. You should immediately recognize an obstructed airway and begin airway procedures. These include opening the airway, assessing for breathing, attempting ventilations, repositioning the airway, attempting to ventilate again, and beginning the foreign body airway obstruction removal method if necessary.

2E. During the neck assessment, look for DCAP-BTLS, cervical spine deformity, tracheal deviation, jugular vein distention, medical identification insignia, signs of increased chest pressure, or signs of airway obstruction.

3A. During the focused history and physical exam of a medical patient, determine whether the patient is responsive or unresponsive. (These two levels of responsiveness are the only categories for medical patients.)

3B. Because the patient responds to verbal questioning, however slowly, she would qualify as responsive. For a responsive patient, the assessment is limited to a focused history and physical exam based on the complaint. It includes a SAMPLE history, focused medical assessment, baseline vital signs, and a decision to transport. (While these are listed in order, several steps can be completed simultaneously.)

For an unresponsive patient, a rapid medical assessment of the entire person is indicated. For a rapid medical assessment, perform a head-to-toe exam, obtain baseline vital signs and a SAMPLE history, and make a decision to transport. (While these steps are listed in order, several steps can be completed simultaneously in many cases.)

3C. Dementia, respiratory disorder or hypoxia, hyperthermia or hypothermia, traumatic head injury, or medical problem such as a stroke, infection, decreased or elevated blood sugar level, cardiac complications, decreased blood volume, shock, medication complications or street drug use

3D. When gathering additional information on the chief complaint of a responsive medical patient, use the OPQRST mnemonic. Questions associated with each letter can include:

- Onset—"When did the symptoms begin?"
- Provocation—"What were you doing when the symptoms began?"
- Quality—"Describe the pain for me."
- Radiation—"Does your pain travel or radiate anywhere?"
- Severity—"On a scale of 1 to 10, 10 being the worst pain you have ever had, how do you rate this pain?"
- Time—"How long have you had these or similar symptoms?"

3E. According to the vital signs chart, the student should list:

- heart rate 60 to 100
- blood pressure 120/80
- respiration rate 12 to 20 per minute

4A. This patient is an unresponsive trauma patient. You should complete an initial assessment, a rapid trauma assessment, package and transport to the closest appropriate facility. While en route to the hospital, the detailed physical exam may be performed. It includes:

- Expose and exam all areas of the body

- Inspect and palpate all areas, looking for DCAP-BTLS
- Manage significant injuries as they are found
- Complete a systematic anatomic survey of the patient from head to toe

4B. It appears that the unresponsive patient is the victim of trauma. Due to the mechanism of injury, a potential spinal injury cannot be ruled out. Therefore, it is critical that spinal precautions be completed prior to movement or transport.

4C. Gloves only, unless the nosebleed is profuse.

5A. The three main goals of the ongoing assessment are to identify any missed or new injuries or conditions, to check for any changes in the patient's condition, and to determine the effectiveness of any and all interventions.

5B. In unstable patients, measure vitals signs at least once every five minutes. In very critical patients or patients receiving a large number of interventions, the blood pressure, pulse, and respiratory rate should be taken as often as necessary. These successive readings help the EMS and hospital crews by providing a valuable history of the patient's condition while on scene and en route to the hospital.

5C. The EMT-Basic must check on each intervention to ensure that the patient's airway, breathing, and circulation status has not changed and that the treatment given is still working properly.

Key Terms Matching

1. Crepitation: (F) A crackling sensation felt and heard beneath the skin; caused by broken bone ends grating against each other or by subcutaneous air
2. Detailed Physical Exam: (I) A careful, comprehensive examination of the body performed on critical patients, usually while en route to the receiving facility
3. Edema: (H) Abnormal accumulation of fluid in the tissues causing swelling
4. Focused History and Physical Exam: (G) Assessment procedure used to identify conditions requiring emergency care; performed after initial assessment and lifesaving interventions
5. Jugular Venous Distention (JVD): (J) Abnormal bulging of the jugular veins indicating injury to the heart or chest
6. Ongoing Assessment: (E) Frequent reevaluation of a patient after initial assessment and primary interventions; to identify changes in patient condition and ensure appropriate care
7. Paradoxical Motion: (D) Chest movement during breathing in which one section of the chest moves in the opposite direction from the rest; indicates multiple rib fractures (flail chest)
8. Rapid Medical Assessment: (A) A physical exam designed to quickly determine the nature and severity of an illness and identify necessary interventions
9. Rapid Trauma Assessment: (B) A physical exam designed to quickly identify critical injuries and emergency interventions
10. Tracheal Deviation: (C) A shifting of the trachea to either side of the midline caused by the pressure of air trapped in the chest cavity

Labeling Diagrams

DCAP-BTLS

D = deformities

C = contusions

A = abrasions

P = punctures/perforations

B = burns

T = tenderness

L = lacerations

S = swelling

Steps in the Assessment of a Medical Patient

A. Initial assessment

B. Baseline vital signs

C. Transport decision

D. Ongoing assessment

CHAPTER 10
Communications and Documentation

Review Questions

1. D	**6.** D	**11.** B	**16.** D	**21.** B
2. A	**7.** A	**12.** D	**17.** A	**22.** A
3. B	**8.** A	**13.** C	**18.** B	**23.** D
4. C	**9.** B	**14.** B	**19.** A	**24.** C
5. B	**10.** C	**15.** C	**20.** B	**25.** C

Case Studies

Documentation

1A. Documentation is designed to provide a complete and accurate record of the nature and extent of the problem and the type and quality of the emergency medical care given. The document functions as both a medical record and a legal record.

1B. Patient data should include the chief complaint, mental status, systolic blood pressure, skin perfusion (color and temperature), pulse rate, and respiratory rate.

1C. To provide the EMS agency with important data, the administrative information includes:

- Time of incident report
- Time the unit was notified
- Time of arrival
- Time of departure
- Time of arrival at the local destination

1D. Areas that seem to create problems for EMT-Basics trying to complete the paperwork include:

- Not drawing a single line through an error
- Repeatedly spelling words incorrectly

Other errors are less common, but have severe legal repercussions. These errors include:

- Documenting skills that were not performed
- Attempting to cover up an error on the patient exam

1E. During mass casualty incidents, paperwork is nearly impossible. The use of simplified documents, such as triage tags, provides an excellent way of tracking patients. Depending on your EMS system and available resources, you may be able to generate the forms in the Emergency Department after you have completed your direct patient care.

1F. Federal and most state laws mandate reporting in the following situations:

- Suspicions of neglect or abuse of children, the elderly, or spouses
- Sexual assault
- Wounds resulting from violent crime
- Animal bite
- Suspicion of infectious diseases

Common Medical Abbreviations

2A. **a)** Alcohol = ETOH
b) Blood pressure = BP
c) Chief complaint = CC
d) Estimated time of arrival = ETA
e) History = HX
f) Loss (Level) of consciousness = LOC
g) Oxygen = O_2
h) Past medical history = PMHx
i) Signs and symptoms = S/S
j) Shortness of breath = SOB
k) Vital signs = VS
l) Year old = Y/O

3A. 46 y/o male pt c/c crushing cp × 1 hr. provoked by mowing the yard increasing in intensity described as 8/10. Pt. Hx. of HD & Htn. Meds: 1 aspirin qd & Nitro prn. VS p 108, respirations 22, BP 150/104. Pt. (–) allergies (+) diaphoresis (+) pale. Tx. O-2 via NRB, 1 Nitro SL which caused a headache. Repeat VS p 104, respirations 22, BP 138/88 with no change in pain from Nitro. En route, the pt's. pain remains unchanged. Vs. stable. ED MD notified.

4A. Some of the strategies you can use include:

- Try again to persuade the patient to go to the hospital.
- Inform the patient why he or she should go to the hospital, and what might happen if he or she does not.
- Ensure that the patient is able to make a rational, informed decision. If you suspect that the patient is under the influence of alcohol or other drugs, or if the patient's thinking is affected by illness or injury, consult medical direction as directed by local protocol. The physician may make a recommendation or talk directly with the patient. Advise law enforcement if appropriate.

4B. Document the following if the patient still refuses to go:

- Document any assessment findings and emergency medical care given, then have the patient sign a refusal of care form (used in most departments).
- Have a law enforcement officer, family member, or bystander sign the form as a witness. If the patient will not sign the refusal form, ask a witness to sign verifying that the patient refused to sign.
- Suggest your willingness to return if the situation changes or the patient changes his or her mind.
- Complete the PCR. Record as much of the patient assessment as possible, including physical exam and vital signs. Document all care given. Also describe the care you wanted to provide for the patient. Include a statement that you explained to the patients the possible consequences of failure to accept care, including the potential for death.

4C. You could be arrested for kidnapping or assault and battery if you actually touched the patient against his will. If he is not in immediate danger of losing his life and he is an adult, he does still have the right to refuse.

Key Terms Matching

1. Base Station: (E) Radio used for central dispatch operations and coordination of emergency services in an EMS communication system
2. Minimum Data Set: (C) Patient and administrative information required to be included in a prehospital care report
3. Mobile Radio: (D) Two-way radios that are usually built into emergency vehicles
4. Prehospital Care Report (PCR): (B) Documentation of the assessment and treatment of a patient in the field
5. Repeaters: (A) Communications devices that receive a low-power transmission and rebroadcast the signal at higher power

Fill-in-the-Blanks

1. unit; providers
2. arrival
3. age
4. complaint
5. illness
6. past
7. mental
8. baseline
9. physical
10. medical care
11. response

CHAPTER 11
General Pharmacology

Review Questions

1. B	6. C	11. C	16. D	21. D
2. B	7. A	12. B	17. A	22. A
3. D	8. A	13. A	18. B	23. D
4. A	9. C	14. A	19. C	24. C
5. A	10. A	15. D	20. B	25. A

Case Studies

General Pharmacology

1A. Ask the patient again if he has any allergies to medications. Ask if the patient understands how to take the medication. (In this case, allow the medication to dissolve instead of chew or swallow.)

1B. Right patient, Right medication, Right dose, Right route of administration

2A. Activated charcoal is a liquid suspension that the patient drinks through a straw.

2B. The route of administration for activated charcoal is drinking by mouth.

2C. Activated charcoal is not given by mouth to patients who do not have a gag reflex.

Key Terms Matching

1. Action: (G) The desired effect of a medication or treatment
2. Contraindication: (I) Condition under which a specific medication or treatment should not be given
3. Dosage: (H) Appropriate amount of a medication to administer; also dose
4. Generic Name: (J) Official common name of a medication
5. Indication: (F) A sign, symptom, or condition for which a specific medication or treatment is given
6. Metered Dose Inhaler (MDI): (A) Hand-held inhalation device for delivering liquid or powdered medication in premeasured doses
7. Nebulizer: (D) Device for administering vaporized liquid medication
8. Route of Administration: (C) Pathway by which a medication is administered: sublingual, oral ingestion, injection, inhalation, etc.
9. Side Effect: (B) Unwanted effect of a medication
10. Trade Name: (E) Manufacturer's brand name for a medication

CHAPTER 12
Respiratory Emergencies

Review Questions

1. B	8. A	15. A	22. A	29. A
2. D	9. D	16. A	23. A	30. C
3. A	10. B	17. A	24. B	31. D
4. B	11. D	18. B	25. A	32. B
5. C	12. D	19. C	26. B	33. A
6. D	13. B	20. A	27. B	34. C
7. B	14. A	21. D	28. C	35. B

Case Studies

1A. The patient's past medical history, the history of the present illness, medication allergies, and current medications are especially important. When discussing medications, it is important to obtain the medication name, strength, frequency, and time of last dose. The effectiveness of many medications is dependent upon dose and timing.

1B. Most inhalers are based upon epinephrine (adrenaline), a compound naturally secreted by the adrenal glands. Epinephrine works to constrict blood vessels (thereby reducing swelling in the bronchial tubes, which are very vascular), but it also increases the heart rate. It may also result in anxiety and nervous tremors.

1C. Initially, you should place the patient on high-flow oxygen and remove the patient from the environment to the ambulance. Be prepared to assist respirations if breathing becomes inadequate. You can assist the patient with additional inhaler doses, as long as the patient is able to use the device, the device is the patient's own, permission is obtained from medical direction, and the patient has not met the maximum prescribed dosage.

1D. The signs of inadequate breathing include:

- A feeling of shortness of breath, chest tightness, or difficulty breathing
- A feeling of anxiousness or restlessness
- An increased pulse rate or very slow rate
- Increased breathing rate
- Irregular breathing pattern
- Skin sign changes (cyanotic, flushing, or paleness)
- Audible sounds from the upper airway (stridor, gurgling, snoring, or crowing)
- Wheezing or other signs of bronchoconstriction
- Abnormal sounds upon auscultation
- Limited or no ability to speak due to respiratory distress
- Use of accessory muscles in breathing
- Abdominal breathing
- Shallow breathing, poor chest wall expansion
- Altered mental status (an early sign)
- Tripod position
- Persistent coughing
- Barrel chest wall
- Paradoxical chest wall motion

1E. A person should be able to breathe without conscious effort. Adequate breathing includes a good tidal volume within the average range for respiratory rates. There should be no evidence of any accessory muscle use.

2A. Expect to find numerous sources of home oxygen, including portable oxygen cylinders, oxygen concentrators, and large backup cylinders. You may also find portable suction units, aerosol nebulizers, and numerous inhalers for self-administration.

2B. The primary intervention should be to maintain oxygen therapy during transport. If necessary, increase the flow rate slightly to compensate for the stressors of movement and transport. Be prepared to assist the patient with the administration of inhaler medications or to assist with ventilation if her condition should deteriorate.

2C. It is important that you recognize the emotional needs of this situation. In some cases, it may be the last time the patient sees her home. Acceptance into a hospice unit has become an important step in dealing with terminal illness. Listen empathetically and provide no false reassurances. Use a gentle and reassuring tone when dealing with the patient and family. Respect the patient's needs with regard to dignity, respect, sharing, communication, privacy, and control. Comfort the family as necessary.

3A. There are several factors that predispose infants and toddlers to foreign body airway obstructions. First, children are naturally curious—they tend to touch, taste, and smell everything in their environment. Airway structures are smaller and more easily obstructed than an adult's. The tongue is proportionally larger than an adult's and can make expelling an obstruction more difficult. Also, a child's smaller structures are more prone to swelling, which can entrap a foreign body.

3B. Follow the American Heart Association, ARC, NSC, guidelines for foreign body airway obstruction. Depending upon the age of the child, this may include abdominal thrusts, chest thrusts, and back blows. Finger sweeps should be avoided unless the object is visualized. Follow these procedures until the object is expelled.

3C. Immediate, rapid transport to the closest medical facility is indicated. If normal foreign body procedures fail, surgical procedures may be necessary to remove the obstruction. Treatment should be initiated even in the absence of parental consent because of the life-threatening nature of the emergency.

4A. Wheezes, both inspiratory and expiratory

4B. Albuterol, Isoetharine, Metaproterenol, Terbutaline

4C. Ask the patient questions to verify that this is the correct medication for the correct patient, which is not expired. Make sure you have the correct route of administrations and find out if she has already taken some medication.

Key Terms Matching

1. Acute Illness: (J) Illness with a severe, rapid onset
2. Asthma: (G) Reactive airway disease caused by spasmodic contraction of the bronchi; characterized by recurrent attacks of dyspnea, coughing, and wheezing
3. Bronchoconstriction: (H) Narrowing of the air passageways due to constriction of the smooth muscle of the bronchi and bronchioles
4. Bronchodilator: (I) Drug that relaxes the smooth muscle of the bronchi and bronchioles, reversing bronchoconstriction
5. Chronic Illness: (B) Long-term illness
6. Chronic Obstructive Pulmonary Disease (COPD): (E) Generic term for emphysema, chronic bronchitis, and other obstructive airway diseases
7. Respiratory Arrest: (D) A complete lack of respiratory drive or pulmonary function
8. Respiratory Distress: (C) Difficulty breathing; increased effort necessary to breathe due to impaired respiratory function
9. Respiratory Failure: (F) When the respiratory system cannot deliver an adequate supply of oxygen to meet the body's current demand
10. Tripod Position: (A) Position that helps keep the airway open and maximizes respiratory effort: sitting, leaning forward with hands on the knees

Labeling Diagram

Causes of Shortness of Breath

A. pulmonary embolism

B. heart attack

C. congestive heart failure

D. asthma

CHAPTER 13
Cardiovascular Emergencies

Review Questions

1. C	**7.** B	**13.** D	**19.** C	**25.** B
2. A	**8.** A	**14.** B	**20.** D	**26.** D
3. A	**9.** C	**15.** C	**21.** A	**27.** A
4. D	**10.** C	**16.** A	**22.** B	**28.** D
5. A	**11.** D	**17.** D	**23.** C	**29.** A
6. B	**12.** A	**18.** B	**24.** D	**30.** A

Case Studies

1A. Upon discovery of a pulseless, apneic patient, the EMT-Basic should apply the AED, stop CPR, clear the patient, and analyze as soon as possible.

1B. Verbalize and visualize that all rescuers are clear of the patient, and that the patient is lying upon a surface suitable for defibrillation (e.g., not in a puddle or on metal bleachers). Administer the shock and immediately reanalyze the rhythm. If an additional shock is advised, clear the patient, deliver the shock, and reanalyze. The EMT-Basic may repeat the shock/analysis sequence one more time, or up to three times in total.

1C. After the third shock, you should check for a pulse. In the absence of a pulse, CPR should be resumed for one minute. Stop after one minute of CPR, clear the patient, and analyze the rhythm. Deliver up to three additional shocks if indicated.

1D. After six shocks, after three consecutive "no shock advised" messages separated by one minute of CPR, and when the patient regains a pulse

2A. Check for a pulse. If present, assess for breathing. If not present, resume CPR for one minute, then reanalyze the rhythm.

2B. The EMT-Basic should immediately begin assisting ventilations with a bag-valve mask and supplemental oxygen. Transport should begin as soon as possible.

3A. No. The patient is not complaining of chest pain, even though her symptoms may be related to a cardiac problem. Nitroglycerin is not indicated.

3B. You should place the patient on high-flow oxygen via non-rebreather mask and prepare for rapid transport to the closest hospital. Ventilatory support should be readied in case the patient's condition worsens.

3C. Explain to the husband that nitroglycerin is for cardiac chest pain and not a treatment for difficulty breathing. Last, you might explain that sharing medications can lead to severe health problems, which is precisely why it is illegal. Do not allow his request to delay the treatment and transport of the patient.

4A. The most common failure of the AED is battery failure.

4B. A routine maintenance program with a checklist and daily battery rotating can help prevent this problem. Also always carry spare batteries with the AED.

5A. The four links in the AHA chain of survival are: early access to the EMS system, early CPR, early defibrillation, and early ACLS.

5B. The first link can be strengthened by training the public how to call 9-1-1.

5C. The second link can be strengthened by training the public to do CPR.

5D. The third link can be strengthened by training all First Responders and EMT-Basics to use an AED.

Key Terms Matching

1. Acute Myocardial Infarction (AMI): (J) Sudden cardiac muscle death or injury due to lack of oxygen; a heart attack
2. Angina Pectoris: (H) Severe pain and constriction about the heart; also called angina or myocardial ischemia; often treated with nitroglycerin
3. Automated External Defibrillator (AED): (E) Defibrillation equipment designed to analyze, shock, and reanalyze cardiac dysfunction after applying electrodes to patient
4. Cardiac Compromise: (F) Any action or factor that reduces the functionality of the cardiac system
5. Chain of Survival: (C) Term used for the four interventions that provide the best chance for successful resuscitation of a patient in cardiac arrest: early access, early CPR, early defibrillation, early ACLS
6. Coronary Artery Disease (CAD): (D) Condition of plaque accumulation causing narrowing within coronary artery walls; leads to decreased oxygen delivery to heart muscle
7. Defibrillation: (I) Electrical shock or current delivered to the heart through the patient's chest wall to help the heart restore a normal rhythm
8. Dysrhythmia: (G) A disturbance in heart rate and/or rhythm; formerly called arrhythmia
9. Nitroglycerin (NTG): (B) Medication that dilates blood vessels and decreases the workload of the heart; taken sublingually by tablet or by spray for relief of chest pain
10. Ventricular Fibrillation (VF): (A) Rapid, uncoordinated movements of the ventricle walls that replace the normal contraction; treated with defibrillation methods

Labeling Diagrams

Structures of the Cardiovascular System

A. plasma
B. heart
C. systemic artery
D. red blood cell

Steps in Using the AED, Two or More Rescuers, Pulseless Patient

A. ALS backup
B. Attaches defibrillator
C. Check pulse
D. Transport

CHAPTER 14
Neurological, Diabetic, and Behavioral Emergencies

Review Questions

1. A	**9.** B	**17.** A	**25.** A	**33.** C
2. B	**10.** A	**18.** D	**26.** C	**34.** B
3. A	**11.** A	**19.** D	**27.** B	**35.** D
4. D	**12.** A	**20.** C	**28.** D	**36.** C
5. A	**13.** D	**21.** B	**29.** A	**37.** A
6. A	**14.** C	**22.** A	**30.** D	**38.** D
7. B	**15.** D	**23.** B	**31.** A	**39.** A
8. B	**16.** A	**24.** A	**32.** A	**40.** B

Case Studies

1A. Accidental overdose of insulin, poor oral intake (not eating enough), and significantly increased activity without modifying glucose/insulin balance.

1B. Oral glucose should not be given to patients with an altered mental status who are not or may not be able to control their own airway. If the possibility exists for Sandra to lose her airway control, using oral glucose should be reconsidered.

1C. The following are signs and symptoms of a patient suffering a diabetic emergency:

- Rapid onset of an altered mental status

- Bizarre behavior, resembling intoxication; staggering gait; slurred speech; etc.
- Elevated heart rate
- Cold, clammy skin
- Significant hunger
- Seizures
- Medications used by diabetics

1D. The response should identify the major assessment and treatment steps and also may include more detail than given here. At a minimum, the treatment steps should include:

- Complete the initial assessment and correct any problems found.
- Look for any medical identification insignias, bracelets, etc.
- Maintain a patent airway, and provide ventilations as required.
- If no spinal injury is suspected, place patient in the recovery position.
- Complete the focused history and physical exam.
- Attempt to gather sample history information.
- Secure baseline vital signs.
- Determine the patient's ability to maintain his or her own airway if patent.
- Provide oral glucose with a physician's order.
- Monitor the patient's airway and mental status.
- Document responses to medication and changes in mental status.

1E. You may feel that it is appropriate to tell the manager what is wrong because it is in Sandra's best interest to clarify the problem and to rule out alcohol on the job. However, it is inappropriate to divulge patient information without consent, regardless of the situation. A more appropriate course is to direct the manager to Sandra's supervisor, who is aware of her medical condition and the circumstances surrounding events in the office.

2A. The list can include any of the following causes:

- Hypoxia
- Head trauma
- Temperature extremes
- Drug or alcohol poisoning
- Infection
- Stroke
- Post-seizure period
- Hypovolemia/shock
- Psychiatric disorders
- Metabolic or hormonal disorders

2B. Alcohol impairs mental status. Since changes in a patient's mental status are a significant indicator in many medical and traumatic emergencies, it can hide findings that could prove to be significant. Alcohol also reacts with certain medications to increase their effect on the body.

2C. The EMT-Basic in this role should focus on maintaining an airway, adequate breathing, and adequate circulation. History taking is also essential.

3A. While many causes of seizure exist, common causes include: noncompliance with seizure medications, fever, infection, hypoxia, hypoglycemia, alcohol or drug withdrawal, poisoning, metabolic disorders, congenital anomalies, preeclampsia, trauma, stroke, tumors, or idiopathic (unknown) causes.

3B. Generally, an EMT-Basic cannot determine whether or not a patient is faking. In the case above, the patient may be trying to delay her trip to jail. However, the EMT-Basic must take the patient at face value. The EMT-Basic's duty is to err on the side of caution, and always assume the worst in forming a treatment plan.

3C. The average duration for a postictal state is 10 to 30 minutes. This is only an average. Some patients may take longer to awake from a particularly violent seizure. When a patient is in a postictal state, the presentation can range from sleepy, confused, and scared to completely unresponsive.

4A. Always treat stroke patients as though they can hear and understand everything that you say or do. Although the patient's ability to communicate may be diminished, his or her sensorium may not have been altered. Transport conscious stroke patients in a position of comfort. Transport unconscious stroke patients on their side. Use a calm, gentle tone when talking with the patient.

4B. Most stroke patients will exhibit one or more of the following signs or symptoms after suffering a stroke:

- Altered mental status
- Paralysis or disability, usually on only one side of the body or the other
- Loss of sensory perception on the affected side
- Speech loss or difficulties
- Unequal pupils
- Vision disturbances

- Severe headaches
- Loss of balance or coordination
- Seizures
- Nausea and vomiting
- Loss of bladder or bowel control

4C. Sonna should receive the following care:

- Ensure scene safety.
- Take spinal precautions since the patient is unable to rule out any possible spinal injury or involvement.
- Complete the initial assessment and correct any problems found.
- Have suction always ready and prevent aspiration.
- Provide adequate levels of oxygenation; assist ventilations if required.
- Position the patient in the appropriate manner to protect the airway and maintain spinal precautions.
- Protect all the patient's extremities.
- Transport to the appropriate facility.

5A. Assure that she has a patent airway.

5B. Profound feelings of discouragement, loss of control, worthlessness, helplessness, and hopelessness. Depression may be a primary factor in most suicides.

5C. Acknowledge that she seems upset and state that you are there to help her. Tell her what you are doing and try to talk her into cooperating with you. Ask questions in a calm and reassuring tone.

5D. Do not lie to her. Avoid making quick or sudden movements.

Key Terms Matching

1. Altered Mental Status (AMS): (N) Broad term indicating a change in normal thinking or clarity of thought; behavior may range from mild confusion to complete unresponsiveness
2. Behavioral emergency: (J) A situation in which the patient exhibits behavior that others consider unacceptable or intolerable
3. Cerebrovascular Accident (CVA): (L) Stroke or brain attack; occurs when a blood vessel in the brain becomes blocked or ruptures
4. Diabetes Mellitus: (K) A disease characterized by inadequate production or use of insulin
5. Glucose: (M) A simple sugar that is the body's basic source of energy
6. Hyperglycemia: (I) Condition in which blood sugar is too high; results from inadequate insulin in the blood for glucose metabolism
7. Hypoglycemia: (E) Condition in which blood sugar is too low; results from too much insulin or not enough glucose in the blood
8. Insulin: (G) Hormone secreted by the pancreas that regulates blood sugar levels
9. Postictal State: (F) A patient's condition after a seizure, during which the patient may appear sleepy, confused, or unresponsive
10. Seizure: (H) Chaotic electrical activity in the brain that can lead to a momentary break in the stream of thought, muscular spasms, or a complete loss of consciousness
11. Status Epilepticus: (D) A state of prolonged seizures or multiple seizures between which the patient does not regain consciousness
12. Stroke: (B) Common term for a cerebrovascular accident
13. Syncope: (C) Sudden onset of a temporary loss of consciousness caused by low blood pressure in the brain; fainting
14. Transient Ischemic Attack (TIA): (A) A sudden loss of neurological functions that clears up within 24 hours; the symptoms are similar to a CVA; also called a ministroke

Labeling Diagram

Causes of Altered Mental Status

A. dementia
B. hyperthermia or hypothermia
C. infection
D. heart rhythm disturbances and heart attack
E. medication related

CHAPTER 15
Allergic Reactions

Review Questions

1. B	5. C	9. A	13. B	17. B
2. C	6. C	10. C	14. C	18. D
3. D	7. D	11. B	15. D	19. C
4. B	8. B	12. A	16. B	20. C

Case Studies

Allergic Reactions

1A. This patient is experiencing anaphylaxis. Remember that it is considered anaphylaxis when either breathing or circulation is compromised.

1B. The treatment for this patient includes: A) administering oxygen at 10 to 15 liters via non-rebreather mask, contacting medical command to get permission to administer epinephrine via her auto-injector, and placing her in a sitting position and elevating her legs. Quickly transport her to the hospital.

2A. The skin, eyes, stomach lining, nose, sinuses, throat, and lungs

2B. Peanuts, eggs, milk, chocolate, cottonseed oil, grains, beans, and fruits

2C. The effect on the respiratory system, cardiovascular system, and the patient's mental status

2D. Treatment for this patient includes: administering oxygen, 10 to 15 liters via non-rebreather mask, contacting medical command to get permission to administer epinephrine via her auto-injector, and quickly transporting her to the hospital.

Key Terms Matching

1. Adrenaline: (J) Another name for epinephrine
2. Allergen: (D) An antigen, such as dust, mold, or pollen, that causes an allergic reaction.
3. Allergic Reaction: (H) An exaggerated immune response to a substance that is normally harmless
4. Anaphylactic Shock: (F) Severe allergic reaction in which blood vessels dilate rapidly, causing a drop in blood pressure and respiratory distress
5. Anaphylaxis: (B) Another name for anaphylactic shock
6. Antibody: (E) A protein produced by the immune system that combines with a specific antigen and helps to destroy it
7. Antigen: (I) A foreign substance that enters the body and cause causes an immune response.
8. Epinephrine: (C) Hormone secreted in response to stress; causes tachycardia and vasoconstriction; used as an injected medication to relieve severe allergic reactions
9. Hives: (G) Raised, red blotches associated with allergic reactions
10. Immune Response: (A) A series of reactions that are the body's defense mechanism against invading viruses, bacteria, and toxins

CHAPTER 16
Poisoning and Overdose

Review Questions

1. B	**7.** C	**13.** A	**19.** D	**25.** C
2. D	**8.** B	**14.** D	**20.** D	**26.** D
3. D	**9.** C	**15.** A	**21.** B	**27.** A
4. B	**10.** B	**16.** B	**22.** B	**28.** B
5. C	**11.** A	**17.** A	**23.** A	**29.** C
6. A	**12.** C	**18.** C	**24.** B	**30.** B

Case Studies

Poisoning

1A. There may be something in the air being inhaled by the patients.

1B. C-O from a poorly vented fireplace

1C. Cherry red skin color

2A. Absorption poisoning

2B. Decontamination

2C. Flush for 20 minutes.

3A. Alert if the charcoal is being administered.

3B. Nausea and vomiting and black stools

3C. 1 gram per kilogram or 25–50 grams for an adult

3D. SuperChar™ InstaChar™ Actidoes™ LiquiChar™

Key Terms Matching

1. Absorbed Poison: (H) A toxic substance taken into the body across unbroken skin or mucous membranes
2. Activated Charcoal: (I) Substance that hinders the absorption of ingested poisons and enhances their elimination from the body, preventing further damage
3. Antidote: (G) An agent that blocks or reverses the effect of a poison
4. Decontamination: (F) The removal or cleansing of dangerous chemicals and other dangerous or infectious materials
5. Ingested Poison: (D) A liquid or solid toxic substance that is swallowed
6. Inhaled Poison: (E) A toxic substance such as a gas, fumes, vapor, or spray that is breathed in
7. Injected Poison: (C) A toxic substance that enters the body through a puncture in the skin; injection may be by needle, animal bite, or insect sting
8. Poison: (A) A food, plant, chemical, or drug that has an adverse effect on the body

9. Toxin: (B) A substance that is poisonous to cells or tissues

CHAPTER 17
Environmental Emergencies

Review Questions

1. A	**6.** B	**11.** A	**16.** D	**21.** A
2. C	**7.** D	**12.** C	**17.** A	**22.** C
3. A	**8.** C	**13.** D	**18.** D	**23.** A
4. C	**9.** B	**14.** A	**19.** B	**24.** A
5. B	**10.** C	**15.** A	**20.** A	**25.** C

Case Studies

Cold-Related Emergencies

1A. The response should include:

- Radiation: body heat is released to the surrounding air
- Conduction: loss of body heat based on direct contact with a cooler object
- Evaporation: body heat lost during the conversion of water (sweat) to gas
- Breathing: body heat lost from the body's core via exhaled air
- Convection: body heat lost as a result of moving air across the body's surface (similar to conduction)

1B. Radiation: body heat is released to the surrounding air; Conduction: loss of body heat based on direct contact with a cooler object (the concrete floor, in this case); Breathing: body heat lost from the body's core via exhaled air

1C. Other contributing factors would include the patient's age and attire. The fact that he is a frequent user of EMS services may indicate a history of health problems.

2A. For the early stage of hypothermia, the response should include:

- Rapid pulse (In late stages, pulse may be slow and barely palpable and/or irregular, or completely absent.)
- Normal blood pressure (In late stages, the blood pressure may decrease or become absent.)
- Rapid breathing (in late stages, shallow, slow or even absent breathing)
- In early hypothermia, the pupils are reactive to light. (In late or more severe hypothermia, the pupils may respond very slowly or not at all when stimulated with light.)
- Shivering may be present or absent.
- In early stages, the skin may be deep red. (In later or more severe cases, the skin may become pale or blue gray.)

2B. Initially, you should determine if the scene is safe and approach the patient with caution. Complete the initial assessment and maintain cervical spine control, as well as a rapid trauma assessment. Because elements of the mechanism are unknown (Did he strike anything underwater?), spinal immobilization is indicated. Remove the patient from the cold environment as soon as possible and protect the patient from further heat loss. Remove wet clothing and cover with blankets. Handle the patient extremely gently. Administer oxygen if not already done as part of the initial assessment. Oxygen administered should be warmed and humidified if possible. Assess pulses for 30–45 seconds before starting CPR. Rewarm passively with warm blankets, and turn the heat up high in the patient compartment of the ambulance. Do not massage the extremities.

2C. The EMT-Basic should mention issues surrounding percentages of body fat, muscle mass, and reduced ability to thermoregulate.

3A. This response should include:

- Pulse—slow and barely palpable, usually irregular
- Blood pressure—low or absent (unable to obtain)
- Breathing—shallow, slow, irregular, or absent
- Skin—pale, cyanotic, stiff, and hard
- Pupils—sluggish or nonreactive

4A. The presence of bruising suggests that the patient has undergone recent trauma. Since she has an altered mental state, err on the side of caution. Treat her as a trauma patient.

4B. You should immediately contact the EMS system and begin a response from the local system. The responder should then complete an initial assessment with c-spine control, and, if possible, provide any lifesaving interventions required. Once additional help arrives, the patient should be immobilized and removed from the environment. Some general treatment considerations include:

- Remove the patient from the harmful environment.
- If the patient is wet, remove all wet clothing and gently dry the patient.
- Wrap the patient is a warm blanket.

- Avoid all rough handling.
- Do not allow the patient to walk or exert herself.
- If available, place warm packs to the patient's groin, axillary and cervical regions.
- Be very slow and careful when checking for a pulse; be absolutely sure no pulse exists before beginning CPR.

5A. Passive rewarming techniques of unresponsive patients includes the following:

- Remove all wet clothing and gently dry off the patients.
- Wrap the patients in warm blankets.
- Establish a heat source in the cabin.
- Do not massage frozen or nearly frozen body tissue.
- Do not allow the patient to eat or drink stimulants (coffee, hot tea, etc.).

5B. Yes, if the site is remote and the patients are showing signs and symptoms of severe cold injury. Rapid transport to a trauma center is vital to survival of these patients.

6A. The response should include the following signs and symptoms:

- White, waxy and almost transparent appearance
- Skin will feel firm.
- Ice crystals under the skin may be palpable.
- Swelling
- Blisters
- Mottled and/or cyanotic in partially thawed skin
- Black or gangrenous tissue in very severe cases
- Various levels of sensation

6B. Treatment for the late or deep localized cold injury should include:

- Removing all the patient's jewelry in the affected area; use a ring cutter if necessary.
- Cover the injured tissue with a dry dressing.
- Do not break blisters or rub or massage injured tissue.
- Do not apply any heat to the damaged tissue.
- Do not rewarm the affected tissue.
- Immobilize the area and do not allow the patient to use the injured tissue.

6C. Ice crystals may present a threat when they move to the central circulation. Such crystals can injure arteries and veins. Also, circulation of ice crystals may drop the body's core temperature.

6D. The proper active/rapid rewarming treatment for the late or deep injuries should include:

- Immerse the affected part in a warm bath (40°C [104° F]) .
- Monitor the water temperature to be sure that it doesn't cool from the frozen part.
- Continuously stir the water.
- Continue to rewarm the tissue part until it is soft and has both color and sensation.
- It is very important to protect the part from freezing again by applying a dry dressing between affected digits.
- There may be significant pain associated with thawing tissue and rewarming.

Heat-Related Emergencies

7A. The response should include the following information:

- Remove the patient from the extreme environment and into a cool environment, preferably a surrounding building or the ambulance.
- Complete the initial assessment and provide any lifesaving interventions as required.
- Place the patient in a supine position and elevate the patient's lower extremities (shock position).
- Loosen any restrictive clothing or any clothing that may retain body heat.
- Provide supplemental cooling; use fanning or evaporation.
- If the patient can protect his airway, allow him to drink cool liquids. If not, take appropriate steps to protect the patient's airway.

7B. The EMT-Basic should recognize the dangers inherent in providing fluids to someone with an unprotected airway. While several different methods might be acceptable, one such method would be to offer a small quantity of fluid in a cup to the patient. If he or she can properly place the cup to the lips and begin drinking, you can allow the patient to take additional fluids. In determining the patency of a conscious patient's airway, be sure to have the patient lean forward in case he or she is not able to keep the airway clear. This will help limit the possibility of aspiration. Keep suction nearby and ready to use.

8A. The response should include the following steps:

- Remove all clothing. (Maintain the patient's dignity and privacy as much as is possible.)
- Apply cool packs to the neck, groin, and axillary points.

- Sponge the skin with cool water, and place a wet, cool towel over and under the patient.
- Begin aggressive fanning to increase evaporation.
- Transport immediately.
- Monitor vital signs, provide airway protection, and notify the receiving facility as early as possible.

Water-Related Emergencies

9A. It is critical that the EMT-Basic immediately confirm that spinal precautions are taken and maintained as the airway is opened and artificial ventilation is progressing. In almost every water emergency, an assumption should be made that the patient has suffered spinal injury until proven otherwise.

9B. Gastric distention occurs when either fluid or gases enter the stomach in quantities that produce expansion or swelling. As the "distention" continues to increase, the stomach organ begins to take up more space in the abdominal cavity and, consequently, begins to place upward pressure on the diaphragm. As the diaphragm moves upwards, the size of the chest cavity decreases, preventing the lungs from expanding at the normal volume.

9C. The patient should be log rolled onto his or her side. While on the side, you should apply firm pressure with a flattened hand over the epigastric region. This pressure will typically induce vomiting of fluids and gases and will reduce the distention. Another common cause of distention is artificial ventilations that are too aggressive. If you suspect this is the case, ventilate slower and more gently at the correct rate for the patient.

Bites and Stings

10A. The EMT-Basic should recognize the signs and symptoms of an allergic reaction and the potentially life-threatening nature of the situation. Aggressive airway protection and rapid transport are the best steps in providing appropriate care for this patient. Oxygen therapy should begin immediately, and the EMT-Basic should closely monitor the patient's airway. Extra effort should be made to remove the stingers as quickly as possible if they are present.

10B. While some controversy exists on the exact nature of removing stingers, be sure to follow local protocols. The basic steps should include:

- Locate the stinger and, using a stiff card or other thin-edged tool, scrape the stinger from the skin.
- Wash the affected area with warm water to remove any remaining venom or toxin.
- Remove any jewelry or other restrictive items before swelling occurs if possible.
- Elevate the area above the level of the patient's heart.
- Contact medical direction for any other possible treatment.

Key Terms Matching

1. Ambient Temperature: (E) The air temperature surrounding the patient
2. Conduction: (D) Transfer of heat from a warmer object in contact with a colder object
3. Convection: (F) Transfer of heat from a warm object to cooler air moving past its surface
4. Drowning: (B) Death resulting from suffocation or cardiac arrest while submerged in water
5. Evaporation: (I) The process of converting a liquid to a gas in which heat is lost
6. Hyperthermia: (C) Abnormally high core body temperature
7. Hypothermia: (J) Abnormally low core body temperature
8. Localized Cold Injury: (K) A cold injury confined to a limited area of the body; more severe cases are called frostbite
9. Near-Drowning: (A) An immersion situation from which the patient is resuscitated and survives for at least 24 hours
10. Radiation: (G) Heat released by an object into the surrounding air as waves of infrared radiation
11. Wind Chill: (H) The combined cooling effect of wind speed and ambient temperature

CHAPTER 18
Obstetrics and Gynecology

Review Questions

1. B	**10.** C	**19.** C	**28.** B	**37.** C
2. A	**11.** B	**20.** B	**29.** C	**38.** A
3. D	**12.** C	**21.** B	**30.** A	**39.** B
4. A	**13.** A	**22.** C	**31.** D	**40.** D
5. C	**14.** D	**23.** B	**32.** B	**41.** A
6. B	**15.** B	**24.** D	**33.** D	**42.** D
7. C	**16.** C	**25.** A	**34.** B	**43.** D
8. B	**17.** D	**26.** B	**35.** B	**44.** B
9. B	**18.** A	**27.** D	**36.** A	**45.** B

Case Studies

Predelivery Emergencies

1A.
- When was your last menstrual period?
- Could you be pregnant?
- When did the bleeding and pain start?
- Did this start after a sexual encounter?
- Does anything make the bleeding or pain better or worse?
- What does the pain feel like?
- Does the pain radiate to other areas?
- How severe is the pain?
- How long have you had the pain and bleeding?
- Is it steady or intermittent?

1B.
- Use standard precautions for body substance isolation.
- Ensure that there is sufficient external padding about the vagina to absorb bleeding. Do not attempt to pack the vagina in order to control bleeding.
- Limit your physical exam to bleeding control and provide emotional support during transport.
- Bring any tissue passed to the hospital.
- Refer the patient to any grief counseling or support personnel available at the receiving facility.
- Treat for shock if the patient develops signs or symptoms of shock.

2A. Pain and vaginal bleeding late in pregnancy can indicate abruptio placenta or placenta previa.

2B. Vaginal bleeding and abdominal pain late in pregnancy represents a potential life-threatening emergency. It is very important that you obtain a detailed history. Rapid transport is indicated. You should notify the receiving facility to ensure they are prepared to receive the patient, who may require an emergency c-section.

3A. The presence of crowning is the principal indicator of imminent delivery. Regular contractions two minutes or less apart should trigger a visual inspection for crowning by the EMT-Basic. If crowning is present, prepare to deliver the infant and contact medical control.

3B.
- First take BSI precautions including gloves, gown, mask, and eye protection. Amniotic fluid, which may contain blood and fecal matter, can be expelled at high pressures during delivery.
- The patient should be positioned to facilitate delivery with buttocks elevated, knees drawn up and thighs spread as far apart as possible. The head of the stretcher can also be elevated to assist with pushing.
- Create a sterile field using the contents of the OB kit. Other contents of the kit should be prepared for ready availability.

4A. Yes. Crowning is the most reliable indicator of imminent delivery. The EMT-Basic should prepare to deliver the fetus and contact medical control.

4B. The green staining indicates that the fetus had a bowel movement inside the amniotic sac. The fecal material, called meconium, can obstruct the newborn's airway and is often the result of fetal distress during the delivery process.

4C. Immediately suction the mouth and nostrils upon delivery of the head. The airway should be cleared as completely as possible before the infant is stimulated to breathe. Aspiration of meconium is a potentially life-threatening complication to newborns. Suctioning, supplemental oxygen, and ventilatory support should be provided as needed after delivery. Rapid transport should begin as soon as possible after delivery. Recognize that the newborn may require advanced airway support and call for advanced providers if available.

Abnormal Deliveries

5A. Due to the length of gestation (about 32 weeks), this will be considered a premature birth. Transport should begin immediately, but you must be prepared to deliver en route to the hospital. Delivery is imminent, but the infant will probably need specialized care you cannot provide. You should request additional resources, such as advanced life support or physician response if your local EMS system has them available.

5B. First, realize that most premature infants require some degree of resuscitation. Clear the airway and thoroughly dry the newborn and wrap it in warm blankets. Pay special attention to the head, making sure that the blankets cover all but the face. Hypothermia is a major concern with preterm infants, and the head is the largest source of heat loss. Stimulate the infant by gently massaging the chest and back. If necessary, you can stimulate the infant by gently flicking the soles of the feet. If the infant still doesn't respond, then provide supplemental oxygen and repeat suctioning, warming, and stimulation. If there is no improvement, provide supplemental ventilation with a bag-valve mask. Continue to warm and stimulate the infant and monitor for spontaneous respiration. Many such infants respond after several minutes of assisted ventilation. Do not spend too much time stimulating the infant. If the infant doesn't respond quickly, begin resuscitation efforts immediately.

Key Terms Matching

1. Abortion: (U) Delivery of the products of conception early in a pregnancy; may be spontaneous or medically induced
2. Amniotic Sac: (T) Sac that holds the fetus suspended in amniotic fluid; also called "bag of waters"
3. APGAR Score: (S) Method for assessing newborns based on five ratings: Appearance, Pulse, Grimace, Activity, and Respiration
4. Breech Presentation: (R) Abnormal delivery in which the infant's buttocks or lower extremities are the presenting part; places infant at high risk for prolapsed cord and oxygen deprivation
5. Crowning: (Q) The stage of delivery in which the head of the fetus is first visible as it stretches the vaginal opening
6. Fetus: (P) Developing, unborn offspring in the uterus; called an embryo for the first eight weeks after conception
7. Gynecology: (K) The medical specialty concerned with conditions of the female reproductive organs
8. Labor: (N) Physical processes of childbirth; begins with uterine contractions and leads to delivery of the fetus and the placenta
9. Limb Presentation: (M) Abnormal delivery in which a limb of the infant is the initial part to deliver through the birth canal
10. Meconium: (L) Dark green fetal waste material that passes into the amniotic fluid; if inhaled, it will cause fetal distress
11. Miscarriage: (O) Delivery of an embryo or fetus prior to viability; spontaneous abortion
12. Obstetrics: (J) The medical specialty concerned with the care of women during pregnancy and child birth
13. Perineum: (I) The area of skin between the vagina and anus in females and between the scrotum and anus in males
14. Placenta: (H) Organ that enables the exchange of nutrients, oxygen, and metabolic wastes between the maternal and fetal circulatory systems
15. Presenting Part: (G) The part of a newborn that comes out of the birth canal first
16. Prolapsed Cord: (F) Presentation of the umbilical cord before the infant's head at delivery; may cause fetal death due to constriction of blood flow through the cord.
17. Show: (E) Discharge of small amount of blood-tinged mucus from the vagina at the onset of labor; also bloody show
18. Supine Hypotensive Syndrome: (D) Maternal hypotension caused when the mother is lying on her back and the weight of the fetus compresses her inferior vena cava
19. Umbilical Cord: (C) Structure that connects the fetus to the placenta; contains arteries and veins responsible for the exchange of materials between fetal and maternal circulation
20. Uterus: (A) Female reproductive organ in which menstruation and fetal development occur; also womb
21. Vagina: (B) Female genital structure; the lower portion of the birth canal

Labeling Diagrams

Newborn Resuscitation Measures: Frequencies and Priorities

A. Medications

B. Establish effective ventilation

C. Dry, warm, position, suction, stimulate

Stages of Labor

A. contractions; dilation

B. canal

C. placenta

CHAPTER 19
Bleeding and Shock

Review Questions

1. C	**7.** A	**13.** C	**19.** D	**25.** B
2. A	**8.** B	**14.** A	**20.** B	**26.** A
3. C	**9.** D	**15.** B	**21.** B	**27.** B
4. D	**10.** D	**16.** A	**22.** C	**28.** A
5. A	**11.** B	**17.** B	**23.** A	**29.** C
6. B	**12.** D	**18.** C	**24.** A	**30.** D

Case Studies

1A.
- Head injuries and lacerations from striking the windshield
- Potential cervical spine injury
- Chest wall injuries (contusions and rib fractures)
- Heart and lung injuries (including pneumothorax, cardiac and pulmonary contusions)

- Transection (tearing) of the aorta (from the rapid deceleration)
- Injuries to the spleen and liver from striking the steering column

1B.
- Place the patient on oxygen via non-rebreather mask at 15 lpm.
- The patient will need to be immobilized on a spine board and carefully removed from the vehicle
- Keep the patient warm.
- You may want to call for ALS assist at the scene or en route to the hospital for this patient.
- Control the bleeding on his forehead with a loose dressing and bandage.

1C. The patient appears to be in shock based on the skin findings and vital signs. He suffered an obvious head (and possible cervical spine) injury. He has obvious blunt chest and abdominal injuries, possibly a ruptured spleen (based on findings of trauma over LUQ and left lower anterior ribs with the presence of shock). The knee injuries are relatively minor compared to the other findings.

1D. The most important thing you can do is transport the patient immediately to the closest facility that can handle major trauma. He needs the "bright lights and cold steel" of the surgical suite for definitive care. Any delay in this will decrease his chance for survival. The ABCs are addressed. The patient is talking so his airway is open. He is breathing, though rapidly, probably due to shock and the chest wall injuries. High-flow oxygen has been placed, and if necessary, breathing can be assisted with a bag-valve mask. The only external bleeding is on the scalp, and the scalp blood is clotted. A rigid cervical collar should be placed on the patient, and the patient should be secured to a long spine board. A blanket can be placed en route to help treat for shock by preventing heat loss. Elevating the extremities is not recommended due to the other injuries (head, neck, chest, abdomen, and knees). Ongoing assessment should be performed en route, including mental status, airway, breathing, circulation, vital signs, etc. If time allows, a more detailed history and physical exam can be performed.

2A.
- Direct nasal trauma
- Environmental factors, such as dry air or dry mucous membranes
- Medical conditions, such as hypertension or blood clotting disorders
- Sinusitis or upper respiratory tract infection
- Digital trauma, caused by nose picking

2B.
- Have the patient sit up and lean forward.
- Pinch the fleshy portion of the nostrils together to apply direct pressure.
- Keep the patient calm, quiet, and reassured.
- Instruct the patient to avoid blowing the nose, even if the bleeding has stopped.

3A.
- Anxiety
- Increased pulse rate
- Pale, cool, clammy skin
- Increased breathing rate
- Nausea

3B.
- Altered mental state
- Dilated pupils
- Decreased BP
- Decreased urinary output
- Shallow, labored, irregular breathing

Key Terms Matching

1. Epistaxis: (D) Hemorrhage from the nose; a nosebleed
2. Hemorrhagic Shock: (E) Hypoperfusion syndrome caused by excessive blood loss; a type of hypovolemic shock; the most common cause of shock in a trauma patient
3. Hypovolemic Shock: (A) Shock caused by inadequate circulatory volume; may be due to loss of blood or depletion of other body fluids
4. Pressure Point: (C) A place where an artery passes near the surface of the body and over a bone; pressure here can stop or reduce bleeding
5. Tourniquet: (B) A device that is wrapped around an extremity to prevent blood flow to or from the distal area

Labeling Diagram

Pressure Points

A. temporal artery
B. brachial artery
C. femoral artery
D. posterior tibial artery

CHAPTER 20
Soft Tissue Injuries

Review Questions

1. B	8. B	15. B	22. A	29. C
2. C	9. C	16. D	23. A	30. B
3. C	10. B	17. C	24. A	31. A
4. C	11. A	18. A	25. D	
5. A	12. B	19. D	26. C	
6. A	13. B	20. C	27. A	
7. D	14. C	21. C	28. A	

Case Studies

Lacerations

1A. Could the airway structures be severed and the potential for an embolism sucking into the large vein?

1B. Bandage, oxygen therapy, supine position, call for ALS, monitor vitals, keep him warm, and transport rapidly.

Burns

2A. 4.5 for front of the head, 9 for each arm, 9 for the chest for a total of 31.5

2B. Yes, due to the overall percentage and the involvement of the hands

2C. Wrap him in a clean burn sheet that is dry.

Amputations

3A. No. Usually the vessels constrict to limit the amount of bleeding.

3B. Focus on MS-ABCs of the initial assessment.

3C. Bandage the stump and find the lost extremity. Treat the patient for shock, oxygenate, and keep him warm. Call for ALS and remove him and his extremity to a trauma center as soon as possible.

Key Terms Matching

1. Abrasion: (P) A superficial scrape injury to the top layer of skin
2. Amputation: (S) Removal of an extremity through trauma or surgery
3. Avulsion: (R) A tearing off or tearing away of a skin flap or body part
4. Bandage: (Q) Holds a dressing in place (self-adherent, gauze rolls, triangular, air splint)
5. Closed Soft Tissue Injury: (A) Damage to muscle, vessels or skin; outer skin remains intact
6. Contusion: (O) Bruise; a wound in which the epidermis remains intact, but the cells and blood vessels in the dermis become damaged
7. Crush Injury: (N) Open or closed soft tissue injury resulting from bilateral blunt trauma forces
8. Dressing: (K) Protective covering applied directly to a soft tissue wound
9. Evisceration: (L) Abdominal organs (viscera) protruding through an open wound
10. Full-Thickness Burn: (M) Burn extending through all dermal layers; may involve the subcutaneous tissues, muscle, bone, or organs; third-degree burn
11. Hematoma: (J) Swelling or mass of blood caused by breaking a blood vessel
12. Impaled Object: (I) An object that pierces the skin
13. Laceration: (H) Wound or irregular tear of the skin
14. Occlusive Dressing: (G) A dressing that forms an airtight seal; often applied to open neck, chest, or abdominal wounds; items commonly used include defibrillation pads or thick plastic wrap
15. Open Soft Tissue Injury: (F) Open wound in which muscle, vessels, and/or skin is damaged
16. Partial-Thickness Burn: (E) Burn involving both the epidermis and the dermis, but not involving underlying tissue; second-degree burn
17. Pneumothorax: (D) Air in the chest cavity between the lung and chest wall
18. Sterile: (C) Free of microorganisms (bacteria, viruses, spores) that can cause infection
19. Superficial Burn: (B) Burn involving only the top layer of the skin (epidermis); first-degree burn

Labeling Diagram

Rule of Nines

Adult:

A. Head and neck – 9%

B. Anterior trunk – 18%

C. Posterior trunk – 18%

D. Each upper extremity – 9%

E. External genitals – 1%

F. Each lower extremity – 18%

Infant:

G. Head and neck – 18%

H. Each lower extremity – 14%

CHAPTER 21
Musculoskeletal Injuries

Review Questions

1. D	**5.** C	**9.** C	**13.** B	**17.** A
2. B	**6.** A	**10.** A	**14.** D	**18.** C
3. A	**7.** A	**11.** B	**15.** D	**19.** D
4. C	**8.** A	**12.** D	**16.** C	**20.** A

Case Studies

1A. After confirming that the injury is localized to the left thigh, complete the spinal immobilization and then assess and splint the injured extremity.

1B. True. Femur fractures can cause significant bleeding into the surrounding tissues. In some cases, this can be as much as a liter of hidden blood loss.

1C. Splinting reduces injuries to surrounding tissues when a broken bone is present. This helps decrease the amount of bleeding at the fracture site and reduces the risk of damage to nerves and muscle. Splinting also helps control pain and allows for easier transport of the patient.

1D. A traction splint is indicated when the patient has a painfully swollen and deformed mid-thigh region with no joint or lower leg injury.

1E. Contraindications to a traction splint include:

- An injury that is close to the knee or involves the knee itself
- An injury to the hip or pelvis
- Partial amputation with the distal limb connected by marginal tissue, such that traction would risk separation
- Lower leg or ankle injury

1F.
- Use body substance isolation (BSI) precautions.
- Assess and record the pulse, motor function, and sensory status distal to the injury.
- Manually stabilize the injured leg.
- Manual traction will be required while applying the splint.
- Adjust the splint to the proper length.
- Position the splint under the injured leg with the ischial pad against the bone.
- Raise the heel stand and secure the ischial (proximal) strap.
- Secure the ankle (distal) strap, with the foot in an upright position.
- Attach the hooks. Apply mechanical traction until it is equal to the manual traction being applied and pain and spasms are reduced. (If the patient is unresponsive, apply mechanical traction until both legs are of equal length.)
- Secure the support straps. Reevaluate the ischial and ankle straps.
- Reassess pulse, motor, and sensory status.
- Secure the patient's torso to a backboard to help immobilize the hip joint and femur. Secure the splint to the board to prevent movement of the injured leg.

2A. Absolutely, so you can assess the injury site

2B. Be sure to assess distal pulses, motor function, and sensation before and after splinting.

2C. Immobilize the adjacent joints (e.g., the knee), apply a cold pack and reassess the patient's vital signs and the splinting en route to the hospital.

3A. The tibia or fibula

3B. Splint the limb by applying a small amount of traction and carefully moving the extremity back to a straight "splintable" position. It is not recommended that the injury be splint in the position as found. Splinting him where he is found (where he lies) as opposed to how he lies is the most appropriate plan of action.

3C. Keep the patient warm, bandage the wound, apply a cold pack to the fracture, administer oxygen if the patient is weak, and reasses the vital signs every few minutes.

4A. When the fracture involves the knee, when the injury involves the hip or pelvis, a partial amputation with the distal limb connected by marginal tissue so that traction would risk separation, or a lower leg or ankle injury

4B. Yes, an uncomplicated femur fracture can bleed up to a liter of blood into the thigh. If it is a complicated fracture, such as one where the femoral artery has been severed, the patient could lose a considerable amount of blood.

4C. The PASG is an acceptable splint for a patient with a femur fracture who also has other things wrong with him or her and is in shock. If the patient just needs a splint applied, air splints or the PASG are not the best and the femur would be better splinted with a rigid immobilization device or a traction splint.

Key Terms Matching

1. Direct Force: (C) A force that causes injury to a body part at the site of impact

2. Indirect Force: (D) A transmitted force that causes

injury some distance away from the point of impact

3. Splint: (A) Equipment used to prevent or reduce movement of body joints or injured tissue
4. Twisting Force: (B) Occurs when one part of an extremity remains in place while the rest moves or twists

Labeling Diagram

Direct Impact Injury

A. humerus

B. radius

C. ulna

CHAPTER 22
Head and Spine Injuries

Review Questions

1. B	**7.** C	**13.** A	**19.** B	**25.** A
2. C	**8.** C	**14.** D	**20.** A	**26.** C
3. A	**9.** A	**15.** A	**21.** C	**27.** A
4. D	**10.** C	**16.** B	**22.** A	**28.** A
5. B	**11.** B	**17.** A	**23.** B	**29.** C
6. B	**12.** D	**18.** C	**24.** D	**30.** D

Case Studies

1A.
- You observe there is a significant mechanism of injury present. Immediately establish and maintain in-line manual immobilization of the cyclist's head and neck. This is done by your partner while you continue your rapid trauma assessment.
- You complete the rapid trauma assessment and find complete paralysis and loss of sensation in the lower extremities.

1B. The helmet should be removed if:
- The EMT-B's ability to assess or manage the airway and breathing is restricted.
- The helmet does not fit properly and allows excessive head movement. (The head must be immobilized to prevent neck injury. If there is an existing neck injury, movement of the head within a loose helmet can lead to further spinal damage.)
- Proper spinal immobilization cannot be performed with the helmet in place.
- The patient is in cardiac arrest.

1C. The helmet should be left in place if:
- The patient has no impending airway or breathing problems and the EMT-B's access to the airway is not restricted.
- The helmet does not interfere with assessment or reassessment of the airway and breathing.
- There is a good fit, with little or no movement of the patient's head inside the helmet.
- Proper spinal immobilization can be performed. This may require padding behind the shoulders to make up for the helmet in the occiput area of the skull.
- Removal of the helmet would cause further injury to the patient.

1D. You elect to remove the helmet because you feel that cervical immobilization may be inadequate and you are having difficulty maintaining an open airway.

1E.
- A two-rescuer procedure is recommended when removal of a helmet is required.
- Only one EMT-Basic should move at a time, while the other EMT-Basic stabilizes the spine.
- EMT-B #1 manually stabilizes the helmet and keeps the neck in a neutral position by kneeling at the patient's head and holding the sides of the helmet in both hands. The EMT-Basic's fingers extend to support the mandibular angle on both sides. This stabilizes the head and neck.
- The second EMT-Basic approaches from below the head and loosens the chin strap or face shield. The face shield or chin straps may have to be cut.
- EMT-Basic #2 uses one hand to stabilize the mandible at the mandibular angle and uses the other hand to support the back of the skull at the cranial occiput.
- While EMT-Basic #2 is supporting the head, the EMT-Basic holding the helmet pulls the sides apart laterally so that it will clear the ears, then gently slips the helmet halfway off the patient's head.
- As the helmet is removed fully, you must stabilize the neck and prevent the head from falling backwards. EMT-B #2 adjusts his hand position, sliding his posterior hand superiorly to secure the head.
- The helmet is removed completely, with EMT-B #1 pulling it straight off to avoid flexion or extension of the neck. Keep the neck in a neutral position to avoid further injury.

- A motorcycle helmet with face mask may have to be rotated slightly to clear the patient's nose, but the neck should never be turned or moved laterally.

2A. No, call for another ambulance since at least two patients will need to be placed on spine boards.

2B. Use the KED or short board to immobilize him in the seated position.

2C.
- Do a rapid takedown onto a long spine board.
- Get some vitals.
- Apply some oxygen by non-rebreather mask.
- Fully immobilize him to the long backboard.
- Use ALS if they are available to you.
- Reassess en route to the hospital.

2D. Based on the mechanism of injury and the fact that the alcohol may be masking the injury, you should not medically clear the patient in the street.

3A. No. If you know how to swim, go to the shallow end and slowly wade over to the patient so you do not created a wave or big splash.

3B. No. The patient should be fully immobilized in the water with plenty of help.

3C. He may have compressed his neck diving onto his head in the shallow water and injured his cervical spine. His prognosis is not good.

3D.
- Assess the airway and ventilations; assist as needed.
- Apply oxygen by non-rebreather mask.
- Make sure he is fully immobilized to the long backboard.
- Call for ALS if they are not yet on the scene.
- Keep the patient warm.
- Transport to the most appropriate emergency department for the patient's problem.

Key Terms Matching

1. Battle's Sign: (E) Bruising behind the ears or mastoid process due to basilar skull fracture
2. Cerebrospinal Fluid (CSF): (C) Fluid that fills the ventricles and cavities of the brain and surrounds the spinal cord
3. Closed Head Injury: (I) Trauma to the head in which the skull remains intact; scalp may or may not be lacerated
4. Compression Injury: (G) Spinal injury caused when a strong force is transmitted up or down the length of the body.
5. Concussion: (A) Temporary disruption of normal brain function; usually caused by blunt trauma to the head
6. Dementia: (B) A loss of cognitive and intellectual functions caused by a variety of disorders
7. Glasgow Coma Scale (GCS): (D) A tool for assessing a patient's level of responsiveness
8. Open Head Injury: (F) A severe traumatic head injury in which the skull is fractured
9. Paresthesia: (H) Abnormal sensations of tingling, numbness, burning, coldness, pain, or tightness in the extremities

Labeling Diagram

The Spinal Column

A. cervical vertebrae
B. thoracic vertebrae
C. lumbar vertebrae
D. sacrum
E. coccyx

CHAPTER 23
Infants and Children

Review Questions

1. B	11. D	21. C	31. C	41. D
2. C	12. B	22. D	32. A	42. D
3. A	13. B	23. B	33. A	43. A
4. A	14. C	24. B	34. A	44. A
5. C	15. B	25. D	35. B	45. B
6. B	16. B	26. B	36. C	46. B
7. D	17. B	27. D	37. A	
8. B	18. A	28. A	38. C	
9. D	19. B	29. D	39. B	
10. A	20. D	30. A	40. A	

Case Studies

General Pediatric Assessment

1A. Your general impression, as well as a baseline respiratory and mental status assessment, can be obtained as you approach the patient. Observe to see how the child is interacting with the caregiver. Allow the father to continue holding the child as you conduct a physical evaluation. Unless you perceive an immediate threat to the airway, breathing, or circulation, allow the child a few moments to become familiar with you. Begin by playing with the child's hands or feet and moving to the abdomen and chest. Examine the head last.

1B. There are several history questions that may be important in this situation. First, ask how long the child has been running the fever. Also ask the father about the child's eating habits over the past few days. You should find out whether the father has been changing diapers with increasing or decreasing frequency.

1C. Depending on the information obtained during the physical examination and history, several factors could alert the EMT-Basic to change the priority of the patient. Discovering a rapid onset and rise of a fever or duration of a fever for a long time period would indicate the need for rapid medical attention. Likewise, children who show signs and symptoms of dehydration should receive rapid medical attention. Such signs might include skin tenting, sunken eyes or fontanelles, decreased diaper count, and presence of vomiting or diarrhea.

Seizures

2A. There are three types of consent that may be involved in this case. First, the school may have written parental permission to access and provide medical care for the child. If so, request a copy to carry with you to the hospital to avoid a delay in treatment. In the absence of such a document, ask the school officials whether the parents have been contacted. If so, permission may have already been given. If not, have someone attempt to contact them as soon as possible. If unable to talk with the parents, you should proceed under implied consent. Lifesaving care should not be withheld under any circumstances.

2B. Your first action should be to secure the scene. There are no threats to yourself or your crew, but the patient is in danger of injuring himself on the furniture. You should move all chairs, tables, or other objects well out of the way. Although you may be unable to open the airway due to muscle spasm, you should consider placing a non-rebreather mask on the patient if possible. A nasopharyngeal airway may also be indicated. While waiting for the seizure to end, you should prepare for immediate transport. Suction and ventilatory support should be readily available.

2C. The EMT-Basic should document the number of seizure episodes, the duration of the episodes, and the nature of body parts or systems affected.

2D. You should ask whether the child has a past history of seizures. If so, how does the current episode compare to previous seizures? Is the child on any anti-seizure medications? If so, has he been taking them appropriately?

Pediatric Trauma

3A. Lower extremity, abdominal, head, neck, and spine injuries are frequently seen in patients who have been struck by vehicles.

3B. Expect this patient to have significant head, neck, and spinal trauma. There may also be bilateral femur fractures from being thrown violently over the handlebars.

3C. First, the airway should be secured using suction and either an oral or a nasal airway as tolerated. Cervical spine precautions should be maintained throughout. Based on the mechanism and suspicion of head injury, assist ventilations appropriately. Immediate transport is indicated and should begin as soon as immobilization is completed.

4A. The child communicates well with you from inside the car. It would be appropriate for you to sit down beside the car seat (if possible) and begin talking with the child. A limited assessment should be performed without removing the toddler from her safety seat.

4B. Yes. The same criteria apply to immobilizing both adults and children. Any patient involved in a motor vehicle collision where force was applied sufficient to significantly damage the vehicle should be immobilized. The best tool for immobilizing the child is the child's own car seat. A cervical collar can be applied without removing the restraints. The head and neck should be surrounded with a blanket roll. Voids on each side of the patient should be filled. Secure all immobilization with tape. Remaining in his or her own seat will hopefully have a calming effect. Be sure to bring along any dependency objects, such as a teddy bear or blanket.

Near-Drowning

5A. Yes, if you know how to swim. Enter from the other side of the pool to limit the waves you might create since you do not know if this could be a possible spine injury also.

5B. Carefully roll the child into the head up position, maintaining manual stabilization of the head and neck. Begin artificial respirations as needed. Float a long backboard up from under the child and immobilize the head, neck, and spine in the pool.

5C. Tilt the board to the side and suction out the child's mouth. Next assist ventilations with high-flow oxygen and consider the need for airway adjuncts.

5D. Yes, ALS at the scene or enroute to the hospital to better manage the airway

Key Terms Matching

1. Adolescent: (E) Child who is 12 to 18 years old
2. Capillary Refill Time: (F) Time required for the capillary beds to refill with blood after blanching; used for assessing perfusion in infants and children
3. Early Respiratory Distress: (D) Respiratory problem in which patient can compensate for decreased oxygenation or circulation by increasing breathing rate and effort
4. Febrile: (B) Having a fever
5. Hydrocephalus: (A) Excessive fluid accumulation inside the brain
6. Preschooler: (C) Child who is 3 to 6 years old
7. School-Aged: (I) Child who is 6 to 12 years old
8. Sudden Infant Death Syndrome (SIDS): (G) Crib death; cause unknown
9. Toddler: (H) Child from 1 to 3 years old

Labeling Diagram

General Impression: Infants and Children

A. Calm, or cries but can be comforted by parent
B. Strong
C. Playful, active
D. Attentive, responds to parents and EMTs, makes eye contact
E. Pink
F. Normal for age
G. Cannot be consoled
H. Whimpering, weak, or high-pitched
I. Lethargic, refuses to play, exhausted
J. Inappropriate or absent
K. Pale or cyanotic
L. Resistant, limp, flaccid

CHAPTER 24
Operations

Review Questions

1. A	11. C	21. D	31. C	41. B
2. A	12. C	22. B	32. C	42. C
3. D	13. D	23. D	33. A	43. A
4. A	14. B	24. A	34. B	44. D
5. D	15. D	25. B	35. D	45. B
6. B	16. A	26. A	36. A	46. B
7. B	17. C	27. A	37. B	47. C
8. D	18. C	28. A	38. D	48. D
9. B	19. B	29. C	39. B	49. B
10. C	20. B	30. B	40. B	50. A

Case Studies

Equipment

1A. While the list can vary with each EMS system, the following is a good start:

- Basic first aid supplies, such as bandages and dressings
- Patient transfer equipment such as backboards
- Airways
- Suction equipment
- Artificial ventilation devices
- Oxygen inhalation equipment
- Basic wound care supplies
- Splinting supplies
- Medications
- Automated external defibrillator batteries and supplies

Phases of an Ambulance Call

2A. The typical phases of an ambulance call are the following:

1) Vehicle maintenance and preparation for each call
2) Dispatch
3) En route
4) Arrival on Scene and Scene Safety
5) Assessment and transfer of the patient to the ambulance
6) En route patient assessment and emergency interventions
7) Arrival at appropriate receiving facility
8) Return to station
9) Post-run follow-up

3A. The EMT-Basic should describe at a minimum the following steps:

- Close and secure all outside compartments.
- Disconnect any external shorelines or other electrical cords.
- Retrieve any necessary equipment (jump kits, special extrication equipment etc.).
- Fasten seatbelts.
- Adjust all mirrors, seats, and other items necessary to safely drive the emergency unit.
- Scan equipment for proper running values.
- Notify dispatch of unit response.
- Confirm exact location of the emergency scene and best route for arrival.
- Reconfirm or request any special information regarding the response.
- Operate the emergency response vehicle in a safe manner at all times.
- Predetermine team member responsibilities en route to the call.
- Notify and request advance or special response teams if necessary.

4A. The crew should take a few moments to lay out some action plan. The lead EMT-Basic should make specific assignments on exactly what each person should do once they arrive on scene.

4B. The operator should consider positioning the ambulance in such a fashion and area that immediate and safe exit from the scene is possible. The operator may also consider advising dispatch of the situation and have all other emergency responders park their vehicles in a location that will allow quick and safe arrival and departure of all ambulances. Some additional consideration may also be given to exactly how the arriving air ambulance can be placed to optimize patient care.

5A. The EMT-Basic should mention at a minimum the components of the ongoing assessment. They include:

- Repeat the initial assessment.
- Reassess and record the vital signs.
- Repeat focused assessment specific to the patient's complaint or injuries.
- Check interventions.

5B. The EMT-Basic should notify the receiving facility of the patient's condition as soon as possible. In many cases, specialized staff will need to be notified within the hospital. Teams of specialists will usually converge on the emergency department prior to the patient's arrival.

Vehicle Escorts

6A. The response should include some mention that the Department of Transportation recommends that all vehicles in an escort response refrain from using their emergency lights or siren. A safe distance (500 feet) must be maintained between all the vehicles in the response and all operators must agree on a communication channel prior to the escort.

Scene and Patient Safety

7A. The EMT-Basic should complete or consider use of appropriate levels of standard precautions or body substance isolation for the situation. The response should always include gloves. The situation may also warrant eyewear, gowns, face masks, and eye protection.

7B. Assess the scene for any evidence of danger (location, approach, emergency moves, and self-evacuation). Based on the mechanism involving the patient, traffic hazards should be a major concern.

8A. The questions should include such examples as:

- Is the patient in a critical or life-threatening condition?
- Can I lift and safely move the patient, given the assistance currently on scene?
- Is the patient's position compromising my ability to maintain his airway?
- Is moving the patient going to aggravate or increase his pain level?
- What type of unique packaging will be required for proper immobilization?

Decontamination

9A. Notify dispatch of your delayed status due to an extended clean-up. In many systems, assistance can be dispatched to the ED to assist the crew in preparing or restocking the ambulance. Refuel the unit if necessary. Inspect the ambulance equipment and restock supplies after cleaning and disinfecting the ambulance as required. Clean and disinfect any equipment prior to replacing in the ambulance. Return and secure equipment into its proper storage area. Collect all equipment you left and may need from previous calls to the facility, and file all the appropriate patient care forms.

10A. The response should include the following information:

- Sterilization is the approved process whereby pressurized steam, gases, or specialized chemical agents destroy all microorganisms, bacteria, and bacterial spores. This process is usually not used in the prehospital setting.

- High-level disinfecting is similar to sterilization in that it is designed to kill all microorganisms yet lacks the function of killing off a large number of bacterial spores. The process usually includes hot-water pasteurization and soaking.
- Disinfection is designed to destroy most viruses, the tuberculosis bacteria, and fungi. Disinfection is accomplished by wiping with an approved germicidal chemical or spray. In the prehospital setting, disinfection is commonly accomplished with a proper mixture of bleach and water (1:100). Disinfection is not capable of destroying bacterial spores.
- Cleaning is the process that is designed to kill off most bacteria, some viruses, and fungi. Cleaning will not destroy the tuberculosis bacteria or bacterial spores. Similar to disinfection, cleaning is accomplished by wiping with a disinfectant.

Driving Safety

11A. The response should include some reference to due regard for the safety of others. The respondent should not only be concerned for the safety of his crew and patient but to the motoring public and pedestrians at large.

11B. Emergency vehicle operation regulations provide exemptions from the normal traffic laws in very specific circumstances. Strict conditions must be met before operators may use these exemptions. If the operator follows these conditions, uses all visual and audible warning devices, and drives with due regard for the safety of others, then an emergency vehicle generally may:

- Exceed posted speed limits
- Proceed through red lights, flashing red lights, stop signs, and stop signals
- Proceed against the "right of way" at uncontrolled intersections
- Proceed through yield or merge signs
- Ignore "no turns" signs (right and left turns)
- Disregard proper traffic lanes
- Drive the wrong way on a divided highway or one-way street
- Drive left of the center line
- Cross solid double or single lines
- Pass on the right side of other moving vehicles
- Change directions
- Continue past a school bus that is loading (but not when unloading, unless directed by a crossing guard)
- Proceed without regard to emergency or disaster routes
- Ignore parking and standing regulations

When operating an ambulance under normal conditions (that is, not responding in an emergency mode), all applicable laws, rules, and regulations must be obeyed.

12A. The response will depend on local and state laws and regulations; however, some mention should be made regarding contacting the appropriate law enforcement agency to have the vehicle stopped. Follow local protocol. The EMT-Basic should not suggest exiting the unit to speak with the driver. If the driver is creating a hazard for other motorists and endangering your response, consider requesting that another unit handle the call and discontinue the response.

Aeromedical Services

13A. Aeromedical evacuation should be considered on any occasion that a patient has a significant mechanism of injury and needs definitive medical care. Consider calling for aeromedical evacuation of these patients if the ground transport time will be longer than the flight time of the aeromedical program. Other factors to consider when evaluating the need for aeromedical evacuation include decreased out of hospital transport time and the enhancement of resources for multi-casualty. Also consider the presence of a suitable landing site and favorable weather conditions. The response may include additions or deletions from this list based on local protocol.

The answers should include as a minimum:

- Vehicle rollover with unrestrained and injured passengers
- Auto vs. pedestrian crashes where the vehicle was traveling in excess of 10 mph
- Falls greater than 15 ft.
- Motorcycle crashes in excess of 10 mph
- Automobile crashes involving a death of one or more occupants of the same vehicle
- Patient ejection from a vehicle
- The response may also include additions or deletions from this list based on local protocol

13B. The response should include at a minimum the following steps:

- Identify the person in charge of landing zone communications. Do not allow that person to become involved in direct patient care.

Contact aeromedical dispatch with vital landing zone information. Set up the landing zone and be sure the area is clear of obstructions and of items that may become airborne.. The landing zone should be at a minimum 100 ft. by 100 ft. The zone should be level and solid ground. No vehicles may be parked within 50 ft. of the zone.

- Set independent lighting systems in each of the four corners. Set a lighting system on the upwind side to help identify wind direction. Warn arriving aeromedical crew of any unusual conditions or tall objects, buildings, or wires. Wet the area down if possible. Keep the patient and crew clear of the air downwash area. Keep spectators at least 200 ft. away from the landing zone. Assign one person to direct the helicopter into position. Have the person stand next to the wind direction marker. The landing director should use hand signals, lighting, and be familiar with movement around the aircraft.

Incident Management Systems

14A. The answer should include a brief discussion on providing basic lifesaving care as soon as possible without compromising personal or crew safety. There should also be mention of being the patient's advocate to reduce or minimize further injury as well as providing patient care as soon as possible.

14B. Responses will vary with the individual's level of rescue training. In general, the EMT-Basic should:

- First, establish a chain of command or incident command system.
- Second, provide as much lifesaving care to patients as possible prior to extrication.
- Third, reduce as much as possible any additional movement that may increase or further existing injuries.
- Finally, patient care takes priority over extrication unless delayed movement is too dangerous or life threatening.

15A. The EMT-Basic should recognize that during extrication situations, at a minimum, PPE should include:

- Impact-resistant protective helmets with ear protection and a chinstrap
- Protective eyewear
- Lightweight, puncture-resistant turnout coat
- OSHA-approved hand protection
- Calf-high boots with steel insoles and steel toes
- BSI protective equipment during patient contact

16A. Initially, it is important to establish an incident command post at a safe distance from the scene. After establishing a command post, additional resources must be requested. Remaining crew members should begin the process of triage. As early as possible, establish the following sectors to aid in organization:

- Extrication
- Treatment
- Transportation
- Staging
- Triage
- Mobile Command Center

16B. While the response can vary slightly, the following major purposes should be identified:

- IMS is designed to assist with control, direction, and coordination of emergency response and resource allocation.
- IMS is also designed to assist in the orderly communication and interaction between all allied agencies using a single command structure.

Extrication

17A. The steps as identified should include:

- Communicate with the patient and explain what is happening. Describe sounds, smells and the reason behind any possible or real movements.
- Protect the patient by placing a blanket or heavy tarp over both you and the patient. Have a small light with you to continue the dialogue.
- Limit the number of people communicating directly with either you or the patient. Reduce the amount of confusion and stress around the patient.
- Limit access to the scene by bystanders.

18A. Disentanglement is a sub-category of extrication involving specialized cutting, spreading, or prying equipment. Many patients will require extrication from an environment with the need for disentanglement.

19A. While the specific answers will differ slightly due to regional or local variations, the common or general types should include:

- A light-duty unit carrying basic rescue equipment. The equipment may include hand tools and basic hydraulic tools. This unit is designed to respond to situations requiring simple disentanglement. Some ambulances also carry light-duty extrication equipment.

- A medium-duty unit carries more specialized extrication equipment including manually operated and hydraulically powered spreaders, cutter, and rams. In addition, the medium-duty unit usually carries all of the equipment found on the light-duty unit.
- The heavy-duty units are designed to carry all necessary equipment or resources for the most complex and difficult extrications. A brief list of equipment might include: high-pressure air bags, arc air welding and cutting torches, dive equipment, rigging, and rappelling gear.

20A. The EMT-Basic should include some basic discussion on personal and crew safety, proper use and upkeep of extrication equipment, and the proper management of all patients. The specifics of the local EMS HAZ-MAT response will be determined by the training, roles, and responsibilities of the EMT-Basic as assigned by the response plan.

Hazardous Materials

21A. The response should include the following steps:

- Park a safe distance away from the scene, upwind and, if possible, uphill.
- Keep all unnecessary people out of the area. Notify law enforcement to help with scene control.
- Isolate the area—do not enter the area unless specially trained and properly protected.
- Avoid contact with the hazardous materials
- After the material is identified and the scene is determined safe to enter, remove patients to a safe zone.

22A. No. The scene may be unsafe, or it is possible that the patient may contaminate the providers and the ambulance. EMS providers should retreat until the material is identified. Hazardous materials personnel should be consulted and/or asked to respond to the scene. Once the material responsible for the burn has been identified, the patient must be decontaminated before further emergency medical care or transportation can take place.

22B. The response should suggest the dispatch of the hazardous materials team. These highly trained professionals can identify and contain any offending materials. If the HAZ-MAT team is not an option, the EMT-Basic should then suggest contacting the CHEMTREC service via an 800 number to help identify the materials.

23A. The four levels of training for hazardous materials include:

1) First Responder Awareness: designed for those who will arrive first on scene and simply recognize a potential problem and are able to notify the proper authorities.
2) First Responder Operations: designed for personnel who will be protecting life, property, and the environment.
3) Hazardous Materials Technician: designed for personnel who will contain and manage the hazardous materials.
4) Hazardous Materials Specialists: advanced-level training including command and control functions on scene of a hazardous materials event. The specialist has advanced knowledge and skills regarding hazardous materials events.

Key Terms Matching

1. Complex Access: (E) A rescue requiring specialized skills and equipment.
2. Disinfection: (F) Removal of germs, bacteria, or other potentially infectious materials. High-level disinfection; used for instruments that have come in contact with mucous membranes and involving a process of hot-water pasteurization (176° to 212° F).
3. Hazardous Material (HAZ-MAT): (G) Substance that is potentially harmful or that presents an unreasonable risk for injury, health problems, or significant property damage if not properly controlled
4. HAZ-MAT Team: (H) Personnel specially trained to manage emergencies involving hazardous materials
5. Incident Management System (IMS): (A) A system designed to control, direct, and coordinate emergency responders and resources in case of a disaster
6. Multiple Casualty Incident (MCI): (B) Response that can involve a few serious injuries or several hundred patients; can place great demands on a local EMS system
7. Self-Contained Breathing Apparatus (SCBA): (C) Equipment that provides clean air to a rescuer and protects him or her from hazardous vapors
8. Simple Access: (D) A rescue that does not require sophisticated equipment

APPENDIX A
Advanced Airway Management

Review Questions

1. A	**6.** D	**11.** A	**16.** C	**21.** A
2. A	**7.** A	**12.** B	**17.** B	**22.** C
3. C	**8.** B	**13.** C	**18.** A	**23.** A
4. A	**9.** B	**14.** D	**19.** B	**24.** D
5. A	**10.** D	**15.** B	**20.** C	**25.** B

Key Terms Matching

1. Barotrauma: (F) Ruptured lung resulting from overaggressive ventilations
2. Endotracheal intubation: (G) Advanced airway technique involving insertion of a tube through the mouth and into the trachea; also orotracheal intubation
3. Laryngoscope: (H) An instrument with a light and interchangeable blades, used for holding the tongue out of the way for intubation
4. Nasogastric (NG) Tube: (E) Tube inserted into the nasal passage for decompression of the stomach or proximal bowel or for gastric lavage
5. Orotracheal Intubation: (B) Advanced airway technique involving insertion of a tube through the mouth and into the trachea; also endotracheal intubation
6. Right Mainstem Intubation: (C) Placement of an endotracheal tube beyond the carina and into the right mainstem bronchus; results in ventilation of the right lung only
7. Sellick's Maneuver: (D) Pressure applied directly over the cricoid cartilage; also cricoid pressure
8. Vagus Nerve: (A) Tenth cranial nerve; controls smooth muscles of the lungs, heart, and abdominal viscera

Labeling Diagram

The Respiratory System

A. oropharynx
B. larynx
C. esophagus
D. trachea
E. nasopharynx
F. tongue
G. epiglottis
H. cricoid cartilage